Optometry Handbook

2nd Edition

by Leroy Rubin

Optometry Handbook

2nd Edition

by Leroy Rubin

Butterworth (Publishers) Inc.
Boston London

Every effort has been made to ensure that the drug dosage schedules within this text are accurate and conform to standards accepted at time of publication. However, as treatment recommendations vary in light of continuing research and clinical experience, the reader is advised to verify drug dosage schedules herein with information found on product information sheets. This is especially true in cases of new or infrequently used drugs.

Library of Congress Cataloging in Publication Data
Main entry under title:

Optometry handbook.

Includes index.
1. Optometry—Handbooks, manuals, etc. I. Rubin, Leroy.
DNLM: 1. Optometry—Tables. WW 16 R8960
RE952.9.067 1981 617.7'5'0202 81-4424
ISCN 0-409-95180-3 AACR2

Published by Butterworth (Publishers) Inc.
10 Tower Office Park
Woburn, MA 01801

Printed in the United States of America

Foreword

Question: What's better than a good thing? Answer: More of a good thing. And that's what is in store for you when you read this second edition of ***Optometry Handbook.***

Enlarged to accommodate a number of new, different, and important areas, the 374 page volume is literally crammed with data and information valuable, and necessary, to today's doctors of optometry.

The ***Handbook*** is a compilation of statistics, tables, charts, definitions, and descriptions — collated, codified, and classified for eacy retrieval. Most are cross-indexed and cross-referenced so it is difficult ***not*** to find what you might be looking for!

How do you get around to compile a book like this? In the first place, you ascertain the need. That's what author Leroy Rubin did. After he consumed futile hours in searching — with volumes to search — when he was in need of data, he decided to put it all together. This second volume contains more "all" then its predecessor.

The bookshelf of the O.D. is incomplete without a number of basic works — a drug reference text, a dictionary of vision terms, volumes on pathology and eye conditions — and, of course, an ***Optometry Handbook.***

Irving Bennett, O.D., *Editor*
Optometric Management

Preface to the 2nd Edition

This handbook presents the basic considerations of current optometric practice in a concise and convenient form. In this revised edition, the primary purpose has been continued and more completely realized.

There have been extensive additions to each segment and new and important sections are now included. The largest of these is devoted to pathology, and in keeping with the clinical nature of the ***Handbook,*** the emphasis is on differential diagnosis.

Most tables have been completely updated, and even those which are apt to change from year to year should remain useful for the forseeable future.

The reader should give the volume a serious perusal and familiarize him- or herself with its contents. Although a book of tables, it is easily readable.

It is not always possible to give recognition to all those who have contributed to the preparation of this work, but I would particularly like to thank Dr. Howard Silverstein of East Northport, New York, for his ideas and constructive criticism, and Mrs. Margaret Lewis, the head librarian at SUNY School of Optometry, for her cooperation and the privileges extended. A special thank you to my wife whose patience was certainly at least as valuable as her typing.

Leroy Rubin
Port Washington, New York

Preface to the 1st Edition

The primary purpose of this book is to provide the practicing optometrist with a convenient single source of clinical data. Although every effort has been made to avoid errors, the possibility of their appearance in a book of this type must be considered. The editor and publishers will be most grateful to readers who call our attention to any that may be discovered. Suggestions for improvement will also be welcome.

I would like to thank the many individuals who offered their kind assistance and consultation, especially the following: Howard Silverstein, OD, Hempstead, N.Y.; Alvin Schiff, OD, N.Y.C. Community College; Douglas R. Williams, OD, Huntington Beach, Cal. and, of course, my wife: typist, proofreader, critic.

Leroy Rubin
Port Washington, New York

Contents

Visual Acuity 1

1.1. Visual Acuity Equivalents

Decimal Notation	*Snellen Imperial*	*Snell Sterling Efficiency*	*Minutes of Arc*	*Metric*	*Points*	*Jaeger*	*14" (35 cm.)*	*16" (40 cm.)*	*Approx. Orthorater Scores*
2.0	20/10	109.4	.5	6/3					
1.5	20/13		.65		2		14/9.1	61.5/40	
1.33	20/15	104.9	.75	6/4.5			14/12	50/40	
1.0	20/20	100.0	1.0	6/6	3	+1	14/14	40/40	10
.80	20/25	95.6	1.3	6/75	4	1	14/17.5	40/50	8
.67	20/30	91.4	1.5	6/9	4.5	2+	14/21	40/60	
.57	20/35	87.4	1.75		5	2		40/70	6
.50	20/40	83.6	2.0	6/12	6	3	14/28	40/80	5
.40	20/50	76.5	2.5	6/15	7.5	5	14/35	40/100	
.33	20/60	70.0	3.0	6/18	8	6	14/42	40/120	4
.29	20/70	63.9	3.5	6/21	10	7		40/140	3
.25	20/80	58.5	4.0	6/24	12	8	14/56	40/160	
.22	20/90	53.4	4.5		12.5	9		40/180	
.20	20/100	48.9	5.0	6/30	13	10	14/70	40/200	
.167	20/120	40.9	6.0		14	11	14/84	40/240	2
.15	20/130				16	12		40/260	
.14	20/140	34.2	7.0					40/280	
.133	20/150				18	13		40/300	
.125	20/160	28.6	8.0				14/112	40/320	
.12	20/170				24	14		40/340	1
.11	20/180	23.9	9.0						
.10	20/200	20.0	16.0	20/60	28	17	14/140	40/400	
.09	20/220		11.0						
.085	20/240		12.0						
.08	20/260	11.0	13.0				14/175	40/500	
.075	20/280	9.8	14.0						
.07	20/300	8.2	15.0	6/90			14/210	40/600	
.06	20/340	5.7	17.0						
.05	20/380	4.0	19.0						
.05	20/400	3.3	20.0	6/120					
.04	20/500	1.4	25.0	6/150					
.03	20/600	.56	30.0	6/180					
.025	20/800	.09	40.0	6/240					
.02	20/1000	.02	50.0	6/300					
.012	20/1200	0.00	60.0	6/360					

1.2. Normal Visual Acuities by Age

Age	*Acuity*
2	20/50
3	20/40
5	20/35
6	20/25–
8	20/25
9	20/25+
11	20/20
27	20/20+
37	20/20
67	20/20–
72	20/25
77	20/40
82	20/60

Adapted by permission from F.J. Slataper, "Age norms of refraction and vision," *Arch. Ophthalmol.* 43:466 (1950).

1.3. Correlation Between Visual Acuity and Refractive Condition

Diopters	*Simple Myopia or Absolute Hyperopia*	*Simple Hyperopic and Myopic Astigmatism*		
		Horizontal Axis	*Oblique Axis*	*Vertical Axis*
.50	20/30	20/25+	20/25	
.75	20/40	20/25	20/30	20/25
1.0	20/50	20/30	20/40	20/30
1.25	20/70			20/40
1.50	20/100	20/40	20/50	
1.75			20/70	20/50
2.0	20/150	20/50	20/80	20/70
2.25			20/100	20/80
2.50	20/200	20/80		20/100
2.75			20/150	
3.0	20/250	20/100	20/200	20/150
3.5	20/300			
4.0		20/150		20/200
4.5	20/400	20/200	20/250	
5.0		20/250	20/300	

1.4. Visual Standards

Table A. United States Government

Agency	*Uncorrected Acuity*	*Corrected Acuity*	*Color Vision*	*Refractive Error*	*Muscle Balance*	*Other*
U.S. Military Academy	Any	20/20,20/20	Red-green	Any meridian −5.50 to +5.50 cyl 3.00, aniso 3.50	Eso .15 Exo to 10 Hyper to 2.0	3,4
U.S. Naval Academy	20/20,20/20	20/20,20/20	Normal	Any meridian −4.50 to +4.50 cyl 3.00, aniso 3.50	None	1,3,4
U.S. Air Force Academy				Any meridian	Eso to 10	1,3,4
Pilot	20/20,20/20	20/20,20/20	Normal	+1.75 to −0.25	Exo to 5	
Non-Flying	20/50,20/50	20/20,20/20		cyl .75	Hyper 1.0	
U.S. Coast Guard Academy	20/40,20/40	20/20,20/20	Normal	None	None	1,4
U.S. Merchant Marine Academy	20/100,20/100	20/20,20/20	Normal	+3.25 to −3.25 cyl 3.00, aniso 3.50	Marked sympt. disqualify	1,4
Armed Forces						1,4
Officer	20/200,20/200	20/20,20/40	Dependent on Specialty	+5.00 to −3.00	Strabismus < 20°	
Medical	20/400,20/400	20/20,20/40		none		
Em	20/400,20/400	20/40,20/70[6]		none		
F.A.A. Licenses						
First Class	20/100,20/100	20/20,20/20	Normal	None	Evaluation if over 10 hyper or eso or exo 6	2
Second Class	20/100,20/100	20/20,20/20				
Third Class	20/50,20/50	20/30,20/30				
Coast Guard Licenses						
Operator, Master, Pilot, etc.	20/40,20/70	20/20,20/40	Normal	None	None	
Engineer, Radio	20/50,20/70	20/30,20/50	Red-green Blue-yellow			
Federal Highway Administration	20/40,20/40	20/40,20/40	Normal	None	None	5
F.B.I.	20/40,20/50	20/20,20/20	Normal	None	None	

[1] Waivers permitted
[2] Near vision requirement
[3] Any strabismus disqualifies
[4] Specific pathologies disqualify
[5] Specific visual field test required
[6] **Also acceptable 20/20, 20/100 corrected or one eye 20/100 to 20/20**

(continued)

1.4. Visual Standards

Table B. Flight Attendants

Airlines	*Uncorrected*	*Corrected*	*Airlines*	*Uncorrected*	*Corrected*
Major U.S. Airlines			TWA	20/200	20/50*
Air California	20/40	20/20	United	20/200	20/30*
Air Florida	none specified		U.S. Air	20/50	20/30
Alaska	20/200	*	Western	20/200	20/20
Aloha		20/50	Wien Air Alaska		20/20
American	20/50	*	World		20/20
Braniff	20/200	20/30	*Minor Airlines*		
Capital	none specified		Airlift Int.		20/20
Continental	20/200	20/40	Air New England		20/50*
Delta	20/100	20/20	Air South	none specified	
Eastern	20/200	20/40*	Altair		20/20*
Evergreen	20/100	20/20	Mackey Int.		20/50
Flying Tiger	none specified		Marco Island		20/20
Frontier	20/200	20/20	N.Y. Airways		20/50
Hawaian		20/50	Reeve Aleutian		20/50
Hughes	20/200	20/30	Seabord World		20/20
National	20/200	20/40	Swift Aire		20/20
Northwest Orient	20/200	20/20	*Canadian Airlines*		
Ozark	20/100	20/20*	Air Canada	20/100	20/50
Pacific S.W.		20/20	C.P. Air	20/100	20/30*
Pan American	20/100	20/40	Eastern Provincial	none specified	
Piedmont	20/200	20/70	Nordair		20/40
Republic		20/50	Pacific Western		20/60
Southwest	20/200	20/50	Quebec Air		20/50
Texas Int.	20/200	20/20	Transair		20/20
Trans Int.		20/20	Wardair Canada	20/80	*

*glasses specifically permitted

1.4. Visual Standards

Table C. Motor Vehicle Operators, U.S. and Canada

State	*Minimum Visual Acuity* — *Without Glasses* — *2 Eyes*	*Without Glasses* — *1 Blind Eye*	*With Glasses* — *2 Eyes*	*With Glasses* — *1 Blind Eye*	*Depth Perception*	*Color Blindness*	*Visual Field*	
ALA.	20/40	20/30	20/70	20/60	✓	✓		x
ALAS.	20/40	20/40	20/40	20/40	✓			
ARIZ.	20/40	20/40	20/40	20/40	✓	✓		x
ARK.	20/40	20/30	20/50	20/40		✓	110°	x
CAL.	20/40	20/40	20/40	20/40				x
COLO.	20/40	20/40	20/40	20/40	✓	✓		
CONN.	20/40	20/30	20/40	20/30	✓	✓	120°	x
DEL.	20/40	20/40	20/40	20/40	✓	✓		
D.C.	20/40	20/40	20/40	20/40	‖	✓	130°	
FLA.	20/70	20/40	20/70	20/40		✓	x	x
GA.	20/60	20/60	20/60	20/60	✓	✓		
HAW.	20/40	20/40	20/40	20/40	✓	✓	140°	
IDA.	20/40	20/40	20/40	20/40	✓	✓	140°	
ILL.	20/40	20/40	20/40	20/40		✓		
IND.	20/40	20/30	20/50	20/40	✓	✓		
IOWA	20/40	20/40	20/40	20/40	✓	‖		
KAN.	20/40	20/30	20/70	20/30		✓	✓	
KY.	20/45	20/33	20/60	20/45				
LA.	20/40	20/40	20/40	20/40	✓	✓		x
ME.	20/40	20/40	20/40	20/40	✓	✓	✓	
MD.	20/40	20/40	20/40	20/40	✓	✓	140°	
MASS.	20/40	20/40	20/40	20/40			120°	x
MICH.	20/40	20/40	20/40	20/40			140°	x
MINN.	20/40	20/30	20/40	20/30	✓	✓	✓	
MISS.	20/40	20/30	20/30	20/30	✓	✓	120°	
MO.	20/40	20/40	20/70	20/70	✓	✓	140°	
MONT.	20/40	20/40	20/40	20/40	✓	✓		x
NEB.	20/40	20/30	20/40	20/30	✓	✓	120°	x
NEV.	20/40	20/30	20/60	20/50	✓	✓		
N.H.	20/40	20/30	20/40	20/30	✓	✓	120°	
N.J.	20/50	20/50	20/50	20/50		✓		x
N.M.	20/40	20/40	20/40	20/40		✓		
N.Y.	20/40	20/40	20/40	20/40		✓	o	x
N.C.	20/40	20/29	20/50	20/40		✓		x
N.D.	20/40	20/30	20/40	20/30	§	§	§	
OHIO	20/40	20/30	20/70	20/60	✓	✓	140°	x
OKLA.	20/40	20/30	20/40	20/30	✓	✓	100°	
ORE.	20/40	20/40	20/40	20/40	✓	✓	‖	x
PA.	20/40	20/40	20/40	20/40	‖	‖	✓	
R.I.	20/40	20/40	20/40	20/40	✓	✓		
S.C.	20/40	20/20	20/40	20/40		✓		x
S.D.	20/40	20/40	20/40	20/40	✓	✓		
TENN.	20/70	20/40	20/70	20/40				
TEXAS	20/40	20/25	20/70	20/70		✓		
UTAH	20/40	20/40	20/40	20/40				
VT.	20/40	20/40	20/40	20/40	✓	✓	120°	
VA.	20/40	20/40	20/40	20/40		✓	100°	
WASH.	20/40	20/40	20/40	20/40	F	✓		x
W.V.	20/40	20/40	20/40	20/40	✓	✓		
WIS.	20/40	20/40	20/40	20/40	✓	✓		
WYO.	20/40	20/40	20/40	20/40	✓	✓		
Canada								
ALBERTA	20/40	20/40	20/60	20/60				
BR. COL.	20/40	20/40	20/50	20/50			100°	
MAN.	20/40	20/40	20/60	20/60		✓	120°	
N. FD.	20/40	20/40	20/40	20/40			140°	
N. BR.	20/40	20/40	20/40	20/40			120°	
NOV. SC.	20/40	20/40	20/40	20/40			120°	
ONT.	20/40	20/40	20/40	20/40			120°	
QUE.	20/40	20/40	20/50	20/50			120°	
P.E.I.	20/40	20/40	20/40	20/30			120° ‡	
SASK.	20/40	20/40	20/40	20/40			120° †	

†Waiver
‡ Guidelines
✓ = STANDARD
§ Optional with examiner
‖ Special cases
F = FUSION
x = Telescopes have been permitted
o = 140° when VA is 20/70

U.S. portion reprinted courtesy American Optical Corp., Southbridge, Mass.

Reprinted with permission of the American Optometric Association, Survey date 1978.

1.5. Percentage Visual Acuity at Some Eccentricities

central	30′	1°	1.5°	2°	2.5°	3.5°	5°	6°	7°
100%	77%	62%	53%	47%	42%	37%	32%	29%	27%

Reprinted from "Foveal and extra Foveal Acuity with and without Stabilized Retinal Images", Millidot, M., *British Journal Phys. Opt.*, Vol. 23 #2, 1966.

1.6. Equivalent Acuities for Nonstandard Viewing Distances

Acuity Measured	*Test Distance*								
	7.5 *25*	*4.8* *16*	*3.8* *12*	*3.0* *10*	*2.4* *8*	*1.9* *6.3*	*1.5* *5*	*1.2* *4*	*meters* *feet*
20/200	160	250	320	400	500	630	800	1000	
20/160	125	200	250	320	400	500	630	800	
20/125	100	160	200	250	320	400	500	630	
20/100	80	125	160	200	250	320	400	500	
20/80	60	100	125	160	200	250	320	400	
20/60	50	80	100	125	160	200	250	320	
20/50	40	60	80	100	125	160	200	250	
20/40	30	50	60	80	100	125	160	200	
20/30	25	40	50	60	80	100	125	160	
20/25	20	30	40	50	60	80	100	125	
20/20	15	25	30	40	50	60	80	100	
20/15	12.5	20	25	30	40	50	60	80	
20/12.5	10.0	15	20	25	30	40	50	60	

This chart is designed with a logarithmic progression in size. The denominator only of the 20-foot Snellan Designation is shown.

Adapted from: "New Design Principles for Visual Acuity Letter Charts." I.L. Bailey, Jan E. Lovie AJO Vol 53, #11 11/76 p. 740

1.7. Distances at Which Jaeger Test Types Can Be Read with Normal Acuity and Accommodation

Type	*Distance in Centimeters*	*Type*	*Distance in Centimeters*
J.1	50	J.8	125
J.2	60	J.10	150
J.4	80	J.12	175
J.6	100	J.14	225

Reprinted by permission from N. Bier, *Correction of Subnormal Vision*, 2nd ed. London: Butterworths, 1970.

1.8. Relative Difficulty of Snellen Letters

Letter	*Visual Acuity*	*Letter*	*Visual Acuity*
B	1.00	P	.81
H	.92	F	.81
G	.89	Y	.80
S	.88	L	.80
R	.85	T	.79
E	.85	V	.79
N	.84	U	.78
Z	.84	C	.74
D	.81	O	.70

Reprinted by permission from C. Sheard, "Some factors affecting visual acuity," *Am. J. Physiol. Optics* 2: 1921.

Ophthalmic Optics 2

2.1. Overcoming Horizontal Prismatic Effects of Oblique Axis Cylinders

Amount to Decenter Each Segment
(Decenter segments inward where imbalance is BASE OUT between the eyes)
(Decenter segments outward where imbalance is BASE IN between the eyes)
Also decenter segments inward 1½ mm. each to allow for convergence.

Prismatic Imbalance to be Balanced	*Reading Additions* 1.00	1.25	1.50	1.75	2.00	2.25	2.50	2.75	3.00	3.25	3.50	3.75	4.00
½△	2.5 mm.	2.0 mm.	1.7 mm.	1.4 mm.	1.2 mm.	1.1 mm.	1.0 mm.	0.9 mm.	0.8 mm.	0.8 mm.	0.7 mm.	0.7 mm.	0.6 mm.
¾	3.7	3.0	2.5	2.1	1.8	1.7	1.5	1.4	1.3	1.2	1.1	1.0	0.9
1	5.0	4.0	3.3	2.8	2.5	2.2	2.0	1.8	1.7	1.5	1.4	1.3	1.2
1¼	6.3	5.0	4.2	3.6	3.1	2.8	2.5	2.3	2.1	1.9	1.8	1.7	1.6
1½	7.5	6.0	5.0	4.3	3.8	3.3	3.0	2.7	2.5	2.3	2.1	2.0	1.9
1¾	Impractical Use Prism Segments	7.0	5.8	5.0	4.4	3.9	3.5	3.2	2.9	2.7	2.5	2.3	2.2
2	"	Impractical	6.7	5.7	5.0	4.4	4.0	3.6	3.3	3.1	2.9	2.7	2.5
2¼	"	"	7.5	6.4	5.6	5.0	4.5	4.1	3.8	3.5	3.2	3.0	2.8
2½	"	"	Impractical	7.1	6.3	5.5	5.0	4.5	4.2	3.8	3.6	3.3	3.1
2¾	"	"	"	Impractical	6.9	6.1	5.5	5.0	4.6	4.2	3.9	3.7	3.4
3	"	"	"	"	Impractical	6.7	6.0	5.5	5.0	4.6	4.3	4.0	3.7
3¼	"	"	"	"	"	7.2	6.5	5.9	5.4	5.0	4.6	4.3	4.1
3½	"	"	"	"	"	Impractical	7.0	6.4	5.8	5.4	5.0	4.7	4.4
3¾	"	"	"	"	"	"	Impractical	6.8	6.3	5.8	5.4	5.0	4.7
4	"	"	"	"	"	"	"	7.3	6.7	6.2	5.7	5.3	5.0

2.2. Compounding of Perpendicular Prisms

Resultant of Combined Prisms and Angle With the 180° Line

Prism Diopters Base Up or Down	*Prism Diopters Base In or Out* 0.5	1.0	1.5	2.0	2.5	3.0	3.5	4.0	4.5	5.0	5.5	6.0
0.5	0.7 45°	1.1 27°	1.6 18°	2.1 14°	2.6 11°	3.0 9°	3.5 8°	4.0 7°	4.5 6°	5.0 6°	5.5 5°	6.0 5°
1.0	1.1 63°	1.4 45°	1.8 34°	2.2 27°	2.7 22°	3.2 18°	3.6 16°	4.1 14°	4.6 13°	5.1 11°	5.6 10°	6.1 9°
1.5	1.6 72°	1.8 56°	2.1 45°	2.5 37°	2.9 31°	3.4 27°	3.8 23°	4.3 21°	4.7 18°	5.2 17°	5.7 15°	6.2 14°
2.0	2.1 76°	2.2 63°	2.5 53°	2.8 45°	3.2 39°	3.6 34°	4.0 30°	4.5 27°	4.9 24°	5.4 22°	5.9 20°	6.3 18°
2.5	2.6 79°	2.7 68°	2.9 59°	3.2 51°	3.5 45°	3.9 40°	4.3 36°	4.7 32°	5.1 29°	5.6 27°	6.0 24°	6.5 23°
3.0	3.0 81°	3.2 72°	3.4 63°	3.6 56°	3.9 50°	4.2 45°	4.6 41°	5.0 37°	5.4 34°	5.8 31°	6.3 29°	6.7 27°
3.5	3.5 82°	3.6 74°	3.8 67°	4.0 60°	4.3 54°	4.6 49°	4.9 45°	5.3 41°	5.7 38°	6.1 35°	6.5 32°	6.9 30°
4.0	4.0 83°	4.1 76°	4.3 69°	4.5 63°	4.7 58°	5.0 53°	5.3 49°	5.7 45°	6.0 42°	6.4 39°	6.8 36°	7.2 34°
4.5	4.5 84°	4.6 77°	4.7 72°	4.9 66°	5.1 61°	5.4 56°	5.7 52°	6.0 48°	6.4 45°	6.7 42°	7.1 39°	7.5 37°
5.0	5.0 84°	5.1 79°	5.2 73°	5.4 68°	5.6 63°	5.8 59°	6.1 55°	6.4 51°	6.7 48°	7.1 45°	7.4 42°	7.8 40°
5.5	5.5 85°	5.6 80°	5.7 75°	5.9 70°	6.0 66°	6.3 61°	6.5 58°	6.8 54°	7.1 51°	7.4 48°	7.8 45°	8.1 43°
6.0	6.0 85°	6.1 81°	6.2 76°	6.3 72°	6.5 67°	6.7 63°	6.9 60°	7.2 56°	7.5 53°	7.8 50°	8.1 47°	8.5 45°

Reprinted by permission from Bausch & Lomb Optical Co., *Job Coach for Prescription Laboratory Operations.* Courtesy Bausch & Lomb, Rochester, N.Y.

2.3. Horizontal Prismatic Effect in Near Work Produced by Spherical Lenses Centered for Distance

P.D. = 60 mm.

	Object 30 cm. beyond lens			*Object 40 cm. beyond lens*		
Power of Lens D	*Effective Decentration x cm.*	*Prism Effect at Lens d △*	*Prism Effect on Eye △*	*Effective Decentration x cm.*	*Prism Effect at Lens d △*	*Prism Effect on Eye △*
+20	0.48	9.60	8.82	0.37	7.50	7.03
18	0.44	7.88	7.24	0.34	6.14	5.75
16	0.40	6.45	5.92	0.31	5.01	4.69
14	0.37	5.22	4.79	0.29	4.03	3.79
12	0.35	4.16	3.82	0.27	3.22	3.01
10	0.32	3.24	2.98	0.25	2.50	2.34
8	0.30	2.44	2.24	0.23	1.87	1.76
6	0.29	1.72	1.58	0.22	1.33	1.24
5	0.28	1.40	1.28	0.21	1.07	1.00
4	0.27	1.08	1.00	0.21	0.83	0.78
3	0.26	0.79	0.73	0.20	0.61	0.57
2	0.26	0.52	0.47	0.20	0.39	0.37
+ 1	0.25	0.25	0.23	0.19	0.91	0.18
0	0.245	0.0	0.0	0.19	0.0	0.0
− 1	0.24	−0.24	−0.22	0.18	−0.18	−0.17
− 2	0.23	−0.47	−0.43	0.18	−0.36	−0.33
− 3	0.23	−0.68	−0.63	0.17	−0.52	−0.49
− 4	0.22	−0.89	−0.82	0.17	−0.68	−0.64
− 5	0.22	−1.09	−1.00	0.17	−0.83	−0.78
− 6	0.21	−1.28	−1.18	0.16	−0.98	−0.92
− 8	0.20	−1.64	−1.50	0.16	−1.25	−1.17
−10	0.20	−1.97	−1.81	0.15	−1.50	−1.41
−12	0.19	−2.27	−2.09	0.14	−1.73	−1.62
−14	0.18	−2.55	−2.34	0.14	−1.95	−1.82
−16	0.18	−2.82	−2.59	0.13	−2.14	−2.01
−18	0.17	−3.06	−2.81	0.13	−2.32	−2.18
−20	0.16	−3.28	−3.02	0.125	−2.50	−2.34

Reprinted by permission from H. Emsley, *Optical Tables and Data.* London: United Kingdom Optical Ltd., 1968.

2.4. Vertical Prismatic Effects of Spheres for Various Depressions

	Sphere Powers																		
Depressions	*0.50*	*0.75*	*1.00*	*1.25*	*1.50*	*1.75*	*2.00*	*2.25*	*2.50*	*2.75*	*3.00*	*3.25*	*3.50*	*3.75*	*4.00*	*4.25*	*4.50*	*4.75*	*5.00*
3 mm.	0.15	0.22	0.30	0.37	0.45	0.52	0.60	0.67	0.75	0.82	0.90	0.97	1.05	1.12	1.20	1.27	1.35	1.42	1.50
4 mm.	0.20	0.30	0.40	0.50	0.60	0.70	0.80	0.90	1.00	1.10	1.20	1.30	1.40	1.50	1.60	1.70	1.80	1.90	2.00
5 mm.	0.25	0.37	0.50	0.62	0.75	0.87	1.00	1.12	1.25	1.37	1.50	1.62	1.75	1.87	2.00	2.12	2.25	2.37	2.50
6 mm.	0.30	0.45	0.60	0.75	0.90	1.05	1.20	1.35	1.50	1.65	1.80	1.95	2.10	2.25	2.40	2.55	2.70	2.85	3.00
7 mm.	0.35	0.52	0.70	0.87	1.05	1.22	1.40	1.57	1.75	1.92	2.10	2.27	2.45	2.62	2.80	2.97	3.15	3.32	3.50
8 mm.	0.40	0.60	0.80	1.00	1.20	1.40	1.60	1.80	2.00	2.20	2.40	2.60	2.80	3.00	3.20	3.40	3.50	3.80	4.00
9 mm.	0.45	0.67	0.90	1.12	1.35	1.57	1.80	2.02	2.25	2.47	2.70	2.92	3.15	3.37	3.60	3.82	4.05	4.27	4.50
10 mm.	0.50	0.75	1.00	1.25	1.50	1.75	2.00	2.25	2.50	2.75	3.00	3.25	3.50	3.75	4.00	4.25	4.50	4.75	5.00

	Sphere Powers																		
Depressions	*5.25*	*5.50*	*5.75*	*6.00*	*6.50*	*7.00*	*7.50*	*8.00*	*8.50*	*9.00*	*9.50*	*10.00*	*10.50*	*11.00*	*11.50*	*12.00*	*13.00*	*14.00*	*15.00*
3 mm.	1.57	1.65	1.72	1.80	1.95	2.10	2.25	2.40	2.55	2.70	2.85	3.00	3.15	3.30	3.45	3.60	3.90	4.20	4.50
4 mm.	2.10	2.20	2.30	2.40	2.60	2.80	3.00	3.20	3.40	3.60	3.80	4.00	4.20	4.40	4.60	4.80	5.20	5.60	6.00
5 mm.	2.62	2.75	2.87	3.00	3.25	3.50	3.75	4.00	4.25	4.50	4.75	5.00	5.25	5.50	5.75	6.00	6.50	7.00	7.50
6 mm.	3.15	3.30	3.45	3.60	3.90	4.20	4.50	4.80	5.10	5.40	5.70	6.00	6.30	6.60	6.90	7.20	7.80	8.40	9.00
7 mm.	3.67	3.85	4.02	4.20	4.55	4.90	5.25	5.60	5.95	6.30	6.65	7.00	7.35	7.70	8.05	8.40	9.10	9.80	10.50
8 mm.	4.20	4.40	4.60	4.80	5.20	5.60	6.00	6.40	6.80	7.20	7.60	8.00	8.40	8.80	9.20	9.60	10.40	11.20	12.00
9 mm.	4.72	4.95	5.18	5.40	5.85	6.30	6.75	7.20	7.65	8.10	8.55	9.00	9.45	9.90	10.35	10.80	11.70	12.60	13.50
10 mm.	5.25	5.50	5.75	6.00	6.50	7.00	7.50	8.00	8.50	9.00	9.50	10.00	10.50	11.00	11.50	12.00	13.00	14.00	15.00

Reprinted by permission from I.B. Lueck, "Bifocal analysis in anisometropia," Bausch & Lomb *Technical Bulletin*, No. 18 (1937).

2.5. Horizontal and Vertical Powers of Oblique Axis Cylinders

Cyl. Power	*Axis of Cylinder for Horizontal Power*								
	90	*80 100*	*70 110*	*60 120*	*50 130*	*40 140*	*30 150*	*20 160*	*10 170*
.25	.25	.24	.22	.19	.15	.10	.06	.03	.01
.50	.50	.49	.44	.38	.30	.21	.13	.06	.02
.75	.75	.73	.66	.58	.44	.31	.18	.09	.02
1.00	1.00	.97	.88	.75	.59	.41	.25	.12	.03
1.25	1.25	1.21	1.10	.94	.74	.51	.31	.15	.04
1.50	1.50	1.45	1.32	1.12	.89	.61	.38	.18	.04
1.75	1.75	1.70	1.54	1.31	1.03	.72	.44	.21	.05
2.00	2.00	1.94	1.76	1.50.	1.18	.82	.50	.24	.06
2.25	2.25	2.18	1.98	1.69	1.33	.92	.56	.27	.07
2.50	2.50	2.42	2.20	1.87	1.47	1.03	.63	.30	.08
2.75	2.75	2.66	2.42	2.06	1.62	1.13	.69	.33	.08
3.00	3.00	2.91	2.64	2.25	1.77	1.23	.75	.36	.09
3.25	3.25	3.15	2.86	2.44	1.92	1.33	.81	.39	.10
3.50	3.50	3.39	3.08	2.62	2.06	1.44	.88	.42	.11
3.75	3.75	3.64	3.30	2.81	2.21	1.54	.94	.45	.11
4.00	4.00	3.88	3.52	3.00	2.36	1.64	1.00	.48	.12
	0 180	*10 170*	*20 160*	*30 150*	*40 140*	*50 130*	*60 120*	*70 110*	*80 100*
	Axis of Cylinder for Vertical Power								

Reprinted by permission from T.H. Calkins, *Essentials of Modern Lens Theory and Practice.* Rochester, N.Y.: Shuron Continental Co.

2.6. Vertical Prismatic Effect of Cylinders at Oblique Axes

Table A. Data: b = 6 mm. i = 2 mm.

Cylinder Axis Given in Prescription: Left Eye	Right Eye	Cylinder Power Given in Prescription: .50	1.00	1.25	1.50	1.75	2.00	2.25	2.50	2.75	3.00	3.25	3.50	3.75	4.00	4.25	4.50	4.75	5.00	5.50	6.00
180	0-180	0.30	0.60	0.75	0.90	1.05	1.20	1.35	1.50	1.65	1.80	1.95	2.10	2.25	2.40	2.55	2.70	2.85	3.00	3.30	3.60
175	5	0.30	0.61	0.76	0.91	1.07	1.22	1.37	1.52	1.68	1.83	1.98	2.13	2.28	2.44	2.59	2.74	2.90	3.05	3.35	3.66
170	10	0.31	0.62	0.77	0.92	1.08	1.23	1.38	1.54	1.69	1.84	2.00	2.15	2.30	2.46	2.62	2.76	2.92	3.08	3.38	3.69
165	15	0.30	0.60	0.75	0.90	1.05	1.20	1.35	1.50	1.65	1.80	1.95	2.10	2.25	2.40	2.55	2.70	2.85	3.00	3.30	3.60
160	20	0.30	0.59	0.74	0.89	1.03	1.18	1.32	1.43	1.62	1.73	1.91	2.06	2.21	2.36	2.50	2.65	2.80	2.95	3.24	3.54
155	25	0.28	0.56	0.70	0.84	0.98	1.12	1.26	1.40	1.54	1.68	1.82	1.96	2.10	2.24	2.38	2.52	2.66	2.80	3.08	3.36
150	30	0.27	0.54	0.67	0.81	0.95	1.08	1.21	1.35	1.48	1.62	1.75	1.89	2.06	2.16	2.29	2.43	2.56	2.70	2.97	3.24
145	35	0.25	0.49	0.61	0.73	0.86	0.98	1.10	1.22	1.35	1.47	1.59	1.71	1.84	1.96	2.08	2.20	2.33	2.45	2.69	2.94
140	40	0.23	0.45	0.56	0.67	0.79	0.90	1.01	1.12	1.24	1.35	1.46	1.57	1.69	1.80	1.91	2.02	2.14	2.25	2.48	2.70
135	45	0.20	0.40	0.50	0.60	0.70	0.80	0.90	1.00	1.10	1.20	1.30	1.40	1.50	1.60	1.70	1.80	1.90	2.00	2.20	2.40
130	50	0.18	0.35	0.44	0.52	0.61	0.70	0.79	0.87	0.96	1.05	1.14	1.22	1.31	1.40	1.49	1.57	1.66	1.75	1.92	2.10
125	55	0.15	0.29	0.36	0.43	0.51	0.58	0.65	0.72	0.80	0.87	0.94	1.01	1.09	1.16	1.23	1.30	1.38	1.45	1.59	1.74
120	60	0.12	0.24	0.30	0.36	0.42	0.48	0.54	0.60	0.66	0.72	0.78	0.84	0.90	0.96	1.02	1.08	1.14	1.20	1.32	1.44
115	65	0.09	0.18	0.22	0.27	0.31	0.36	0.41	0.45	0.49	0.54	0.58	0.63	0.67	0.72	0.76	0.81	0.85	0.90	0.99	1.08
110	70	0.06	0.13	0.16	0.19	0.23	0.26	0.29	0.32	0.36	0.39	0.42	0.45	0.49	0.52	0.55	0.58	0.62	0.65	0.71	0.78
105	75	0.05	0.09	0.11	0.13	0.16	0.18	0.20	0.22	0.25	0.27	0.29	0.31	0.34	0.36	0.38	0.40	0.43	0.45	0.49	0.54
100	80	0.02	0.05	0.06	0.07	0.09	0.10	0.11	0.12	0.14	0.15	0.16	0.17	0.19	0.20	0.21	0.22	0.24	0.25	0.27	0.30
95	85	0.01	0.02	0.02	0.03	0.03	0.04	0.04	0.05	0.05	0.06	0.06	0.07	0.07	0.08	0.08	0.09	0.09	0.10	0.11	0.12
90	90	0.00	0.00	0.00	0.00	0.00	0.00	0.00	0.00	0.00	0.00	0.00	0.00	0.00	0.00	0.00	0.00	0.00	0.00	0.00	0.00
85	95	0.00	0.01	0.01	0.01	0.02	0.02	0.02	0.02	0.03	0.03	0.03	0.03	0.04	0.04	0.04	0.04	0.05	0.05	0.05	0.06
80	100	0.01	0.02	0.02	0.03	0.03	0.04	0.04	0.05	0.05	0.06	0.06	0.07	0.07	0.08	0.08	0.09	0.09	0.10	0.11	0.12
75	105	0.02	0.04	0.05	0.06	0.07	0.08	0.09	0.10	0.11	0.12	0.13	0.14	0.15	0.16	0.17	0.18	0.19	0.20	0.22	0.24
70	110	0.03	0.06	0.07	0.09	0.10	0.12	0.13	0.15	0.16	0.18	0.19	0.21	0.22	0.24	0.25	0.27	0.28	0.30	0.33	0.36
65	115	0.03	0.06	0.07	0.09	0.10	0.12	0.13	0.15	0.16	0.18	0.19	0.21	0.22	0.24	0.25	0.27	0.28	0.30	0.33	0.36
60	120	0.03	0.06	0.07	0.09	0.10	0.12	0.13	0.15	0.16	0.18	0.19	0.21	0.22	0.24	0.25	0.27	0.28	0.30	0.33	0.36
55	125	0.05	0.10	0.12	0.15	0.17	0.20	0.22	0.25	0.27	0.30	0.32	0.35	0.37	0.40	0.42	0.45	0.47	0.50	0.55	0.60
50	130	0.07	0.15	0.19	0.22	0.26	0.30	0.34	0.37	0.41	0.45	0.49	0.52	0.56	0.60	0.64	0.67	0.71	0.75	0.82	0.90
45	135	0.10	0.20	0.25	0.30	0.35	0.40	0.45	0.50	0.55	0.60	0.65	0.70	0.75	0.80	0.85	0.90	0.95	1.00	1.10	1.20
40	140	0.12	0.25	0.31	0.37	0.44	0.50	0.56	0.62	0.69	0.75	0.81	0.87	0.94	1.00	1.06	1.12	1.19	1.25	1.37	1.50
35	145	0.15	0.30	0.37	0.45	0.52	0.60	0.67	0.75	0.82	0.90	0.97	1.05	1.12	1.20	1.27	1.35	1.42	1.50	1.65	1.80
30	150	0.18	0.36	0.45	0.54	0.63	0.72	0.81	0.90	0.99	1.08	1.17	1.26	1.35	1.44	1.53	1.62	1.71	1.80	1.98	2.16
25	155	0.20	0.41	0.51	0.61	0.72	0.82	0.92	1.02	1.13	1.23	1.33	1.43	1.54	1.64	1.74	1.84	1.95	2.05	2.25	2.46
20	160	0.23	0.47	0.59	0.70	0.82	0.94	1.06	1.17	1.29	1.41	1.53	1.64	1.76	1.88	2.00	2.11	2.23	2.35	2.58	2.82
15	165	0.25	0.51	0.64	0.76	0.89	1.02	1.15	1.27	1.40	1.53	1.65	1.78	1.91	2.04	2.16	2.29	2.42	2.55	2.80	3.06
10	170	0.27	0.55	0.69	0.82	0.96	1.10	1.24	1.37	1.51	1.65	1.78	1.92	2.06	2.20	2.34	2.47	2.61	2.75	3.02	3.30
5	175	0.28	0.57	0.71	0.85	1.00	1.14	1.28	1.42	1.56	1.71	1.85	1.99	2.14	2.28	2.42	2.56	2.70	2.85	3.13	3.42

b = distance below optical center; i = inset.

2.6. Vertical Prismatic Effect of Cylinders at Oblique Axes

Table B. Data: b = 8 mm. i = 2 mm.

Cylinder Axis Given in Prescription

Left Eye	Right Eye	*Cylinder Power Given in Prescription* .50	1.00	1.25	1.50	1.75	2.00	2.25	2.50	2.75	3.00	3.25	3.50	3.75	4.00	4.25	4.50	4.75	5.00	5.50	6.00
180	0-180	0.40	0.80	1.00	1.20	1.40	1.60	1.80	2.00	2.20	2.40	2.60	2.80	3.00	3.20	3.40	3.60	3.80	4.00	4.40	4.80
175	5	0.40	0.80	1.00	1.20	1.40	1.60	1.80	2.00	2.20	2.40	2.60	2.80	3.00	3.20	3.40	3.60	3.80	4.00	4.40	4.80
170	10	0.40	0.81	1.01	1.21	1.42	1.62	1.82	2.02	2.22	2.43	2.63	2.83	3.04	3.24	3.44	3.64	3.84	4.05	4.45	4.86
165	15	0.40	0.79	0.99	1.18	1.38	1.58	1.78	1.97	2.17	2.37	2.56	2.76	2.96	3.16	3.36	3.55	3.75	3.95	4.35	4.74
160	20	0.39	0.77	0.96	1.15	1.35	1.54	1.73	1.92	2.12	2.31	2.50	2.69	2.88	3.08	3.27	3.46	3.66	3.85	4.24	4.62
155	25	0.36	0.73	0.91	1.09	1.28	1.46	1.64	1.82	2.01	2.19	2.37	2.56	2.74	2.92	3.10	3.28	3.47	3.65	4.01	4.38
150	30	0.34	0.69	0.86	1.03	1.21	1.38	1.55	1.72	1.90	2.07	2.24	2.51	2.68	2.76	2.93	3.10	3.28	3.45	3.79	4.14
145	35	0.31	0.63	0.79	0.95	1.10	1.26	1.42	1.57	1.73	1.89	2.04	2.20	2.36	2.52	2.68	2.83	2.99	3.15	3.46	3.78
140	40	0.28	0.57	0.71	0.85	1.00	1.14	1.28	1.42	1.57	1.71	1.85	1.99	2.14	2.28	2.42	2.56	2.71	2.85	3.14	3.42
135	45	0.25	0.50	0.62	0.75	0.87	1.00	1.12	1.25	1.37	1.50	1.62	1.75	1.87	2.00	2.12	2.25	2.37	2.50	2.75	3.00
130	50	0.21	0.43	0.54	0.64	0.75	0.86	0.97	1.07	1.18	1.29	1.40	1.50	1.61	1.72	1.83	1.93	2.04	2.15	2.36	2.58
125	55	0.18	0.36	0.45	0.54	0.63	0.72	0.81	0.90	0.99	1.08	1.17	1.26	1.35	1.44	1.53	1.62	1.71	1.80	1.98	2.16
129	60	0.15	0.29	0.36	0.43	0.51	0.58	0.65	0.72	0.80	0.87	0.94	1.01	1.09	1.16	1.23	1.30	1.38	1.45	1.59	1.74
115	65	0.12	0.23	0.29	0.34	0.40	0.46	0.52	0.57	0.63	0.69	0.75	0.80	0.86	0.92	0.98	1.03	1.09	1.15	1.26	1.38
110	70	0.08	0.16	0.20	0.24	0.28	0.32	0.36	0.40	0.44	0.48	0.52	0.56	0.60	0.64	0.68	0.72	0.76	0.80	0.88	0.96
105	75	0.05	0.11	0.14	0.16	0.19	0.22	0.25	0.27	0.30	0.33	0.36	0.38	0.41	0.44	0.47	0.49	0.52	0.55	0.60	0.66
100	80	0.03	0.06	0.07	0.09	0.10	0.12	0.13	0.15	0.16	0.18	0.19	0.21	0.22	0.24	0.25	0.27	0.28	0.30	0.33	0.36
95	85	0.01	0.03	0.04	0.04	0.05	0.06	0.07	0.07	0.08	0.09	0.09	0.10	0.11	0.12	0.13	0.13	0.14	0.15	0.16	0.18
90	90	0.00	0.00	0.00	0.00	0.00	0.00	0.00	0.00	0.00	0.00	0.00	0.00	0.00	0.00	0.00	0.00	0.00	0.00	0.00	0.00
85	95	0.00	0.01	0.01	0.01	0.02	0.02	0.02	0.02	0.03	0.03	0.03	0.03	0.04	0.04	0.04	0.04	0.05	0.05	0.05	0.06
80	100	0.00	0.01	0.01	0.01	0.02	0.02	0.02	0.02	0.03	0.03	0.03	0.03	0.04	0.04	0.04	0.04	0.05	0.05	0.05	0.06
75	105	0.01	0.02	0.02	0.03	0.03	0.04	0.04	0.05	0.05	0.06	0.06	0.07	0.07	0.08	0.08	0.09	0.09	0.10	0.11	0.12
70	110	0.01	0.03	0.04	0.04	0.05	0.06	0.07	0.07	0.08	0.09	0.10	0.10	0.11	0.12	0.13	0.13	0.14	0.15	0.16	0.18
65	115	0.03	0.07	0.09	0.10	0.12	0.14	0.16	0.17	0.19	0.21	0.23	0.24	0.26	0.28	0.30	0.31	0.33	0.35	0.38	0.42
60	120	0.06	0.11	0.14	0.16	0.19	0.22	0.25	0.27	0.30	0.33	0.36	0.38	0.41	0.44	0.47	0.49	0.52	0.55	0.60	0.66
55	125	0.09	0.17	0.21	0.25	0.30	0.34	0.38	0.42	0.47	0.51	0.55	0.59	0.64	0.68	0.72	0.76	0.81	0.85	0.93	1.02
50	130	0.12	0.23	0.29	0.34	0.40	0.46	0.52	0.57	0.63	0.69	0.75	0.80	0.86	0.92	0.98	1.03	1.09	1.15	1.26	1.38
45	135	0.15	0.30	0.37	0.45	0.52	0.60	0.67	0.75	0.82	0.90	0.98	1.05	1.12	1.20	1.27	1.35	1.42	1.50	1.65	1.80
40	140	0.18	0.37	0.46	0.55	0.65	0.74	0.83	0.92	1.02	1.11	1.20	1.29	1.39	1.48	1.57	1.66	1.76	1.85	2.04	2.22
35	145	0.22	0.44	0.55	0.66	0.77	0.88	0.99	1.01	1.21	1.32	1.43	1.54	1.65	1.76	1.87	1.98	2.09	2.20	2.42	2.64
30	150	0.25	0.51	0.64	0.76	0.89	1.02	1.15	1.27	1.40	1.53	1.66	1.78	1.91	2.04	2.17	2.29	2.42	2.55	2.80	3.06
25	155	0.29	0.58	0.72	0.87	1.01	1.16	1.30	1.45	1.60	1.74	1.88	2.03	2.17	2.32	2.46	2.61	2.75	2.90	3.19	3.48
20	160	0.32	0.64	0.80	0.96	1.12	1.28	1.44	1.60	1.76	1.92	2.08	2.24	2.40	2.56	2.72	2.88	3.04	3.20	3.52	3.84
15	165	0.34	0.69	0.86	1.03	1.21	1.38	1.55	1.72	1.90	2.07	2.24	2.51	2.68	2.76	2.93	3.10	3.28	3.45	3.79	4.14
10	170	0.37	0.74	0.96	1.11	1.29	1.48	1.66	1.85	2.03	2.22	2.40	2.59	2.77	2.96	3.14	3.33	3.52	3.70	4.07	4.44
5	175	0.38	0.77	0.96	1.15	1.35	1.54	1.73	1.92	2.12	2.31	2.50	2.69	2.88	3.08	3.27	3.46	3.66	3.85	4.24	4.62

2.6. Vertical Prismatic Effect of Cylinders at Oblique Axes

Table C. Data: b = 10 mm. i = 2 mm.

Cylinder Axis Given in Prescription: Left Eye	Right Eye	Cylinder Power Given in Prescription: .50	1.00	1.25	1.50	1.75	2.00	2.25	2.50	2.75	3.00	3.25	3.50	3.75	4.00	4.25	4.50	4.75	5.00	5.50	6.00
180	0-180	0.50	1.00	1.25	1.50	1.75	2.00	2.25	2.50	2.75	3.00	3.25	3.50	3.75	4.00	4.25	4.50	4.75	5.00	5.50	6.00
175	5	0.50	1.00	1.25	1.50	1.75	2.00	2.25	2.50	2.75	3.00	3.25	3.50	3.75	4.00	4.25	4.50	4.75	5.00	5.50	6.00
170	10	0.50	1.00	1.25	1.50	1.75	2.00	2.25	2.50	2.75	3.00	3.25	3.50	3.75	4.00	4.25	4.50	4.75	5.00	5.50	6.00
165	15	0.49	0.98	1.22	1.47	1.71	1.96	2.20	2.45	2.69	2.94	3.18	3.43	3.67	3.92	4.17	4.41	4.65	4.90	5.39	5.88
160	20	0.47	0.95	1.19	1.42	1.66	1.90	2.14	2.37	2.61	2.85	3.09	3.32	3.56	3.80	4.04	4.27	4.52	4.75	5.22	5.70
155	25	0.45	0.90	1.12	1.35	1.57	1.80	2.02	2.25	2.47	2.70	2.92	3.15	3.37	3.60	3.83	4.05	4.27	4.50	4.95	5.40
150	30	0.42	0.84	1.05	1.26	1.47	1.68	1.89	2.10	2.31	2.52	2.73	2.94	3.15	3.36	3.57	3.78	3.99	4.20	4.62	5.04
145	35	0.38	0.77	0.96	1.15	1.35	1.54	1.73	1.92	2.12	2.31	2.50	2.70	2.89	3.08	3.27	3.46	3.66	3.85	4.24	4.62
140	40	0.34	0.69	0.86	1.03	1.21	1.38	1.55	1.72	1.90	2.07	2.24	2.42	2.57	2.76	2.93	3.10	3.28	3.45	3.80	4.14
135	45	0.30	0.60	0.75	0.90	1.05	1.20	1.35	1.50	1.65	1.80	1.95	2.10	2.25	2.40	2.55	2.70	2.85	3.00	3.30	3.60
130	50	0.25	0.51	0.64	0.76	0.89	1.02	1.15	1.27	1.40	1.53	1.66	1.78	1.91	2.04	2.17	2.30	2.42	2.55	2.80	3.06
125	55	0.21	0.42	0.52	0.63	0.73	0.84	0.94	1.05	1.15	1.26	1.36	1.47	1.57	1.68	1.78	1.89	2.00	2.10	2.31	2.52
120	60	0.17	0.34	0.42	0.51	0.59	0.68	0.76	0.85	0.93	1.02	1.11	1.19	1.27	1.36	1.44	1.53	1.61	1.70	1.87	2.04
115	65	0.13	0.26	0.33	0.39	0.45	0.52	0.58	0.65	0.71	0.78	0.85	0.91	0.98	1.04	1.10	1.17	1.23	1.30	1.43	1.56
110	70	0.09	0.18	0.22	0.27	0.31	0.36	0.40	0.45	0.49	0.54	0.58	0.63	0.67	0.72	0.76	0.81	0.85	0.90	0.99	1.08
105	75	0.06	0.12	0.15	0.18	0.21	0.24	0.27	0.30	0.33	0.36	0.39	0.42	0.45	0.48	0.51	0.54	0.57	0.60	0.66	0.72
100	80	0.03	0.06	0.07	0.09	0.10	0.12	0.13	0.15	0.16	0.18	0.19	0.21	0.22	0.24	0.25	0.27	0.28	0.30	0.33	0.36
95	85	0.01	0.03	0.04	0.04	0.05	0.06	0.07	0.07	0.08	0.09	0.10	0.10	0.11	0.12	0.13	0.14	0.14	0.15	0.16	0.18
90	90	0.00	0.00	0.00	0.00	0.00	0.00	0.00	0.00	0.00	0.00	0.00	0.00	0.00	0.00	0.00	0.00	0.00	0.00	0.00	0.00
85	95	0.00	0.01	0.01	0.01	0.02	0.02	0.02	0.02	0.03	0.03	0.03	0.03	0.04	0.04	0.04	0.04	0.05	0.05	0.05	0.05
80	100	0.00	0.00	0.00	0.00	0.00	0.00	0.00	0.00	0.00	0.00	0.00	0.00	0.00	0.00	0.00	0.00	0.00	0.00	0.00	0.00
75	105	0.01	0.02	0.02	0.03	0.03	0.04	0.04	0.05	0.05	0.06	0.06	0.07	0.07	0.08	0.08	0.09	0.09	0.10	0.11	0.12
70	110	0.03	0.05	0.06	0.08	0.09	0.10	0.11	0.13	0.14	0.15	0.16	0.18	0.19	0.20	0.21	0.22	0.24	0.25	0.27	0.30
65	115	0.05	0.10	0.12	0.15	0.17	0.20	0.22	0.25	0.27	0.30	0.32	0.35	0.37	0.40	0.42	0.45	0.47	0.50	0.55	0.60
60	120	0.08	0.16	0.20	0.24	0.28	0.32	0.36	0.40	0.44	0.48	0.52	0.56	0.60	0.64	0.68	0.72	0.76	0.80	0.88	0.96
55	125	0.11	0.23	0.29	0.34	0.40	0.46	0.52	0.57	0.63	0.68	0.75	0.80	0.86	0.92	0.98	1.03	1.09	1.15	1.26	1.38
50	130	0.15	0.31	0.39	0.46	0.54	0.62	0.70	0.77	0.85	0.93	1.00	1.08	1.16	1.24	1.32	1.39	1.47	1.55	1.70	1.86
45	135	0.20	0.40	0.50	0.60	0.70	0.80	0.90	1.00	1.10	1.20	1.30	1.40	1.50	1.60	1.70	1.80	1.90	2.00	2.20	2.40
40	140	0.25	0.49	0.61	0.74	0.86	0.98	1.10	1.22	1.35	1.47	1.59	1.71	1.83	1.96	2.08	2.20	2.32	2.45	2.69	2.94
35	145	0.29	0.58	0.72	0.87	1.01	1.16	1.30	1.45	1.59	1.74	1.88	2.03	2.17	2.32	2.46	2.61	2.75	2.90	3.19	3.48
30	150	0.34	0.67	0.84	1.00	1.17	1.34	1.51	1.67	1.84	2.01	2.18	2.34	2.51	2.68	2.84	3.01	3.18	3.35	3.68	4.02
25	155	0.37	0.75	0.94	1.12	1.31	1.50	1.69	1.87	2.06	2.25	2.44	2.62	2.81	3.00	3.19	3.38	3.56	3.75	4.12	4.50
20	160	0.41	0.82	1.02	1.23	1.43	1.64	1.85	2.05	2.25	2.46	2.66	2.87	3.08	3.28	3.48	3.69	3.90	4.10	4.51	4.92
15	165	0.44	0.88	1.10	1.32	1.54	1.76	1.98	2.20	2.42	2.54	2.86	3.08	3.30	3.52	3.74	3.96	4.18	4.40	4.84	5.28
10	170	0.47	0.94	1.17	1.41	1.64	1.88	2.12	2.35	2.59	2.82	3.06	3.29	3.52	3.76	4.00	4.23	4.47	4.70	5.17	5.65
5	175	0.49	0.98	1.22	1.47	1.71	1.96	2.20	2.45	2.69	2.94	3.18	3.43	3.67	3.92	4.16	4.41	4.65	4.90	5.39	5.88

Reprinted by permission from I. B. Lueck, "Bifocal analysis in anisometropia," Bausch & Lomb *Technical Bulletin* No. 18 (1937).

2.7. Compensations for Tilting High Plus or Minus Lenses

(A) Where Distance From Top of Lens to Plane of Sight is . . .	*(B) And Where Degree of Tilt of Lenses (Angle of End Piece) is . . .*									
	2°	*4°*	*6°*	*8°*	*10°*	*12°*	*14°*	*16°*	*18°*	*20°*
	(C) Place Optical Center DOWN From Top of Lens									
0 mm.	0.9 mm.	1.9 mm.	2.8 mm.	3.8 mm.	4.8 mm.	5.7 mm.	6.7 mm.	7.7 mm.	8.8 mm.	9.8 mm.
1 mm.	1.9	2.9	3.8	4.8	5.8	6.7	7.7	8.7	9.8	10.8
2 mm.	2.9	3.9	4.8	5.8	6.8	7.7	8.7	9.7	10.8	11.8
3 mm.	3.9	4.9	5.8	6.8	7.8	8.7	9.7	10.7	11.8	12.8
4 mm.	4.9	5.9	6.8	7.8	8.8	9.7	10.7	11.7	12.8	13.8
5 mm.	5.9	6.9	7.8	8.8	9.8	10.7	11.7	12.7	13.8	14.8
6 mm.	6.9	7.9	8.8	9.8	10.8	11.7	12.7	13.7	14.8	15.8
7 mm.	7.9	8.9	9.8	10.8	11.8	12.7	13.7	14.7	15.8	16.8
8 mm.	8.9	9.9	10.8	11.8	12.8	13.7	14.7	15.7	16.8	17.8
9 mm.	9.9	10.9	11.8	12.8	13.8	14.7	15.7	16.7	17.8	18.8
*10 mm.**	10.9	11.9	12.8	13.8	14.8	15.7	16.7	17.7	18.8	19.8
11 mm.	11.9	12.9	13.8	14.8	15.8	16.7	17.7	18.7	19.8	20.8
12 mm.	12.9	13.9	14.8	15.8	16.8	17.7	18.7	19.7	20.8	21.8
13 mm.	13.9	14.9	15.8	16.8	17.8	18.7	19.7	20.7	21.8	22.8
14 mm.	14.9	15.9	16.8	17.8	18.8	19.7	20.7	21.7	22.8	23.8
15 mm.	15.9	16.9	17.8	18.8	19.8	20.7	21.7	22.7	23.8	24.8
16 mm.	16.9	17.9	18.8	19.8	20.8	21.7	22.7	23.8	24.8	25.8
17 mm.	17.9	18.9	19.8	20.8	21.8	22.7	23.7	24.7	25.8	26.8
18 mm.	18.9	19.9	20.8	21.8	22.8	23.7	24.7	25.7	26.8	27.8
19 mm.	19.9	20.9	21.8	22.8	23.8	24.7	25.7	26.7	27.8	28.8
20 mm.	20.9	21.9	22.8	23.8	24.8	25.7	26.7	27.7	28.8	29.8

*Example: Where the distance from the top of the lens to plane of sight is found to be 10 mm.; and the lenses are angled at 8°, then place the optical center down from the top of the lens 13.8 mm.

Reprinted by permission from Univis Lens Co., *Cataract Prescription Handbook.* Courtesy Univis Lens Co., No. Attleboro, Mass.

2.8. Effect of Tilting a Cylinder

Degrees	*Original Cylinder* 1.0	2.0	3.0	4.0	5.0	6.0	7.0	8.0
10°	1.04	2.04	3.12	4.16	5.20	6.24	7.28	8.32
15°	1.1	2.2	3.3	4.4	5.5	6.6	7.7	8.8
20°	1.18	2.36	3.54	4.72	5.9	7.08	8.26	9.44
25°	1.29	2.58	3.87	5.76	7.74	8.34	9.03	
30°	1.45	2.90	4.35	5.80	7.25	8.70		
35°	1.67	3.34	5.01	6.68	8.45			
40°	2.07	4.1	6.15	8.2				
	Resultant Cylinder							

2.9. Effect of Tilting a Sphere*

Degrees	*Original Sphere* 100	200	300	400	500	600	700	800	900	1000	1100	1200
10°	1.01	2.02	3.03	4.04	5.05	6.06	7.07	8.08	9.09	10.10	11.11	12.12
	.04	.08	.12	.16	.20	.24	.28	.32	.36	.40	.44	.48
15°	1.02	2.04	3.06	4.08	5.10	6.12	7.14	8.16	9.18	10.20	11.22	12.24
	.07	.14	.21	.28	.35	.42	.49	.56	.63	.70	.77	.84
20°	1.04	2.08	3.12	4.16	5.20	6.24	7.28	8.32	9.36	10.40	11.44	12.48
	.13	.26	.39	.52	.65	.78	.91	1.04	1.17	1.30	1.43	1.56
25°	1.06	2.12	3.28	4.24	5.30	6.36	7.42	8.48	9.54	10.60	11.66	12.72
	.23	.46	.69	.92	1.15	1.38	1.61	1.84	2.07	2.30	2.53	2.76
30°	1.09	2.18	3.27	4.36	5.45	6.54	7.63	8.72	9.81	10.90	11.99	13.08
	.36	.72	1.08	1.44	1.80	2.16	2.52	2.88	3.24	3.60	3.96	4.32
35°	1.12	2.24	3.36	4.48	5.60	6.72	7.84	8.96	10.08	11.20	12.32	13.44
	.55	1.10	1.65	2.20	2.75	3.30	3.85	4.40	4.95	5.50	6.05	6.60
40°	1.16	2.32	3.48	4.64	5.80	6.96	8.12	9.28	10.44	11.60	12.76	13.92
	.83	1.66	2.49	3.32	4.15	4.98	5.81	6.64	7.47	8.30	9.13	9.96

***Resultant Power: Upper value is the new sphere. Lower value is the induced cylinder.**

2.10. Resultant of Obliquely Crossed Cylinders

Values of θ and C are obtained from the table for various values of $\propto$ and $\kappa = F_1/F_2$. Opposite each value of κ and $\propto$ the upper number gives θ; the lower number, multiplied by F_2, gives C.

	κ Negative								*κ Positive*								
κ / ∝	*4*	*3*	*2.5*	*2*	*1.75*	*1.5*	*1.25*	*−1*	*+1*	*1.25*	*1.5*	*1.75*	*2*	*2.5*	*3*	*4*	κ / ∝
10	−3 −3.12	−4½ −2.12	−6½ −1.62	−9 −1.12	−11 −.82	−16 −.62	−25 −.5	−40 −.37	5 2	4½ 2.25	4 2.5	3½ 2.75	3½ 3	3 3.5	2½ 4	2 5	*10*
20	−5½ −3.25	−8 −2.37	−11 −1.87	−14 −1.37	−17 1.12	−20 −1	−28 −.75	−35 −.62	10 1.87	9 2.12	8 2.37	7 2.62	6½ 2.87	5½ 3.37	5 3.87	4 4.75	*20*
30	−7 −3.62	−9½ −2.62	−12 −2.25	−15 −1.75	−17 −1.5	−20 −1.37	−24 −1.12	−30 −1	15 1.75	13 2	12 2.12	10 2.37	9½ 2.62	8 3.12	7 3.62	5½ 4.62	*30*
40	−7 −4	−9½ −3	−11 −2.5	−14 −2.12	−16 −1.87	−18 −1.62	−21 −1.5	−25 −1.25	20 1.5	17 1.75	15 2	13 2.12	12 2.37	10 2.87	8½ 3.37	6½ 4.25	*40*
45	−6½ −4.12	−9 −3.12	−11 −2.62	−13 −2.25	−14 −2	−16 −1.75	−19 −1.62	−22½ −1.37	22½ 1.37	19 1.62	16 1.75	14 2	13 2.25	11 2.62	9 3.12	6½ 4.12	*45*
50	−6½ −4.25	−8½ −3.37	−10 −2.87	−12 −2.37	−13 −2.12	−15 −2	−17 −1.75	−20 −1.5	25 1.25	21 1.5	18 1.62	16 1.87	14 2.12	11 2.5	9½ 3	7 4	*50*
60	−6 −4.62	−7 −3.62	−8 −3.12	−9½ −2.62	−10 −2.37	−12 −2.12	−13 −2	−15 −1.85	30 1	24 1.12	20 1.37	17 1.5	15 1.75	12 2.25	9½ 2.62	7 3.62	*60*
70	−4 −4.75	−5 −3.87	−5½ −3.37	−6½ −2.87	−7 −2.62	−8 −2.37	−9 −2.12	−10 −1.87	35 .62	28 .75	20 1	17 1.12	14 1.37	11 1.87	8 2.37	5½ 3.25	*70*
80	−2 −5	−2½ 4	−3 −3.5	−3½ −3	−3½ −2.75	−4 −2.5	−4½ −2.25	−5 −2	40 .37	25 .5	16 .62	11 .87	9 1.12	6½ 1.62	4½ 2.12	3 3.12	*80*
90	0 −5	0 −4	0 −.5	0 −3	0 −2.75	0 −2.5	0 −2.25	0 −2	— 0	0 .25	0 .5	0 .75	0 1	0 1.5	0 2	0 3	*90*
∝ / κ	*4*	*3*	*2.5*	*2*	*1.75*	*1.5*	*1.25*	*−1*	*+1*	*1.25*	*1.5*	*1.75*	*2*	*2.5*	*3*	*4*	∝ / κ

(continued)

2.10. Resultant of Obliquely Crossed Cylinders (continued)

κ / α	κ Negative 4	3	2.5	2	1.75	1.5	1.25	−1	κ Positive +1	1.25	1.5	1.75	2	2.5	3	4	κ / α
100	2 −5	2½ −4	3 − 3.5	3½ − 3	3½ − 2.75	4 − 2.5	4½ − 2.25	5 − 2	−40 .37	−25 .5	−16 .62	−11 .87	− 9 1.12	− 6½ 1.62	− 4½ − 2.12	− 3 3.12	100
110	4 −4.75	5 −3.87	5½ − 3.37	6½ − 2.87	7 − 2.62	8 − 2.37	9 − 2.12	10 − 1.87	−35 .62	−28 .75	−20 1	−17 1.12	−14 1.37	−11 1.87	− 8 2.37	− 5½ 3.25	110
120	5½ −4.62	7 −3.62	8 − 3.12	9½ − 2.62	10 − 2.37	12 − 2.12	13 − 2	15 − 1.75	−30 1	−23 1.12	−20 1.37	−17 1.5	−15 1.75	−12 2.25	− 9½ 2.62	− 7 3.62	120
130	6½ −4.25	8½ −3.37	10 − 2.87	12 − 2.37	13 − 2.12	15 − 2	17 − 2.75	20 − 1.5	−25 1.25	−21 1.5	−18 1.62	−16 1.87	−14 2.12	−11 2.5	− 9½ 3	− 7 4	130
135	6½ −4.12	9 −3.12	11 − 2.62	13 − 2.25	14 − 2	16 − 1.75	19 − 1.62	22½ − 1.37	−22½ 1.37	−19 1.62	−16 1.75	−14 2	−13 2.25	−11 2.62	− 9 3.12	− 6½ 4.12	135
140	7 −4	9½ −3	11 − 2.5	14 − 2.12	16 − 1.87	18 − 1.62	21 − 1.5	25 − 1.25	−20 1.5	−17 1.75	−15 2	−13 2.12	−12 2.37	−10 2.87	− 8½ 3.37	− 6½ 4.25	140
150	7 −3.62	9½ −2.62	12 − 2.25	15 − 1.75	17 − 1.5	20 − 1.37	24 − 1.12	30 − 1	−15 1.75	−13 2	−12 2.12	−10 2.37	− 9½ 2.62	− 8 3.12	− 7 3.62	− 5½ 4.62	150
160	5½ −3.25	8 −2.37	11 − 1.87	14 − 1.37	17 − 1.12	20 1	28 − .75	35 −62	−10 1.87	− 9 2.12	− 8 2.37	− 7 2.62	− 6½ 2.87	− 5½ 3.37	− 5 3.87	− 4 4.75	160
170	3 −3.12	4½ −2.12	6½ − 1.62	9 − 1.12	11 − .87	15 − .62	25 − .5	40 − .37	− 5 2	− 4½ 2.25	− 4 2.5	− 3½ 2.75	− 3½ 3	− 3 3.5	− 2½ 4	− 2 5	170
180	0 −3	0 −2	0 − 1.5	0 − 1	0 − .75	0 − .5	0 − .25	— 0	0 2	0 2.25	0 2.5	0 2.75	0 3	0 3.5	0 4	0 5	180
α / κ	4	3	2.5	2	1.75	1.5	1.25	−1	+1	1.25	1.5	1.75	2	2.5	3	4	α / κ

Sample Use of Table

θ = the angle between F_1 and the resultant cylinder.
α = angular difference between axes.

Sample Solution: Combine +4.00 x 20 with +2.00 x 60
$F_1/F_2 = +4.00/+2.00 = +2.00$ $\theta = 12°$ (from table)
Cylinder = 2 x +2.37 (from table) = +4.74
Sphere = ½ $(F_1 + F_2 - C)$
Sphere = ½ (+4.00 + 2.00 − 4.74) = +.63 DS
+.63 DS ⟡ +4.74 x 20° + 12° = +.63 DS ⟡ +4.74 x 32°

Values of θ to the nearest degree (above 10°) and nearest half degree (below 10°). Values of C to nearest eighth diopter.
Reprinted by permission from H. Emsley and W. Swaine, *Ophthalmic Lenses*, 5th ed. London: Hatton Press, 1949.

Prescription Design 3

3.1. Plano Lenses Designed for Magnification

% Mag.	1.53 D_1	2.00	2.50	3.00	3.50	4.00	4.50	5.00	5.50	6.00	6.50	7.00	7.50	8.00	8.50
0.50	t	3.84	3.07	3.56	2.19	1.92	1.71	1.54	1.40	1.28	1.18	1.10	1.02	0.96	0.90
	D_2	2.01	2.51	3.02	3.52	4.02	4.52	5.03	5.53	6.03	6.53	7.04	7.54	8.04	8.54
0.75	t	5.74	4.60	3.83	3.28	2.87	2.55	2.30	2.09	1.91	1.77	1.64	1.53	1.44	1.35
	D_2	2.02	2.52	3.02	3.53	4.03	4.53	5.04	5.54	6.05	6.55	7.05	7.56	8.06	8.56
1.00	t	7.64	6.11	5.09	4.37	3.82	3.39	3.06	2.78	2.55	2.35	2.18	2.04	1.91	1.80
	D_2	2.02	2.53	3.03	3.54	4.04	4.55	5.05	5.56	6.06	6.57	7.07	7.58	8.08	8.59
1.25	t	9.52	7.62	6.35	5.44	4.76	4.23	3.81	3.46	3.17	2.93	2.72	2.54	2.38	2.24
	D_2	2.03	2.53	3.04	3.54	4.05	4.56	5.06	5.57	6.08	6.58	7.09	7.59	8.10	8.61
1.50	t	11.4	9.12	7.60	6.52	5.70	5.07	4.56	4.15	3.80	3.51	3.26	3.04	2.85	2.68
	D_2	2.03	2.54	3.05	3.55	4.06	4.57	5.08	5.58	6.09	6.60	7.11	7.61	8.12	8.63
1.75	t	13.3	10.6	8.85	7.58	6.63	5.90	5.31	4.83	4.42	4.08	3.79	3.54	3.32	3.12
	D_2	2.04	2.54	3.05	3.56	4.07	4.58	5.09	5.60	6.11	6.61	7.12	7.63	8.14	8.65
2.00	t	15.1	12.1	10.1	8.64	7.56	6.72	6.05	5.50	5.04	4.65	4.32	4.03	3.78	3.56
	D_2	2.04	2.55	3.06	3.57	4.08	4.59	5.10	5.61	6.12	6.63	7.14	7.65	8.16	8.67
2.25	t	17.0	13.6	11.3	9.70	8.49	7.55	6.79	6.17	5.66	5.22	4.85	4.53	4.24	3.99
	D_2	2.05	2.56	3.07	3.58	4.09	4.60	5.11	5.62	6.14	6.65	7.16	7.67	8.18	8.69
2.50	t	18.8	15.1	12.5	10.8	9.41	8.36	7.53	6.84	6.27	5.79	5.38	5.02	4.70	4.43
	D_2	2.05	2.56	3.08	3.59	4.10	4.61	5.13	5.64	6.15	6.66	7.18	7.69	8.20	8.71
2.75	t	20.7	16.5	13.8	11.8	10.3	9.18	8.26	7.51	6.88	6.35	5.90	5.51	5.16	4.86
	D_2	2.06	2.57	3.08	3.60	4.11	4.62	5.14	5.65	6.17	6.68	7.19	7.71	8.22	8.73
3.00	t	22.5	18.0	15.0	12.8	11.2	9.99	8.99	8.17	7.49	6.91	6.42	5.99	5.62	5.29
	D_2	2.06	2.58	3.09	3.61	4.12	4.64	5.15	5.67	6.18	6.70	7.21	7.73	8.24	8.76
3.25	t	24.3	19.4	16.2	13.9	12.1	10.8	9.71	8.83	8.09	7.47	6.94	6.48	6.07	5.71
	D_2	2.07	2.58	3.10	3.61	4.13	4.65	5.16	5.68	6.20	6.71	7.23	7.74	8.26	8.78
3.50	t	26.1	20.9	17.4	14.9	13.1	11.6	10.4	9.49	8.70	8.03	7.45	6.96	6.52	6.14
	D_2	2.07	2.59	3.11	3.62	4.14	4.66	5.18	5.69	6.21	6.73	8.25	7.76	8.28	8.80
3.75	t	27.9	22.3	18.6	15.9	13.9	12.4	11.2	10.1	9.30	8.58	7.97	7.44	6.97	6.56
	D_2	2.08	2.59	3.11	3.63	4.15	4.67	5.19	5.71	6.23	6.74	7.26	7.78	8.30	8.82
4.00	t	29.7	23.7	20.8	17.0	14.8	13.2	11.9	10.8	9.89	9.13	8.48	7.91	7.42	6.98
	D_2	2.08	2.60	3.12	3.64	4.16	4.68	5.20	5.72	6.24	6.76	7.28	7.80	8.32	8.84
4.25	t	31.5	25.2	21.0	18.0	15.7	14.0	12.6	11.4	10.5	9.69	8.99	8.39	7.86	7.40
	D_2	2.09	2.61	3.13	3.65	4.17	4.69	5.21	5.73	6.26	6.78	7.30	7.82	8.34	8.86
4.50	t	33.2	26.6	22.2	19.0	16.6	14.8	13.3	12.1	11.1	10.2	9.49	8.86	8.31	7.82
	D_2	2.09	2.61	3.14	3.66	4.18	4.70	5.23	5.75	6.27	6.79	7.32	7.84	8.36	8.88
4.75	t	35.0	28.0	23.3	20.0	17.5	15.6	14.0	12.7	11.7	10.8	10.0	9.33	8.75	8.23
	D_2	2.10	2.62	3.14	3.67	4.19	4.71	5.24	5.76	6.29	6.81	7.33	7.86	8.38	8.90
5.00	t	36.7	29.4	24.5	21.0	18.4	16.3	14.7	13.4	12.3	11.3	10.5	9.80	9.18	8.64
	D_2	2.10	2.63	3.15	3.68	4.20	4.73	5.25	5.78	6.30	6.83	7.35	7.88	8.40	8.93

(continued)

3.1. Plano Lenses Designed for Magnification (continued)

% Mag.	1.53 D_1	9.00	9.50	10.00	10.50	11.00	11.50	12.00	12.50	13.00	13.50	14.00	14.50
0.50	t	0.85	0.81	0.77	0.73	0.70	0.67	0.64	0.61	0.59	0.57	0.55	0.53
	D_2	9.05	9.55	10.05	10.55	11.06	11.56	12.06	12.56	13.07	13.57	14.07	14.57
0.75	t	1.28	1.21	1.15	1.09	1.04	1.00	0.96	0.92	0.88	0.85	0.82	0.79
	D_2	9.07	9.57	10.08	10.58	11.08	11.59	12.09	12.59	13.10	13.60	14.11	14.61
1.00	t	1.70	1.61	1.53	1.45	1.39	1.33	1.27	1.22	1.18	1.13	1.09	1.05
	D_2	9.09	9.60	10.10	10.61	11.11	11.62	12.12	12.63	13.13	13.64	14.14	14.65
1.25	t	2.12	2.01	1.90	1.81	1.73	1.66	1.59	1.52	1.47	1.41	1.36	1.31
	D_2	9.11	9.62	10.13	10.63	11.14	11.64	12.15	12.66	13.16	13.67	14.18	14.68
1.50	t	2.53	2.40	2.28	2.17	2.07	1.98	1.90	1.82	1.75	1.69	1.63	1.57
	D_2	9.14	9.64	10.15	10.66	11.17	11.67	12.18	12.69	13.20	13.70	14.21	14.72
1.75	t	2.95	2.79	2.65	2.53	2.41	2.31	2.21	2.12	2.04	1.97	1.90	1.83
	D_2	9.16	9.67	10.18	10.68	11.19	11.70	12.21	12.72	13.23	13.74	14.25	14.75
2.00	t	3.36	3.18	3.03	2.88	2.75	2.63	2.52	2.42	2.33	2.24	2.16	2.09
	D_2	9.1	9.69	10.20	10.71	11.22	11.73	12.24	12.75	13.26	13.77	14.28	14.79
2.25	t	3.77	3.57	3.40	3.23	3.09	2.95	2.83	2.72	2.61	2.52	2.43	2.34
	D_2	9.20	9.71	10.23	10.74	11.25	11.76	12.27	12.78	13.29	13.80	14.32	14.83
2.50	t	4.18	3.96	3.76	3.58	3.42	3.27	3.14	3.01	2.89	2.79	2.69	2.60
	D_2	9.23	9.74	10.25	10.76	11.28	11.79	12.30	12.81	13.33	13.84	14.35	14.86
2.75	t	4.59	4.35	4.13	3.93	3.75	3.59	3.44	3.30	3.18	3.06	2.95	2.85
	D_2	9.25	9.76	10.28	10.79	11.30	11.82	12.33	12.84	13.36	13.87	14.39	14.90
3.00	t	4.99	4.73	4.49	4.28	4.09	3.91	3.75	3.60	3.46	3.33	3.21	3.10
	D_2	9.27	9.79	10.30	10.82	11.33	11.85	12.36	12.88	13.39	13.91	14.42	14.94
3.25	t	5.40	5.11	4.96	4.63	4.42	4.22	4.05	3.89	3.74	3.60	3.47	3.35
	D_2	9.29	9.81	10.33	10.84	11.36	11.87	12.39	12.91	13.42	13.94	14.46	14.97
3.50	t	5.80	5.49	5.22	4.97	4.74	4.54	4.35	4.17	4.01	3.87	3.73	3.60
	D_2	9.32	9.83	10.35	10.87	11.39	11.90	12.42	12.94	13.46	13.97	14.49	15.01
3.75	t	6.20	5.87	5.58	5.31	5.07	4.85	4.65	4.46	4.29	4.13	3.98	3.85
	D_2	9.34	9.86	10.38	10.89	11.41	11.93	12.45	12.97	13.49	14.01	14.53	15.04
4.00	t	6.59	6.25	5.93	5.65	5.40	5.16	4.95	4.75	4.57	4.40	4.24	4.09
	D_2	9.36	9.88	10.40	10.92	11.44	11.96	12.48	13.00	13.52	14.04	14.56	15.08
4.25	t	6.99	6.62	6.29	5.99	5.72	5.47	5.24	5.03	4.84	4.66	4.49	4.34
	D_2	9.38	9.90	10.43	10.95	11.47	11.99	12.51	13.03	13.55	14.07	14.60	15.12
4.50	t	7.38	6.99	6.64	6.33	6.04	5.78	5.54	5.32	5.11	4.92	4.75	4.58
	D_2	9.41	9.93	10.45	10.97	11.50	12.02	12.54	13.06	13.59	14.11	14.63	15.15
4.75	t	7.77	7.37	7.00	6.66	6.36	6.08	5.83	5.60	5.38	5.18	5.00	4.83
	D_2	9.43	9.95	10.48	11.00	11.52	12.05	12.57	13.09	13.62	14.14	14.67	15.19
5.00	t	8.16	7.73	7.35	7.00	6.68	6.39	6.12	5.88	5.65	5.44	5.25	5.07
	D_2	9.45	9.98	10.50	11.03	11.55	12.08	12.60	13.13	13.65	14.18	14.70	15.23

Plano Power Lenses with Desired % Magnification. Required Center Thickness (t) in mm. and inside 1.53 Curve (D_2) for a selected 1.53 Front Curve (D_1).

Ideal thicknesses are included between the two black lines.

Reprinted by permission from A.W. Raynor, "Aniseikonia and magnification in ophthalmic lenses: problem and solutions," *Am. J. Opt.* **43** (1966).

3.2. Design of Iseikonic Prescriptions

Table A. Approximate Magnification (Percent) Changes for Eyewire Distance Changes of Various Lens Powers

△ Eyewire Distance (h)	*Power (Vo) 1D*	*2D*	*4D*	*6D*	*8D*	*10D*
1 mm.	0.1	0.2	0.4	0.6	0.8	1.0
2 mm.	0.2	0.4	0.8	1.2	1.6	2.0
3 mm.	0.3	0.6	1.2	1.8	2.4	3.0
4 mm.	0.4	0.8	1.6	2.4	3.2	4.0
5 mm.	0.5	1.0	2.0	3.0	4.0	5.0

Minus Lens — Moved *closer* to the eye *increases*; moved *farther* from the eye *decreases* magnification.

Plus Lens — Moved *closer* to the eye *decreases*; moved *farther* from the eye *increases* magnification.

Table B. Approximate Magnification (Percent) Changes by Changing Lens Bevel From Center to 1/3–2/3 or 2/3–1/3 (2.1 mm. Center Thickness)

Eye Size (mm.)	*Power (D) −1.00*	*−2.00*	*−4.00*	*−6.00*	*−8.00*	*−10.00*
36	0.03	0.10	0.22	0.37	0.56	0.77
38	0.03	0.10	0.23	0.40	0.61	0.84
40	0.04	0.10	0.24	0.43	0.67	0.92
42	0.04	0.10	0.25	0.46	0.72	1.05
44	0.04	0.10	0.26	0.49	0.78	1.13
46	0.04	0.11	0.28	0.52	0.82	1.19
48	0.04	0.11	0.29	0.54	0.87	1.26
50	0.05	0.11	0.30	0.57	0.92	1.36
52	0.05	0.11	0.31	0.60	0.96	1.44

Minus Lens — Move *closer* to the eye *increases*; move *farther* from the eye *decreases* magnification.

Table C. Approximate Magnification (Percent) Changes Associated With Various Lens Powers And Changes in Front Surface Curvature

Δ Base Curve (D_1)	Power (D) −10 t = 2.1	−8 t = 2.1	−6 t = 2.1	−4 t = 2.1	−2 t = 2.1	−1 t = 2.1	0 t = 2.1	+1 t = 2.6	+2 t = 3.1	+4 t = 4.1	+6 t = 5.1	+8 t = 6.1	+10 t = 7.1
−4	+1.46	+1.04	+0.64	+0.24	−0.16	−0.36	−0.56	−0.90	−1.23	−1.90	−2.56	−3.24	−3.88
−2	+0.72	+0.52	+0.32	+0.12	−0.08	−0.18	−0.28	−0.45	−0.61	−0.95	−1.28	−1.62	−1.94
+2	−0.72	−0.52	−0.32	−0.12	+0.08	+0.18	+0.28	+0.45	+0.61	+0.95	+1.28	+1.62	+1.94
+4	−1.46	−1.04	−0.64	−0.24	+0.16	+0.36	+0.56	+0.90	+1.23	+1.90	+2.56	+3.24	+3.88
+6	−2.18	−1.56	−0.96	−0.36	+0.24	+0.54	+0.84	+1.35	+1.84	+2.85	+3.84	+4.86	+5.82
+8	−2.92	−2.08	−1.28	−0.48	+0.32	+0.72	+1.12	+1.80	+2.46	+3.80	+5.12	+6.48	+7.76

(Side label: ↑ Decrease / Increase ↓)

Table D. Magnification Changes by Changing Thickness (Base Curve)

Δ Thickness (mm.)	Base Curve 0.50	1.50	2.50	3.50	4.50	5.50	6.50	7.50	8.50	9.50	10.50	11.50	12.50	13.50
−1.5	−0.048	−0.150	−0.250	−0.349	−0.450	−0.549	−0.649	−0.750	−0.847	−0.945	−1.050	−1.149	−1.248	−1.348
−1.0	−0.032	−0.100	−0.167	−0.233	−0.300	−0.366	−0.433	−0.500	−0.565	−0.630	−0.700	−0.766	−0.832	−0.898
−0.5	−0.016	−0.050	−0.083	−0.166	−0.150	−0.183	−0.216	−0.250	−0.282	−0.315	−0.350	−0.383	−0.416	−0.450
+0.5	+0.016	+0.050	+0.083	+0.116	+0.150	+0.183	+0.216	+0.250	+0.282	+0.315	+0.350	+0.383	+0.416	+0.450
+1.0	+0.032	+0.100	+0.167	+0.233	+0.300	+0.366	+0.433	+0.500	+0.565	+0.630	+0.700	+0.766	+0.832	+0.890
+1.5	+0.048	+0.150	+0.250	+0.349	+0.450	+0.549	+0.649	+0.750	+0.847	+0.945	+1.050	+1.149	+1.248	+1.348
+2.0	+0.064	+0.200	+0.334	+0.466	+0.600	+0.72	+0.866	+1.00	+1.130	+1.260	+1.400	+1.532	+1.664	+1.798
+2.5	+0.080	+0.250	+0.417	+0.582	+0.750	+0.915	+1.082	+1.250	+1.412	+1.575	+1.750	+1.915	+2.080	+2.245
+3.0	+0.96	+0.300	+0.501	+0.699	+0.900	+1.100	+1.299	+1.500	+1.700	+1.890	+2.100	+2.298	+2.496	+2.694
+3.3	+0.112	+0.350	+0.584	+0.815	+1.050	+1.283	+1.515	+1.750	+1.982	+2.205	+2.450	+2.681	+2.912	+3.143
+4.0	+0.128	+0.400	+0.668	+0.922	+1.200	+1.464	+1.732	+2.00	+2.260	+2.520	+2.800	+3.064	+3.328	+3.587
+4.5	+0.144	+0.450	+0.841	+1.029	+1.350	+1.647	+1.949	+2.250	+2.542	+2.835	+3.150	+3.447	+3.744	+4.031

(Side label: ↑ Decrease Thickness / Increase Thickness ↓)

Table E. Magnification Changes by Changing Thickness (Power)

△ Thickness (mm.)		Lens Power (D) −10	−8	−6	−4	−2	0	+2	+4	+6	+8	+10
−1.5	↑ Decrease Thickness	+0.75	+0.60	+0.45	+0.30	+0.15	0.0	−0.15	−0.30	−0.45	−0.60	−0.75
−1.0		+0.50	+0.40	+0.30	+0.20	+0.10	0.0	−0.10	−0.20	−0.30	−0.40	−0.50
−0.5		+0.25	+0.20	+0.15	+0.10	+0.05	0.0	−0.05	−0.10	−0.15	−0.20	−0.25
+0.5	Increase Thickness ↓	−0.25	−0.20	−0.15	−0.10	−0.05	0.0	+0.05	+0.10	+0.15	+0.20	+0.25
+1.0		−0.50	−0.40	−0.30	−0.20	−0.10	0.0	+0.10	+0.20	+0.30	+0.40	+0.50
+1.5		−0.75	−0.60	−0.45	−0.30	−0.15	0.0	+0.15	+0.30	+0.45	+0.60	+0.75
+2.0		−1.00	−0.80	−0.60	−0.40	−0.20	0.0	+0.20	+0.40	+0.60	+0.80	+1.00
+2.5		−1.25	−1.00	−0.75	−0.50	−0.25	0.0	+0.25	+0.50	+0.75	+1.00	+1.25
+3.0		−1.50	−1.20	−0.90	−0.60	−0.30	0.0	+0.30	+0.60	+0.90	+1.20	+1.50
+3.5		−1.75	−1.40	−1.05	−0.70	−0.35	0.0	+0.35	+0.70	+1.05	+1.40	+1.75
+4.0		−2.00	−1.60	−1.20	−0.80	−0.40	0.0	+0.40	+0.80	+1.20	+1.60	+2.00
+4.5		−2.25	−1.80	−1.35	−0.90	−0.45	0.0	+0.45	+0.90	+1.35	+1.80	+2.25

A-B = △ m% for a given base curve, thickness change, and lens power.

Table F. Approximate Changes in Magnification (Percent) by Changing Lens Bevel From Center to 1/3–2/3 or 2/3–1/3 When the Thickness Has Been Changed in Fixed Steps From Standard (2.1 mm. Minimum) Thickness (Based on 46 mm. Eye Size Minus Lenses)

△ Thickness (mm.)	*Power (D)* −10	−8	−6	−4	−2	−1	0	+1	+2	+4	+6	+8	+10
−1.5 ↑ Decrease Thickness	0.94	0.62	0.36	0.18	0.05	0.02	0.00	0.01	0.02	0.04	0.06	0.08	0.10
−1.0	1.02	0.68	0.41	0.21	0.07	0.03	0.00	0.02	0.04	0.07	0.11	0.14	0.18
−0.5	1.11	0.75	0.46	0.24	0.09	0.04	0.00	0.03	0.05	0.11	0.16	0.22	0.27
+0.5	1.28	0.89	0.56	0.31	0.12	0.05	0.00	0.04	0.09	0.18	0.26	0.35	0.44
+1.0	1.36	0.95	0.61	0.34	0.14	0.06	0.00	0.05	0.10	0.21	0.31	0.42	0.52
+1.5	1.45	1.02	0.67	0.38	0.15	0.07	0.00	0.06	0.12	0.24	0.36	0.48	0.60
+2.0	1.52	1.09	0.71	0.41	0.17	0.08	0.00	0.07	0.14	0.28	0.41	0.55	0.69
+2.5	1.61	1.16	0.77	0.44	0.19	0.09	0.00	0.08	0.16	0.31	0.46	0.62	0.77
+3.0	1.68	1.22	0.82	0.48	0.20	0.09	0.00	0.09	0.17	0.34	0.51	0.68	0.85
+3.5	1.78	1.29	0.87	0.51	0.22	0.10	0.00	0.09	0.19	0.38	0.56	0.75	0.94
+4.0	1.85	1.35	0.91	0.54	0.24	0.11	0.00	0.10	0.20	0.41	0.61	0.82	1.02
+4.5 Increase Thickness ↓	1.94	1.42	0.96	0.57	0.26	0.11	0.00	0.10	0.21	0.44	0.66	0.89	1.10

Minus Lens — Moved *closer* to the eye *increases*; moved *farther* from the eye *decreases* magnification.
Plus Lens — Moved *closer* to the eye *decreases*; moved *farther* from the eye *increases* magnification.

Sample Use of Table 3.2 (A–F)

I. *Rx:* −1.00 Thickness 2.1 Base Curve +5.25 O.D.
−4.00 Thickness 2.1 Base Curve +3.50 O.S.
Eyewire Distance 15 mm. Center Bevels

This anisometropia is assumed to be dioptric in origin. The expected amount is approximately 1.5 percent per diopter of anisometropia. Since some aniseikonia may be axial, 3 percent of this expected 4.5 percent is to be corrected (see also **Table 4.13**).

a. Change eyewire distance **(Table 3.2 A)**.
If eyewire distance is decreased to 10 mm., magnification is increased to +0.5 percent O.D. and 2 percent O.S. There is a relative increase of 1.5 percent O.S.
b. Change base curve **(Table 3.2 C)**.
In this example very little improvement would result and the base curves are left unchanged.
c. Change thickness **(Tables 3.2 D and E)**.
For a +3.50 base curve, a thickness change of 2.5 mm. produces an increase in magnification of +0.582 (Table D). (Table E) A minification of .50 percent is indicated. When this is subtracted, the total is an increase of 1.082 percent.
d. Change the bevel **(Table 3.2 B or F)**.
Modifying the bevel of a −4.00 lens that has been made 2.5 mm. thicker changes the vertex distance and yields an increase of .44 percent O.S.

O.S. (a) 1.5% + (b) 0 + (c) 1.08% + (d) .44% = overall 3.02% O.S.

Final Rx: −1.00 Thickness 2.1 Base Curve +5.25 O.D.
−4.00 Thickness 4.6 Base Curve +3.50 O.S.
Eyewire Distance 10 mm. Bevel 1/3 – 2/3

Antireflective and edge coats are recommended, as steep base curves and thick lenses are often required.

(continued)

Table 3.2. Design of Iseikonic Prescriptions

II. Bitoric

Rx:	+1.00	Thickness 2.6	Base Curve +6.25 O.D.
	−1.00 −2.00 × 180	Thickness 2.1	Base Curve +4.50 O.S.
	Eyewire Distance 14.5 mm.		Center Bevels

The desired aniseikonic correction is: 1.25 percent overall ⊖ 1.75 percent × 180 O.S. (by eikonometry or estimation).

The principal meridians will have to be considered separately.

O.D.	Vertical Meridian	+1.00	Horizontal	+1.00
O.S.	Vertical Meridian	−3.00	Horizontal	−1.00

Vertical Meridian

a. Change eyewire distance (Table 3.2 A).
If the eyewire distance is decreased from 14.5 mm. to 10.5 mm., O.D. decreases .4 percent, O.S. increases 1.2 percent. The total increase is 1.6 percent O.S.

b. Change base curve (Table 3.2 C).
If the base curve is changed to a steeper one, more substantial effects are obtained with thickness changes. In this case the changes are O.D. by 2D = −0.45 percent : O.S. by 4D = −0.04 percent : Relative increase = +0.41 percent.

c. Change thickness (Tables 3.2 D and E).
An increase of O.S. (−3.00 D, +8.50 Base: see step b. above) by 1.5 mm. yields a magnification of +.847 − (−.225) = 1.072 percent O.S.

d. A bevel change is the last choice and can be left until the other steps are evaluated.

Horizontal Meridian

a. Change eyewire distance (Table 3.2 A).
If the change discussed above (4.00 mm.) is made, the O.S. is increased by 0.4 percent and the O.D. is decreased by 0.4 percent with a relative increase of .8 percent O.S.

b. Change base curve (Table 3.2 C).
Since only a small amount remains to be corrected, magnifications produced by the thickness change already made for the vertical meridian should be evaluated before changing the base curve.

c. Change thickness (Tables 3.2 D and E).
When the vertical meridian was analyzed the lens was increased 1.5 mm. which results in changes in the horizontal meridian as well:
+.45 percent − (−0.07) = +.52 percent This change proves to be adequate.

O.S. Vertical (a) 1.6% + (b) .41% + (c) 1.072% + (d) 0 = 3.082%
Horizontal (a) .8% + (b) 0 + (c) .52% + (d) 0 = 1.32%
Total = 1.32% overall ⊖ 1.76% × 180

Final Rx:

+1.00	Thickness 2.6	Base Curve +6.25 (180)	+4.25 (90) O.D.
−1.00 ⊖ −2.00 × 180	Thickness 3.6	Base Curve +4.50 (180)	+8.50 (90) O.S.
Eyewire Distance 10.5 mm.		Center Bevel	

Antireflective and edge coats are recommended as steep base curves and thick lenses are often required.

3.3. Lens Sag (mm.) for Various Lens Sizes and Surface Curvature

Eye Size (mm.)	*Surface Curvature 1.50*	*2.50*	*3.50*	*4.50*	*5.50*	*6.50*	*7.50*	*8.50*	*9.50*	*10.50*	*11.50*	*12.50*	*13.50*	*14.50*	*15.50*
36	0.4	0.7	1.0	1.4	1.7	2.0	2.3	2.6	2.9	3.3	3.6	3.9	4.2	4.5	4.7
38	0.4	0.8	1.1	1.5	1.9	2.2	2.6	2.9	3.3	3.6	4.0	4.3	4.7	5.0	5.3
40	0.5	0.9	1.3	1.7	2.1	2.5	2.9	3.3	3.7	4.1	4.4	4.8	5.2	5.6	6.0
42	0.5	1.0	1.5	1.9	2.3	2.7	3.2	3.6	4.0	4.5	4.9	5.3	5.8	6.2	6.6
44	0.5	1.1	1.5	2.0	2.5	3.0	3.5	4.0	4.4	4.9	5.4	5.9	6.4	6.9	7.4
46	0.6	1.2	1.8	2.2	2.8	3.3	3.8	4.4	4.9	5.4	6.0	6.5	7.1	7.6	8.1
48	0.7	1.3	1.9	2.4	3.0	3.6	4.2	4.7	5.3	5.9	6.5	7.1	7.8	8.3	9.0
50	0.7	1.4	2.1	2.6	3.2	3.9	4.5	5.2	5.8	6.5	7.1	7.8	8.5	9.2	9.9
52	0.8	1.5	2.2	2.8	3.5	4.2	4.9	5.6	6.3	7.1	7.8	8.6	9.3	10.1	10.9
54	1.0	1.7	2.4	3.1	3.8	4.6	5.3	6.1	6.9	7.7	8.4	9.3	10.1	11.0	11.9

This table is used to determine the magnification changes induced by changing the eye size. The effect on the image size of the new eyewire distance is given in Table 3.2. A.

Reprinted with permission from B. Wick, "Iseikonic considerations for today's eyewear — addendum," *Am. J. Opt.* **51**: (1974).

Sample Use of Table 3.3

Rx OD +1.00 Base Curve + 6.50 Back Curve –5.50
OS +4.00 Base Curve +10.50 Back Curve –6.50

Present frame is 42 × 40 and at an eyewire distance of 14 mm. The lenses have center bevels.

A new frame is selected: 52 × 48.

To determine the magnification change induced by the new sag distances of the lenses use Table 3.3. For minus lenses, the smaller measurement is used; for plus lenses, use the larger measurement.

In this case the change in measurement is from 42 to 52 mm.

OD sag increases form 2.3 to 3.5 (Table 3.3). (The consequent magnification increase is .12% (Table 3.2A).

OS sag increases from 2.7 to 4.2, or 1.5 mm. The magnification increase is .6%.

The difference in magnification between the two eyes is now increased by .6–.12 or .48%.

The remedy is a reduction in overall vertex distance from 14 mm to 12.5 mm. This introduces a decrease in magnification.

OD .15% OS .6% (Table 3.2A)

The relative decrease of .45% negates the increase caused by the new sag.

This table is used to determine the magnification changes induced by changing the eye size. The effect on the image size of the new eyewire distance is given in Table 3.2. A.

Reprinted with permission from B. Wick, "Iseikonic considerations for today's eyewear — addendum," *Am. J. Opt.* 51:(1974).

3.4. Amount to Decenter to Achieve a Given Prismatic Effect

Table A. Positive Lenses

Back Vertex Power D	*When required prismatic effect on the eye, in △, is* 0.5	1	1.5	2	2.5	3	3.5	4	5	6	7	8	9	10
	amount of lens decentration, in mm., is													
+ 0.5	10.0	20.0												
1	4.8	9.7	14.1	18.2										
1.5	3.35	6.5	9.5	12.5	15.7	18.9								
2	2.35	4.7	7.0	9.35	11.5	13.65	15.7	17.8						
2.5	1.85	3.7	5.5	7.35	9.15	11.0	12.75	14.4	17.9					
3	1.5	3.0	4.5	6.0	7.5	9.0	10.5	12.0	14.7	17.1				
3.5	1.3	2.55	3.85	5.1	6.35	7.65	8.95	10.2	12.6	14.8				
4	1.1	2.2	3.3	4.4	5.5	6.6	7.7	8.75	10.8	12.8	14.7	16.5		
5	0.9	1.75	2.6	3.5	4.35	5.2	6.05	6.85	8.5	10.1	11.6	13.1	14.5	15.9
6	0.7	1.4	2.1	2.8	3.5	4.2	4.9	5.55	6.85	8.2	9.45	10.7	11.9	13.0
7	0.6	1.2	1.8	2.4	2.95	3.5	4.05	4.6	5.7	6.8	7.9	8.95	10.0	11.0
8	0.5	0.95	1.45	1.95	2.4	2.9	3.4	3.9	4.8	5.75	6.65	7.6	8.45	9.35
9	0.4	0.85	1.3	1.7	2.1	2.55	2.95	3.35	4.2	5.0	5.75	6.5	7.3	8.05
10	0.35	0.75	1.1	1.45	1.8	2.2	2.6	2.95	3.7	4.4	5.05	5.7	6.35	7.0
11	0.35	0.7	0.95	1.25	1.55	1.9	2.25	2.55	3.15	3.75	4.4	4.95	5.55	6.15
12	0.3	0.6	0.9	1.15	1.4	1.7	2.0	2.25	2.8	3.35	3.85	4.4	4.95	5.55
13	0.25	0.5	0.75	1.0	1.25	1.5	1.75	2.0	2.45	3.95	3.45	4.0	4.45	4.95
14	0.25	0.45	0.7	0.95	1.15	1.35	1.55	1.75	2.2	2.65	3.1	3.55	3.95	4.4
+15	0.2	0.4	0.6	0.8	1.0	1.2	1.4	1.6	1.95	2.35	2.75	3.15	3.5	3.9

3.4. Amount to Decenter to Achieve a Given Prismatic Effect

Table B. Negative Lenses

Back Vertex Power D	When required prismatic effect on the eye, in △, is													
	0.5	*1*	*1.5*	*2*	*2.5*	*3*	*3.5*	*4*	*5*	*6*	*7*	*8*	*9*	*10*
	amount of lens decentration, in mm., is													
− *0.5*	10.0	20.0												
− *1*	5.0	10.0	14.5	18.5										
− *1.5*	3.4	6.7	10.0	13.3	16.5	19.7								
− *2*	2.6	5.2	7.75	10.3	12.6	14.8	16.9	19.0						
− *2.5*	2.15	4.15	6.25	8.3	10.2	12.1	14.0	16.0	19.8					
− *3*	1.8	3.55	5.3	7.05	8.8	10.5	12.15	13.8	16.7	19.5				
− *3.5*	1.6	3.15	4.65	6.15	7.6	9.1	10.55	12.05	14.9	17.8				
− *4*	1.4	2.75	4.15	5.5	6.85	8.15	9.45	10.7	13.2	15.6	17.8	20.0	21.9	
− *5*	1.15	2.3	3.4	4.45	5.55	6.65	7.75	8.8	10.95	12.95	14.8	16.7	18.4	20.1
− *6*	1.0	1.95	2.9	3.85	4.8	5.75	6.7	7.6	9.45	11.2	12.85	14.5	16.1	17.6
− *7*	0.85	1.7	2.55	3.35	4.2	5.0	5.85	6.65	8.3	9.85	11.35	12.85	14.3	15.7
− *8*	0.75	1.5	2.25	3.0	3.75	4.5	5.3	6.05	7.55	8.95	10.3	11.65	12.95	14.2
− *9*	0.7	1.35	2.05	2.75	3.45	4.15	4.85	5.5	6.8	8.1	9.4	10.65	11.85	13.0
−*10*	0.65	1.3	1.95	2.55	3.2	3.8	4.45	5.05	6.3	7.5	8.7	9.8	10.95	12.15
−*11*	0.6	1.2	1.8	2.35	2.95	3.55	4.15	4.7	5.85	7.0	8.1	9.2	10.25	11.25
−*12*	0.55	1.1	1.65	2.2	2.75	3.3	3.85	4.4	5.45	6.5	7.55	8.6	9.6	10.6
−*13*	0.5	1.0	1.55	2.05	2.55	3.1	3.6	4.1	5.15	6.1	7.1	8.1	9.05	10.05
−*14*	0.5	1.0	1.5	1.95	2.45	2.9	3.4	3.85	4.85	5.8	6.8	7.7	8.6	9.45
−*15*	0.5	0.95	1.4	1.85	2.35	2.8	3.25	3.7	4.6	5.5	6.4	7.3	8.2	9.05

Reprinted by permission from H. Emsley, *Optical Tables and Data*. London: UK Optical Ltd, 1968.

3.5. Segment Decentration to Make Reading Fields Coincide at 16 Inches

Table of Bifocal Insets for 16″ Reading Distance
Showing amount of inset required for each bifocal segment to make reading fields coincide at 16″ reading distance

Distance From Center of Nose to Center of Pupil When Eyes Are Adapted to Distance Vision

Power of Distance Lenses in 180° Meridian	*27*	*28*	*29*	*30*	*31*	*32*	*33*	*34*	*35*	*36*
+15.00	2.5	2.5	2.6	2.7	2.8	2.9	3.0	3.1	3.2	3.3
+14.00	2.4	2.5	2.5	2.6	2.7	2.8	2.9	3.0	3.1	3.2
+12.00	2.2	2.3	2.4	2.5	2.5	2.6	2.7	2.8	2.9	3.0
+10.00	2.1	2.2	2.2	2.3	2.4	2.5	2.5	2.6	2.7	2.8
+ 9.00	2.0	2.1	2.2	2.2	2.3	2.4	2.5	2.5	2.6	2.7
+ 8.00	2.0	2.0	2.1	2.2	2.2	2.3	2.4	2.5	2.5	2.6
+ 7.00	1.9	2.0	2.0	2.1	2.2	2.3	2.3	2.4	2.5	2.5
+ 6.00	1.9	1.9	2.0	2.1	2.1	2.2	2.3	2.3	2.4	2.5
+ 5.00	1.8	1.9	1.9	2.0	2.1	2.1	2.2	2.3	2.3	2.4
+ 4.00	1.8	1.8	1.9	2.0	2.0	2.1	2.1	2.2	2.3	2.3
+ 3.00	1.7	1.8	1.8	1.9	2.0	2.0	2.1	2.2	2.2	2.3
+ 2.00	1.7	1.7	1.8	1.9	1.9	2.0	2.0	2.1	2.2	2.2
+ 1.00	1.6	1.7	1.7	1.8	1.9	1.9	2.0	2.0	2.1	2.2
0	1.6	1.6	1.7	1.8	1.8	1.9	1.9	2.0	2.1	2.1

Power of Distance Lenses in 180° Meridian	*27*	*28*	*29*	*30*	*31*	*32*	*33*	*34*	*35*	*36*
– 1.00	1.6	1.6	1.7	1.7	1.8	1.8	1.9	2.0	2.0	2.1
– 2.00	1.5	1.6	1.6	1.7	1.7	1.8	1.9	1.9	2.0	2.0
– 3.00	1.5	1.5	1.6	1.6	1.7	1.8	1.8	1.9	1.9	2.0
– 4.00	1.5	1.5	1.6	1.6	1.7	1.7	1.8	1.8	1.9	1.9
– 5.00	1.4	1.5	1.5	1.6	1.6	1.7	1.7	1.8	1.8	1.9
– 6.00	1.4	1.4	1.5	1.5	1.6	1.6	1.7	1.8	1.8	1.9
– 7.00	1.4	1.4	1.5	1.5	1.6	1.6	1.7	1.7	1.8	1.8
– 8.00	1.3	1.4	1.4	1.5	1.5	1.6	1.6	1.7	1.7	1.8
– 9.00	1.3	1.4	1.4	1.5	1.5	1.6	1.6	1.7	1.7	1.7
–10.00	1.3	1.3	1.4	1.4	1.5	1.5	1.6	1.6	1.7	1.7
–12.00	1.2	1.3	1.3	1.4	1.4	1.5	1.5	1.6	1.6	1.7
–14.00	1.2	1.2	1.3	1.3	1.4	1.4	1.5	1.5	1.5	1.6
–16.00	1.2	1.2	1.2	1.3	1.3	1.4	1.4	1.5	1.5	1.5
–18.00	1.1	1.2	1.2	1.2	1.3	1.3	1.4	1.4	1.4	1.5
–20.00	1.1	1.1	1.2	1.2	1.2	1.3	1.3	1.4	1.4	1.4

For distances from 12″ to 16″ add 0.1 mm. to amount of inset for each inch of reading distance nearer than 16″. For distances from 16″ to 20″ deduct 0.1 mm. from amount of inset for each inch of reading distance greater than 16″.

Reprinted by permission from Bausch & Lomb, *Theory and Application of Ophthalmic Lenses.* Rochester, N.Y.: Bausch & Lomb, 1970.

3.6. Bifocal Design in Anisometropia

Table A. Pole Location of Some Bifocal Segments

Lens	*Location of segment pole below top edge of segment (r)*
Executive, Bifield, Dualens	0.0 mm
Panoptik, Titmus CT	3.5 mm
Univis IS22, Univis R, Vision-Ease R	4.0
Sovereign 15.4 × 22	4.4
Tillyer S 17 × 25, Ultex K, Univis B, Vision-Ease B	4.5
Univis F 15¾ × 22	4.75
Univis D series, Sovereign 17.5 × 25, Univis R, Vision-Ease R, Panoptik St, Tillyer S 19 × 28, Vision-Ease D & C	5.0
Tillyer S 16.5 × 22	5.5
Vision-Ease R	6.0
Univis R	7.0
Orthogon C 16, Univis R, Vision-Ease R, Kryptok 16	8.0
Univis R, Vision-Ease R, Kryptok 18	9.0
Tillyer D 20, Univis R, Vision-Ease R, Kryptok 20	10.0
Kryptok 22, Ultex B	11.0
Ultex E, L	16.0
Ultex A, AL, AA	19.0

Table B. "R" Style Compensated Segments

By varying the top and bottom segment lines, the optical center (o.c.) is raised or lowered through positioning of the segment optical centers. The shape numbers in the following illustrations indicate, in millimeters, the positioning of the optical center in relation to the top segment line.

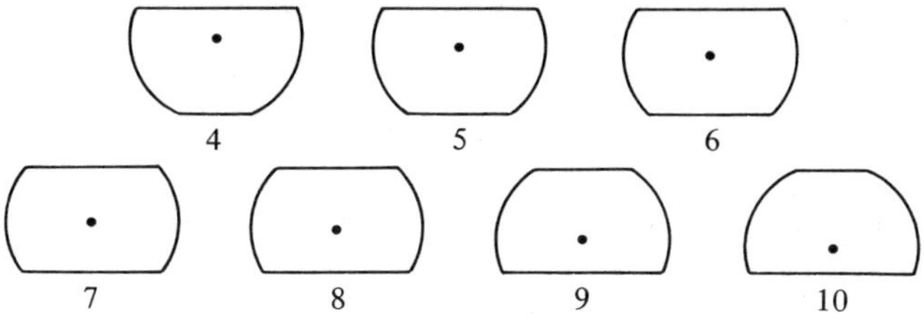

The standard "R" segment has its optical center 7 mm below the top line. This is known as shape #7. Shape #9 has the optical center 9 mm below, shape #5's optical center is 5 mm below, etc.

The following chart shows the prismatic effect obtained for different additions, with a 1 to 6 mm variation in placement of optical centers.

Add	*1 mm*	*2 mm*	*3 mm*	*4 mm*	*5 mm*	*6 mm*
+1.00	.10	.20	.30	.40	.50	.60
+1.25	.13	.25	.38	.50	.63	.75
+1.50	.15	.30	.45	.60	.75	.90
+1.75	.18	.35	.53	.70	.88	1.05
+2.00	.20	.40	.60	.80	1.00	1.20
+2.25	.23	.45	.68	.90	1.13	1.35
+2.50	.25	.50	.75	1.00	1.25	1.50
+2.75	.28	.55	.83	1.10	1.38	1.65
+3.00	.30	.60	.90	1.20	1.50	1.80
+3.25	.33	.65	.98	1.30	1.63	1.95
+3.50	.35	.70	1.05	1.40	1.75	2.10

Reprinted by permission from Univis Lens Co. Aniso Rx, *The Correction of Vertical Imbalance*, 1964. Courtesy Univis Lens Co., No. Attleboro, Mass.

3.7. Ophthalmic Lens Decentration as a Function of Reading Distance

Inset in mm. as a Function of Reading Distance for Various P.D.s.

Far P. D. (mm.)	Reading Distance (cm.)										
	100.0	*50.0*	*40.0*	*33.3*	*25.0*	*20.0*	*16.7*	*14.3*	*12.5*	*11.1*	*10.0*
50.0	0.7	1.4	1.7	2.0	2.6	3.1	3.7	4.2	4.7	5.2	5.6
55.0	0.8	1.5	1.8	2.2	2.8	3.4	4.0	4.6	5.1	5.6	6.1
60.0	0.8	1.6	2.0	2.4	3.1	3.8	4.4	5.0	5.6	6.1	6.7
65.0	0.9	1.8	2.2	2.6	3.3	4.1	4.8	5.4	6.1	6.7	7.2
70.0	1.0	1.9	2.3	2.8	3.6	4.4	5.1	5.8	6.5	7.2	7.8
75.0	1.0	2.0	2.5	3.0	3.8	4.7	5.5	6.3	7.0	7.7	8.3
	1.00	*2.00*	*2.50*	*3.00*	*4.00*	*5.00*	*6.00*	*7.00*	*8.00*	*9.00*	*10.00*
	Dioptric Demand										

Reprinted by permission from D. B. Gerstman, "Opthalmic lens decentration as a function of reading distance," *Br. J. Physiol. Optics* **28:** 1973.

3.8. Standards for First Quality Prescription Ophthalmic Lenses

Lens Characteristic	*Tolerance*	
Refractive Power		
Sphere	0.00 to 6.50 D	±0.13 D
	> 6.50 D	±2%
Cylinder	0.00 to 2.00 D	±0.13 D
	2.12 to 4.00 D	±0.15 D
	>4.50 D	±4%
Cylinder Axis	0.125 to 0.275 D	±7°
	0.500 to 0.750 D	±5°
	0.975 to 1.500 D	±3°
	>1.625 D	±2°
Addition	For distance lens powers 0.00 to 8.00 D	±0.13 D
	For distance lens powers >8.00 D	±.18 D
Prism		
Single lenses	1/3 Δ in any direction (Placement error of 1 mm)	
Mounted lenses (provisional)		
Vertical	1/3 Δ imbalance (Placement error of 1 mm in levels of major reference points)	
Horizontal	2/3 Δ imbalance (Maximum of 2.5 mm difference in horizontal placement of lenses)	
Segment Location		
Single lenses	± 1 mm of specification, horizontal and vertical	
Mounted lenses (provisional)		
Vertical	Within 1 mm	
Horizontal	Within 2.5 mm of specified near interpupillary distance	
Thickness	±0.3 mm of specification	
Base Curve	±0.75 D of specification	
Warpage	1.00 D except within 6 mm of eyewire	

3.9. Choosing the Base Curve for an Ophthalmic Lens

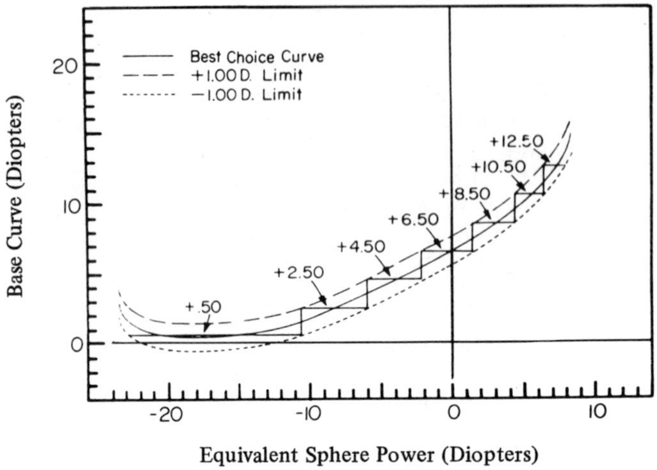

Reprinted from "Choosing the Base Curve for an Ophthalmic Lens," Fry, G.A., *American Journal of Optometry*, April, 1978.

3.10. Largest Blank Sizes Available

Table A. Bifocals (Glass)

Flatop		
22	Lantz, Meyer, Univis, Vision-Ease, X-Cel	71
25	AO, B & L, Lantz, Meyer, Shu, Titmus, Univis, Vision-Ease. X-Cel	71
28	B & L, Lantz, Meyer, Shu, Titmus, Vision-Ease, X-Cel	71
35	Lantz, Meyer, Titmus, X-Cel	71
Curve Top		
22	Meyer	58
25	X-Cel	66
P Top		
24	B & L	71
28	B & L	65
Executive		
	AO, Titmus, X-Cel	65
Kryptok		
	Titmus, Meyer	71
Nochrome		
	B & L, Lantz, Vision-Ease, X-Cel	71
Ultex		
A	Vision-Ease	72
AL	Phillips, Robinson-Houchin	72
B	Phillips	65
Redrite		
	Phillips	65
B Seg		
	Vision-Ease	68
R Seg		
	Vision-Ease	68
Dual Flattop		
22	Lantz, Vision-Ease	71
25	Lantz, Vision-Ease	71
28	Lantz, Vision-Ease	71
Dual Exec		
	AO, Shuron, Meyer, Robinson-Houchin	60
Dual Nochrome		
	Vision-Ease	71
Dual Kryptok		
	Meyer	60

Table B. Trifocals (Glass)

Flattop		
6 × 22	Lantz	71
6 × 28	Vision-Ease	68
7 × 23	Vision-Ease	68
7 × 25	Lantz, Titmus, Univis	71
7 × 28	Lantz, Univis	71
7 × 35	Lantz	71
8 × 22, 25, 28	Vision-Ease	68
9 × 35	Titmus	65
10 × 28	Vision-Ease	68
10 × 35	Vision-Ease	64
Ribbon		
	Vision-Ease	68
P Top		
	B & L	60
Curve Top		
	Vision-Ease	68
Executive		
	AO, Shuron, Titmus, Vision-Ease	60
Quadri		
7 × 23, 25, 28	Lantz, Vision-Ease	71
Ultex X		
	Phillips	65

Table C. Plastic Multifocals

Flattop		
23	Coburn	71
25	Silor	75
28	Silor	75
35	Armorlite, Signet	75
40	X-Cel	71
Ultex A		
	Sola	68
Executive		
	Optical Radiation	71
Round		
22	Armorlite, Signet, Sola	75
40	Armorlite, Signet	65
Flattop Trifocal		
7 × 25	Armorlite, Univis	75
7 × 28	Armorlite, Univis	75
Round	Armorlite	60
8 × 35	Signet	71
Executive Trifocal		
	Optical Radiation	71
ED Trifocal		
	Sola	68
Dual		
Flattop 25		
	Vision-Ease	71
Exec		
	Sola	68
Round		
	Aire-O-Lite	65

Table D. Photochromic Bifocals

Flattop		
22	Lantz, Meyer, Shuron, X-Cel, Prec-Cosmet	71
25	B & L, Lantz, Meyer, Shuron, Titmus, X-Cel, Prec-Cosmet	71
28	Lantz, Meyer, Shuron, Titmus, Prec-Cosmet	71
35	Lantz, Meyer, Titmus, X-Cel	71
Executive		
	AO, Titmus, Vision-Ease, X-Cel	65
Kryptok		
	Lantz, Meyer	71
Nochrome		
	X-Cel	71
Ultex		
A	Robinson-Houchin	72
AL	Robinson-Houchin	72
B	Phillips	65

Table E. Photochromic Trifocals

6 × 23, 28	X-Cel	71
7 × 25	Lantz, X-Cel, Titmus	
7 × 28, 35	Lantz, X-Cel	71
8 × 25, 28	X-Cel	71
Exec	Shuron, Titmus, Vision-Ease, Benson	60
Ultex K	Phillips	65

For progressive adds and seamless lenses, see Table 3.18; for miscellaneous forms see Table 3.13.

3.11. Multifocals Available with Base Curves Less than 2.50 D

Table A. Glass

		Blank Size
Flattop	Vision-Ease	68
	Unicis	68
22	Vision-Ease	68
	Univis	66
25	Meyer	71
	Vision-Ease	68
	Univis	66
28	Vision-Easė	68
	Univis	66
35	Vision-Ease	68
Curve Top		
22, 25, 28	Vision-Ease	68
P-Top		
24	B & L	71
	Titmus	60
Kryptok	Meyer	71
Nochrome	B & L	71
Ultex		
A	Phillips	64 (Hi-Lite)
B	Phillips	65 (Hi-Lite)
TRIFOCAL		
Flattop		
7 × 25, 28	Univis	66
Progressive	Silor (3.00 D)	65

Table B. Plastic

		Blank Size
Flattop		
22	Armorlite, Coburn, Signet, Titmus, Univers, Vision-Ease	65
25	AO	62
	Armorlite, Coburn, Titmus, Univis, Vision-Ease	65
	Signet	75
	Sola	68
28	Armorlite, Coburn, Titmus, Univirs, Vision-Ease	65
	Signet	68
	Sola	65
35	Coburn	65
40	Armorlite	
Progressive	Younger	75
Executive	Coburn, AO	62
	Sola	68
	Univis, Optical Radiation	65
Trifocal		
7 × 25	Coburn, Signet, Univis, Vision-Ease	65
Round		
22	Armorlite, Coburn, Signet, Titmus, Univis, Vision-Ease	65
	Sola	68
40	Coburn	65
	Younger	68

3.12. Indices of Refraction

Material	*Mean Refractive Index* n_4	*Specific Gravity (g cm*^{3}*)*
Crown glass	1.523	2.54
Dense flint	1.654	3.90
Extra dense flint	1.700	4.33
Double extra dense flint	1.748	4.76
CR39	1.499	1.32
Polymethyl methacrylate	1.491	1.19
Tital	1.706	2.99
High-Lite	1.701	2.99

3.13. Specialized Ophthalmic Lenses

Table A. Lenses

All-Around Bifocal
Benson
Anti-Radiation
Nuclear Associates (Radiglass)
Benson (Ray Guard) (63)* +8.00 to −8.00
Anti-Ultraviolet
Hoya (UV) (65, 70)
Orcolite (UV 400)
Anti-Ultraviolet, Anti-Infra Red
Spectra Shield (Human II)
Hoya (UI) Mild Amber (65)
Button Seg Bifocal
Benson
Cataract, Temporary
Universal Resin: 22 mm Round Seg, Ultex, or Multi Aspheric $+8^{00}$ to $+14^{50}$
Vision-Ease Glass: $+9^{00}$ to $+16^{00}$ Bifocal D18 (34)
Trifocal R-20 (34) SV includes to -3^{00} cyl (34, 46, 55)
Cataract, Glass SV
Hoya: 1.8 index (55) Aspheric
Younger: Hi-Lite (58, 63) Aspheric
Vision-Ease: Lenticular (54)
Extra Thick SV
Aire-O-Light: Resin: (65) also minus bases
Precision-Cosmet: Glass: (58, 63, 71)
Exotic Tints (Glass)
Glassblowers: Fish-Schurman (Neophan)
Purple: Robinson-Houchin (71); Precision-Cosmet (58, 63,71)
Crookes: Meyer SV (67); Ultex (71) Benson
Shooters: Benson
Therminon: SV (65) Benson (Vermillion, Limon)
Full Spectrum Transmission
Armorlite: 22 Round, Flattops, 7 mm Trifocals, 3 gray shades, clear
Hilite Bifocal
Phillips: Ultex A (68), Ultex B (65)
Hoya: Executive $+7^{00}$ to -10^{00} (65) Adds .75 to 3.00 (finished); semifinished available
High Adds See Table 6.1E
High Index
Hoya THI (1.806) (60)
Industrial Thickness
Shuron (65)
Titmus (62)

*Blank size in parentheses

(continued)

Table A. Lenses (continued)

Low Transmission
- Recreational Innovations (no IR); Shade #107 (62)

Myodisc Bifocal
- Benson

Night Driving
- Hoya (Neo) Mild Blue (65)

Photochromics – Colored
- Brown
  - Hoya (65, 70)
  - B & L (65)
  - Prec-Cosmet (58, 63, 71)
- Blue
  - Hoya (65, 70)
- Pink
  - Hoya
- Variable
  - B & L (Ambermatic) (71) –0.25 to –2.00 with cyl to 1.00; Sph +1.00 to –2.00
  - Melibrad (Reacto, Pol SF) Laminated Yellow, Green, Brown (65)

Polarized Cataract
- Melibrad Aspheric lenticular (70) Kryptok (70) Flattop (65, 71)

Polarized SV Resin
- Shane Michael: Gray (70)
- Vigor: Gray (70)
- Melibrad: Laminated Yellow (70) Gray, Brown (70)

Polaroid Mirrored
- Melibrad (65) Laminated

Polycarbonate High Impact
- Techsight $+4^{00}$ to -6^{00}, Cyl to -2^{00} (70) No tints, Bifocal: Executive

Reverse Slab Bifocal
- Aire-O-Lite: Resin adds $+1^{00}$ to $+4^{00}$

Scratch Resistant (Finished)
- Armorlite (RL X) (65, 75)
- Hoya (Hi-Quartz) (65, 75) No executives or flattops
- Lens Man (Quartzlite) $+5^{00}$ to -6^{00} spheres $\pm 4^{00}$ with -2^{00} cyl (72)

Ski Tint Coating
- Pacific Universal Vuernet Tint

Thinline Flattop
- Benson

Thin Acrylic
- Optimum Optics

Trifocals Critical Ranges
- Vision Ease: 40%, 60%, 70%, 7 mm intermediates

*** Blank size in parentheses**

Table B. Sources

Aire-O-Lite
Rte. One Industrial Park
Alma, GA 31510

Armorlite Inc.
130 N. Bingham Drive
San Marcos, CA 92062

Benson Optical
6600 France Ave. So.
Minneapolis, MN 55435

Hoya Lens
970 Knox St.
Torrance, CA 90502

Melibrad
333 S. Beverly Drive
Suite 202
Beverly Hills, CA 90212

Meyer Optical
2501 W. Pennway
P.O. Box 1066
Kansas City, MO 64141

Nuclear Associates
100 Voice Road
Carle Place, NY 11514

Optimum Optics
P.O. Box 330
Rochelle Park, NJ 07662

Orcolite
6352 No. Irwindale Ave.
Azusa, CA 91702

Pacific Universal
695 S. Raymond Ave.
Pasadena, CA 91105

Phillips Lens Co.
700 Cedar Ave.
Middlesex, NJ 08846

Precision-Cosmet
811 5th Ave. So.
Minneapolis, MN 55404

Recreational Innovations
P.O. Box 159
South Lyon, MI 48175

Robinson-Houchin
1266 Dublin Road
Columbus, OH 43215

Shane-Michael Optical Co.
70 Elmira St.
San Francisco, CA 94124

Sola Optical
3600 Lakeview Highway
Petaluma, CA 94952

Spectra Shield
201 N. Elmolino
Pasadena, CA 91101

Techsight
3323 W. Warner Ave.
Santa Ana, CA 92702

Therminon
Box 1176
Des Moines, IA

Titmus
Box 191
Petersburg, VA

Universal Opthalmic
P.O. Box 3144
Houston, TX 77001

Vigor Optical
53 W. 23 Street
New York, NY 10010

Vision-Ease
P.O. Box 986
Industrial Park
St. Cloud, MN 56301

3.14. Fitting Guides

Table A. Progressive and Invisible Adds

Company	*Brand Name*	*Seg or Progressive Corridor Placement*
American Optical	Ultravue	0–2 mm below center of pupil
Coburn	E-22	2–4 mm above lower lid
Silor	Noline	2 mm below center of pupil
	Varilux 2	4 mm below center of pupil ("fitting line" falls on pupil)
Univis	Unison	2 mm below center of pupil
Younger	10/30	0–2 mm below center of pupil
	Seamless	1.5–2 mm higher than a flattop

Table B. Distance Decentration Allowable per Welsh Four Drop Aspheric Lens*

	Power in 180° Meridian			
Eye Size	*+9.00 D to +10.75 D*	*+11.00 D to +12.75 D*	*+13.00 to +14.75 D*	*+15.00 D to +16.75 D*
42	6	5	4	3
44	4	4	4	3
46	4	3	3	2
48	2	2	2	1
50	2	2	2	1
52	1.5	1.5	1	1
54	1	1	0	0

***The values shown in this table are "Allowable." They are the limit and should not be the norm. Many professionals prefer 1 mm to 1.5 mm less decentration as the maximum limit.**

Table C. Hyperaspheric

Rx Power	*HyperAsphericity*	*Adds Available All Powers*
Up to ±12.00 D	2.50 D (Specify 12 Base)	2.00 2.25 2.50
+12.25 D to +14.00 D	3.25 D (Specify 13.50 Base)	2.75 3.00 3.50
+14.25 D to +16.50 D	4.00 D (Specify 15.00 Base)	4.00 Special Adds Low Vision
+16.75 D and above	5.00 D (Specify 16.50 Base)	4.50 5.00

Recommended Segment Types:
Round Top (22 mm) seg placement: 3 mm below
Flattop (22 × 16) seg placement: 3 mm below 2.5 mm inset

Table D. Executive Lens Decentration Table

If Eyesize Is	*Total Amount of Decentration Available* (Column A) from 56 × 60 mm blank	(Column B) from 60 × 65 mm blank
46	7 mm	9.5 mm
48	6 mm	8.5 mm
50	5 mm	7.5 mm
52	4 mm	6.5 mm
54	3 mm	5.5 mm
56	2 mm	6.5 mm

How to Use
Determine from the Rx the amount of distance decentration per lens.
Add the segment decentration, this equals total decentration.
Find the eyesize that is to be used in the left column.
Check Column A to see if the amount listed is greater than the total decentration computed from the Rx. If greater, this blank size can be used to fabricate the Rx.
If the amount listed is not greater, check the amount under Column B. If this is greater, this blank size can be used.
These computations do not permit any edging allowance.

3.15. Transmission of Photochromics

Percent Transmission of Photochromic Lenses in Their Lightened and Darkened States

Color	*Lightened State*	*Darkened State*
Light Gray	83	43
Light Brown	88	42
Blue	85	45
Pink	88	45
Dark Gray	67	23
Dark Brown	64	22
Light Fused Multifocal lens	88	38
Dark fused Multifocal lens	66	16
Photogray Extra*	87	16
Supergray†	90	16

***TM Corning Glass Works**
†TM Wesley-Jessen
Also see Table 3.20

3.16. Differences in Edge Thickness Between High Index (1.70) and Crown Ophthalmic Lenses

	Minus Power					
*Semi diameter**	*−6.00*	*−8.00*	*−10.00*	*−12.00*	*−14.00*	*−16.00*
20	.60	.80	1.00	1.20	1.40	1.60
22	.66	.88	1.10	1.32	1.54	1.76
24	.84	1.12	1.40	1.68	1.96	2.24
26	1.02	1.36	1.70	2.04	2.38	2.72
28	1.14	1.52	1.90	2.28	2.66	3.04
30	1.30	1.76	2.20	2.64	3.08	3.52

*The semi diameter is one half the datum length plus the decentration

The difference between plastic and high index is approximately 7% greater than the figures above

Reprinted from Grosvenor, T.P.: *New Lens Materials,* Optometric Monthly (November 13, 1978, pp. 29—31), published by Professional Press, Inc., 101 East Ontario Street, Chicago, Illinois 60611.

3.17. Powers and Diameters at which Lenses Made in Crown or High Index Glass Are Equal in Weight

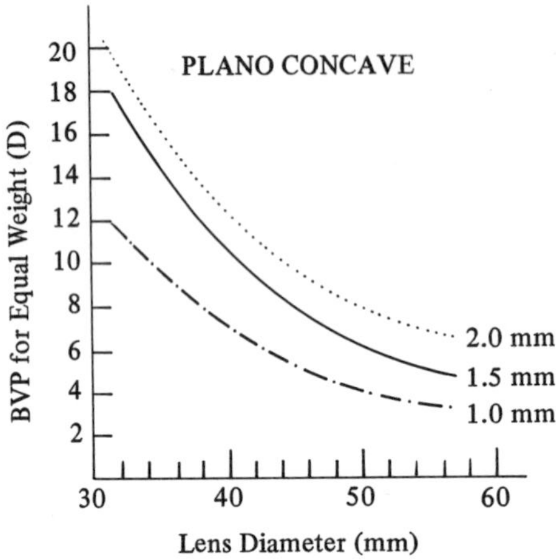

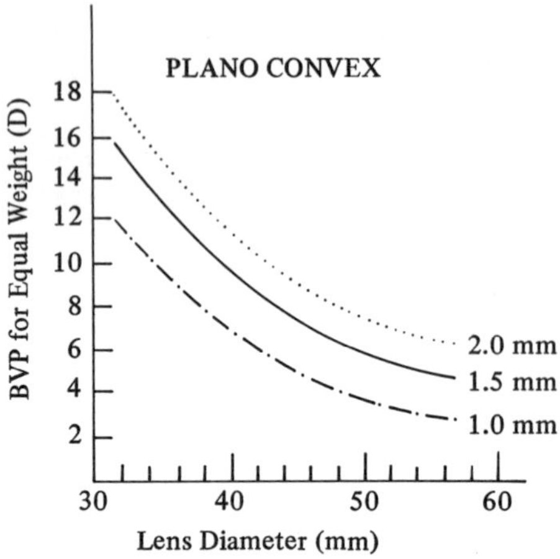

The back vertex powers at which the weights of lenses made in high index glass and crown glass are equal, plotted against lens diameter for plano concave/convex lenses. The dotted, continuous, and chain dotted curves refer to minimum edge thicknesses (convex) or center thickness (concave) of 2.0 mm, 1.5 mm, and 1.0 mm, respectively.

It can be seen that a +10.00 DS lens with edge thickness 1.5 mm will be lighter in high index glass if its diameter exceeds 43 mm, and so on.

For a given lens diameter there is a particular back vertex power at which the weights of the lens in crown or high index glass are equal, the so-called crossover value. This value decreases as the lens size increases. For back vertex powers above this value, a high index glass lens would be lighter than a crown glass lens.

Reprinted from Jill Tucker, The use of high index glass, *The Ophthalmic Optician.* Hatton Press, October 2, 1976.

3.18. Availability of Specialized Lenses

Table A. Progressive Adds and Seamless (Semifinished Unless Noted)

Manufacturer	*Diameter*	*Bases*	*Notes*
Progressive Adds: Plastic			
American Optical			
Ultravue 25	75	4.5 to 8.5	Powers: −5.0 to +4.25 to −3.00 cyl Adds .50 to 3.00 Segs: 25 mm
28	75	4.5 to 8.5	Powers: −5.0 to +4.25 to −3.00 cyl Adds 1.00 to 2.50 Segs: 40 mm
Younger 10/30	76[1]	2.25 to 10.25	Powers: −10.0 to +8.00 Segs: 30 mm Adds .75 to 3.00
Multioptics Varilux 2	75	4.5 to 7.25	Also Uncut +5.50 to −6.00 Cyl to 4.00 Adds .50 to 3.50. Seg: 15 mm
Silor Supernoline	72, 78	4.5 to 8.75	Segs: 28 mm. Adds 1.00 to 3.00 Powers +5.50 to −6.00
Univis Unison	75	4.25 to 8.25	Segs: 25 mm. Adds 1.00 to 3.00 Powers −6.00 to +3.25
Progressive Adds: Glass			
Multioptics Varilux 2	65[1]	4.5 to 7.75[4]	Photogray, Photo-X +5.50 to −6.00 Cyl to 4.00 Adds .50 to 3.00
Silor			
Noline	60, 65	3.5 to 9.5[2]	Clear Photo-X −8.00 to +6.00 Cyl to 4.00 Adds .50 to 3.00
Noline +	65,	4.25 to 7.5[1]	Photo-X Adds 1.00 to 3.00
Seamless: Plastic			
Younger	66, 71, 75[1]	6.25 to 8.25	Segs: 22 mm −8.00 to +10.00 cyl to 6.00
Coburn, EZ 2 Vue	71	4.25 to 8.25	Segs: 25 mm Adds .75 to 2.75
American Optical Ultravue Blended	75	4.5 to 8.5	Segs: to 24 mm +4.25 to −5.00 cyl to 3.00 Adds .50 to 3.00
Sola, Blend 2000	68	4.00 to 6.00	Segs: 22 mm
Silor Super Blend	76	4.00 to 8.00	Segs: 25 mm
Seamless: Glass			
Younger, Plus	71	4.25 to 10.25	−8.00 to +10.00 cyl to 6.00 Photochromics: pink, green, Highlite
Younger Hi-Lite	63	2.25, 4.25	To −16.00 cyl to 4.00 Also pink
Silor	76		

[1] Decentered blanks
[2] 60 mm blanks only
[3] Hi-Lites also
[4] Refractionist should add —0.25 to the DV and +0.50 to the add

Table B. Availability of Fresnel Press on Prisms and Lenses

Plus Lenses	+0.50 to +2.50 in ¼ D steps (except +0.75) +3.00 to +4.00 in ¼ D steps +5.00 to +14.00 in 1 D steps also +16.00, +20.00
Minus Lenses	−1.00 to −14.00 in 1 D steps
Prisms	.50, 1.00, 1.50 2.00 to 10.00 in 1 D steps, also 12.00 D, and from 15.00 to 30.00 D in 5 D steps
Flat Top 25 mm. *Precut Segments*	+.50 to +2.50 in ½ D steps, also +1.25 and +1.75 +3.00 to +8.00 in 1 D steps (includes base in prism)

Reprinted by permission from Codman and Shurtleff, Inc., *Catalogue*. Courtesy Codman and Shurtleff, Inc., Randolph, Mass.

3.19. Typical Base Curve Series

Sphere Power ↓ / Minus Cylinder Power →	0.00	0.12	0.25	0.37	0.50	0.62	0.75	0.87	1.00	1.12	1.25	1.37	1.50	1.62	1.75	1.87	2.00	2.25	2.50	2.75	3.00	3.25	3.50	3.75	4.00	4.25	4.50	4.75	5.00	5.25	5.50	5.75	6.00
+7.00																																	
+6.75																																	
+6.50																																	
+6.25																	12.00																
+6.00																																	
+5.75																																	
+5.50																																	
+5.25																																	
+5.00																																	
+4.75																																	
+4.50																																	
+4.25																	10.25																
+4.00																																	
+3.75																																	
+3.50																																	
+3.25																																	
+3.00																																	
+2.75																																	
+2.50																																	
+2.25																	8.25																
+2.00																																	
+1.87																																	
+1.75																																	
+1.62																																	
+1.50																																	
+1.37																	7.25																
+1.25																																	
+1.12																																	
+1.00																																	
+0.87																																	
+0.75																																	
+0.62																																	
+0.50																																	
+0.37																																	
+0.25																																	
+0.12																	6.25																
Plano																																	

← Minus Cylinder Power

(continued)

3.19. Typical Base Curve Series (continued)

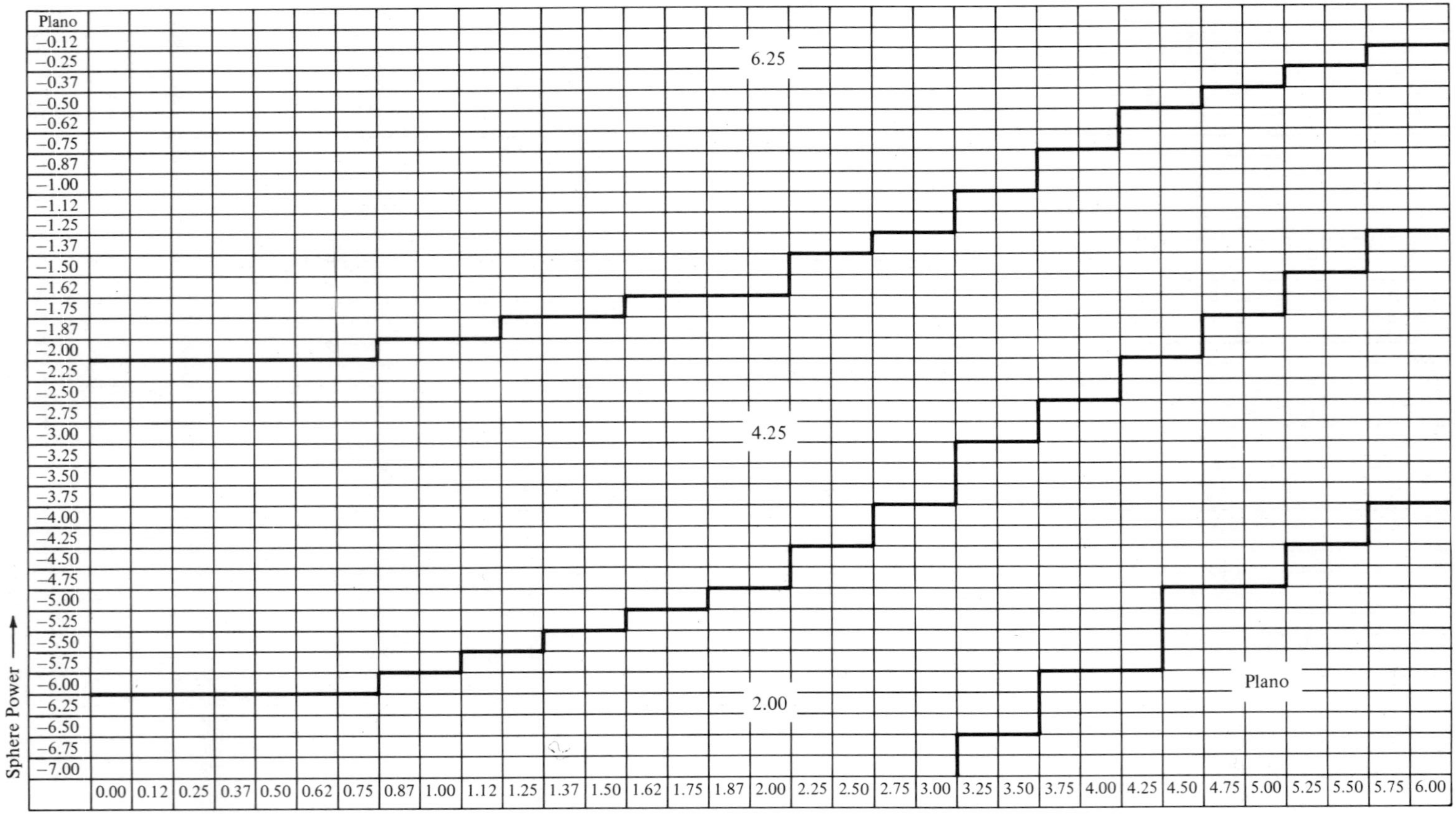

Courtesy of the Vision-Ease Corp.

3.20. Typical Transmission Curves: Tinted Lenses

Legend for Tables A-F

Shades

- **A** ———— (heavy solid)
- **B** — — —
- **C** ———— (light solid)
- **D** —·—·—
- **E** — ·· —

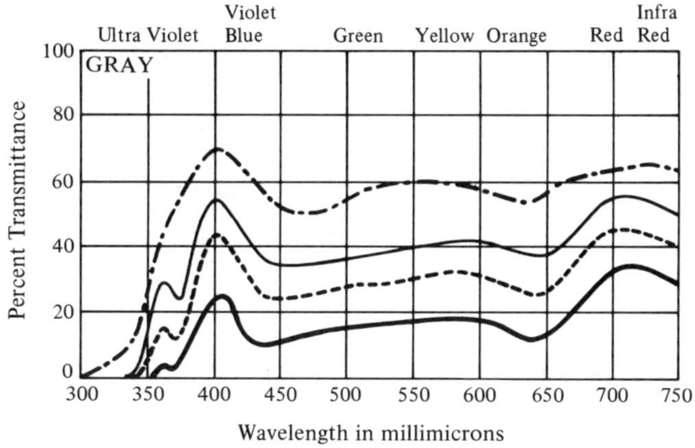

Table A. Gray

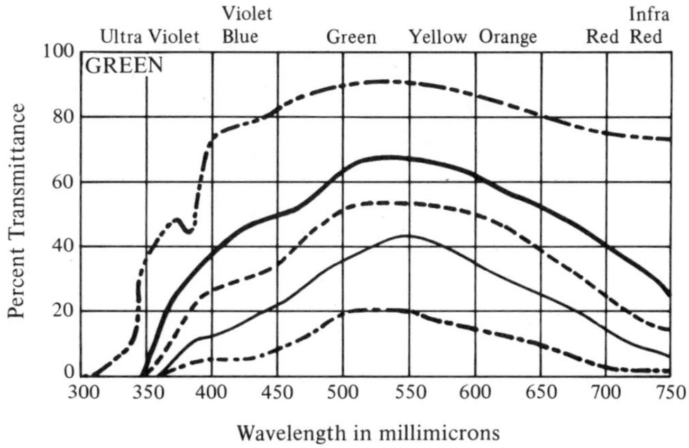

Table B. Green

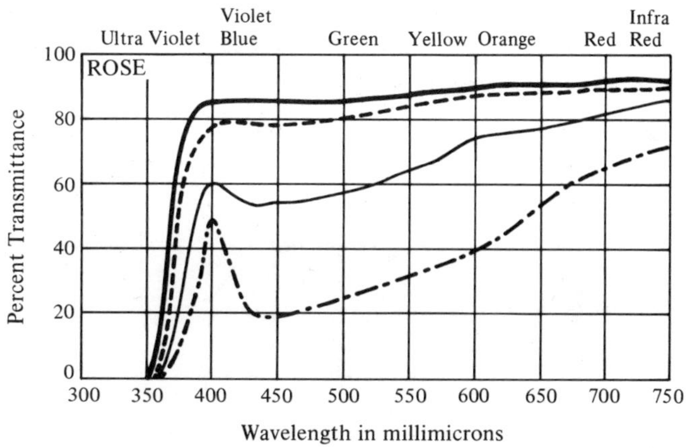

Table C. Rose

3.20. Typical Transmission Curves: Tinted Lenses

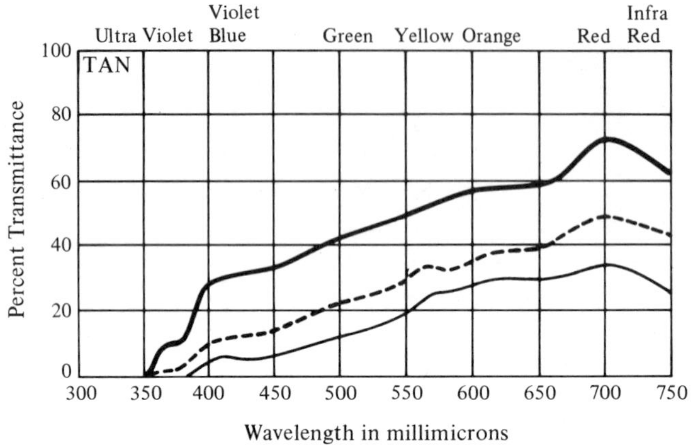

Table D. Tan

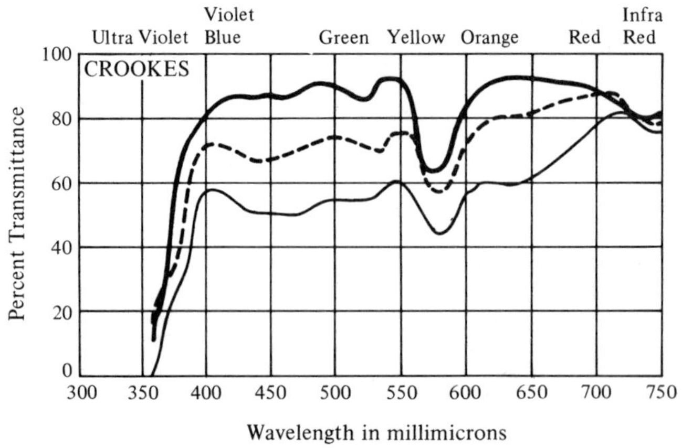

Table E. Crookes

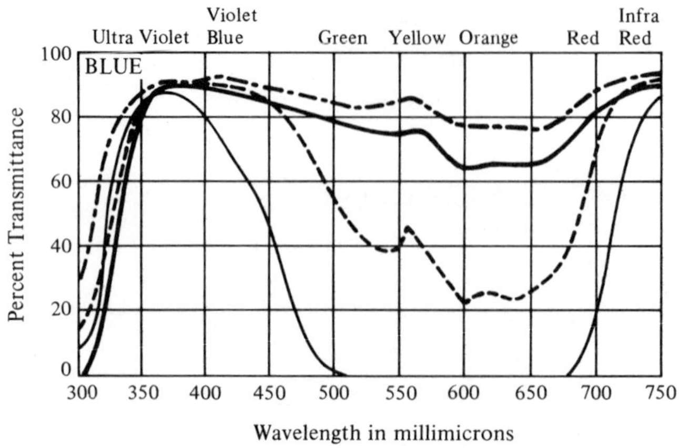

Table F. Blue

3.20. Typical Transmission Curves: Tinted Lenses

Table G. Therminon

Standard Green: – – – – –

Therminon: ———

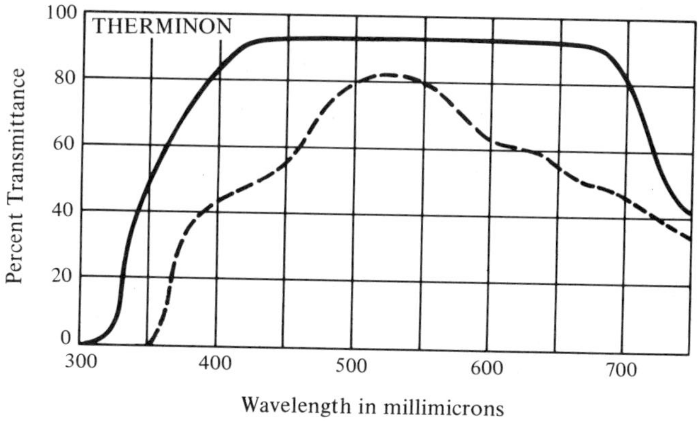

Table H. Photogray

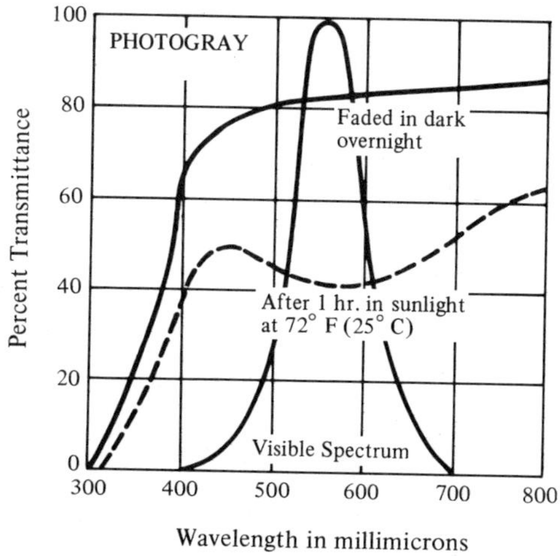

Table I. Photosun

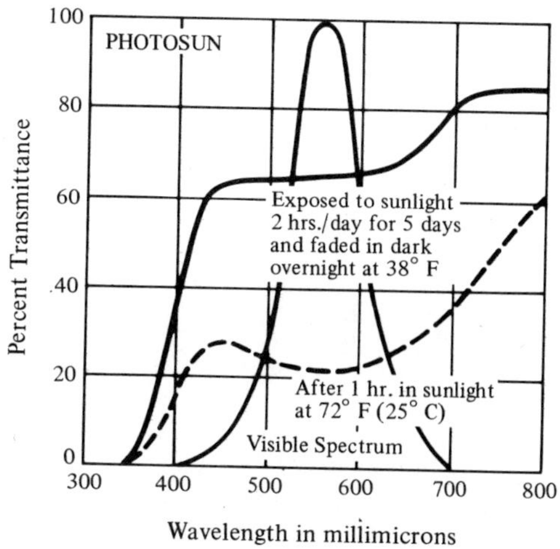

3.20. Typical Transmission Curves: Tinted Lenses

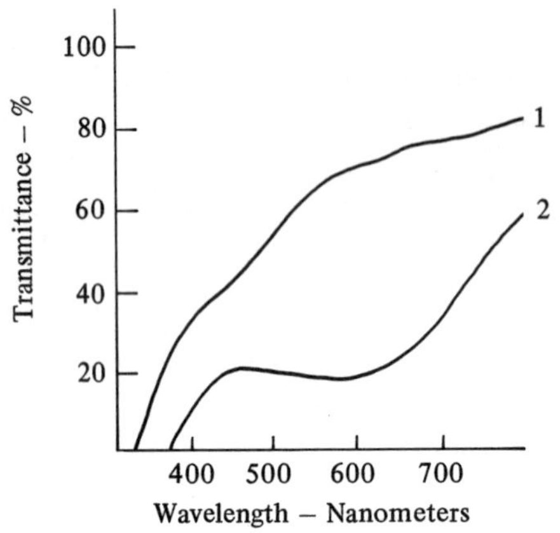

Table J. Dark Brown Photochromic

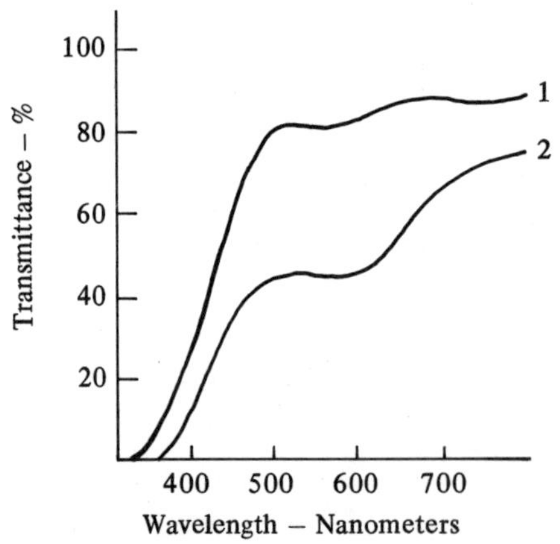

Table K. Light Brown Photochromic

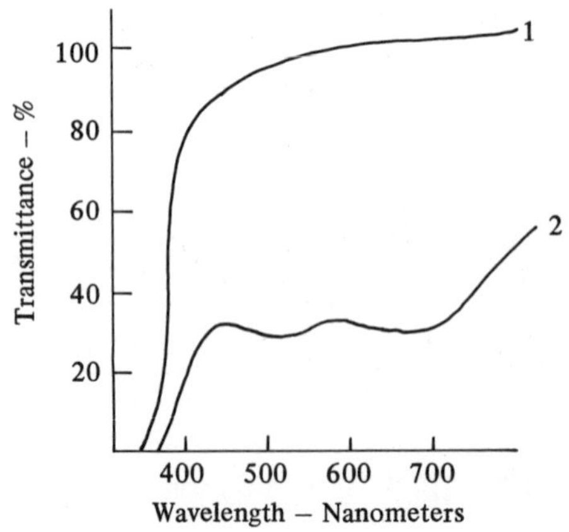

Table L. Photogray Extra

Legend for J, K and L:
1—Faded in dark overnight
2—After one hour in sunlight at 25°C (77°F)

3.20. Typical Transmission Curves: Tinted Lenses

Table M. Photogray Darkening and Fading

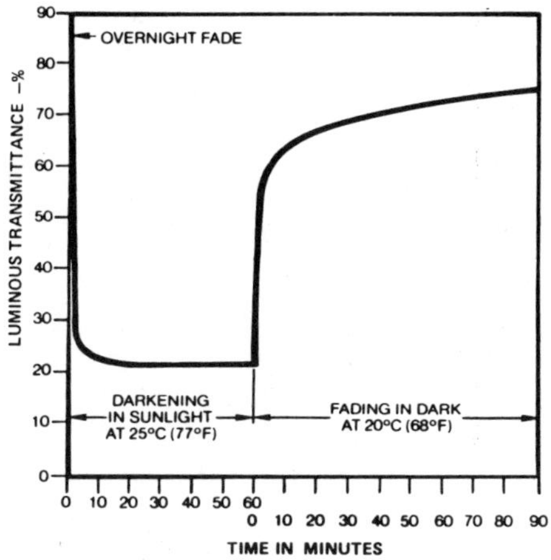

Table N. Kalichrome and Fashion Gray

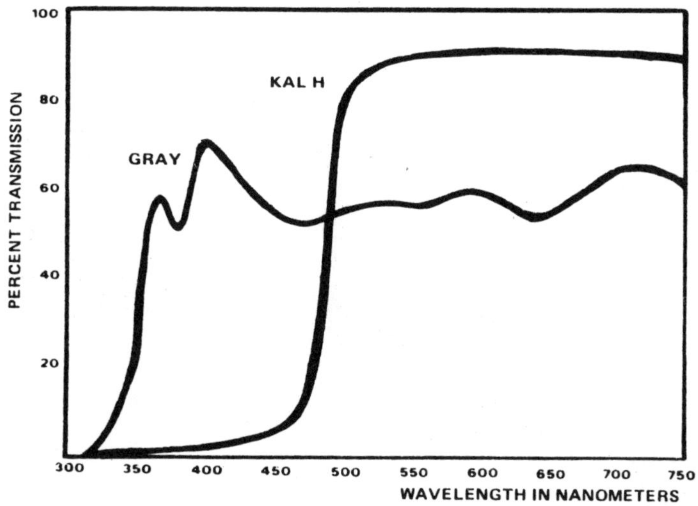

Table O. Dark True-Tone

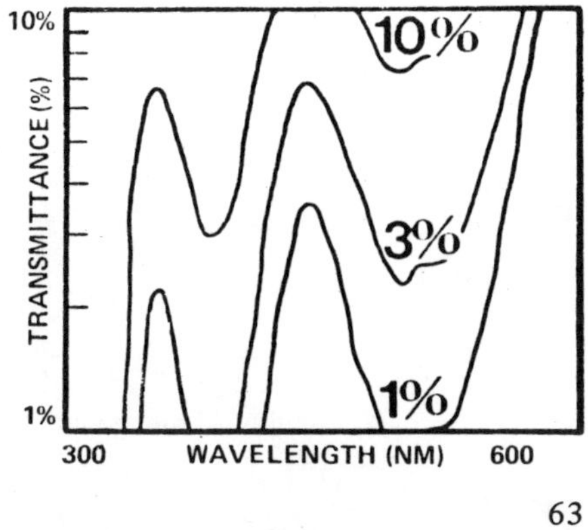

3.20. Typical Transmission Curves: Tinted Lenses

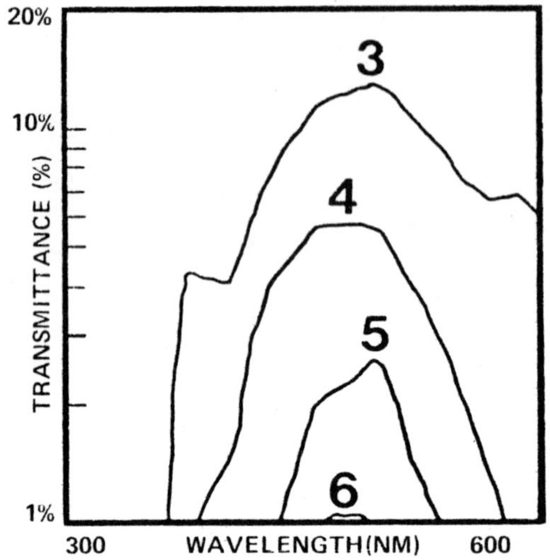

Table P. Filterweld Plano

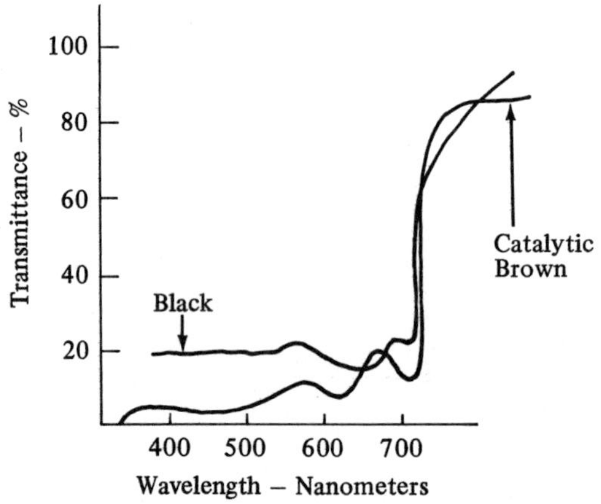

Table Q. Plastics

BPI[r] Catalytic[tm] and Molecular Catalytic[tm] are registered trademarks of Brain Power Incorporated.

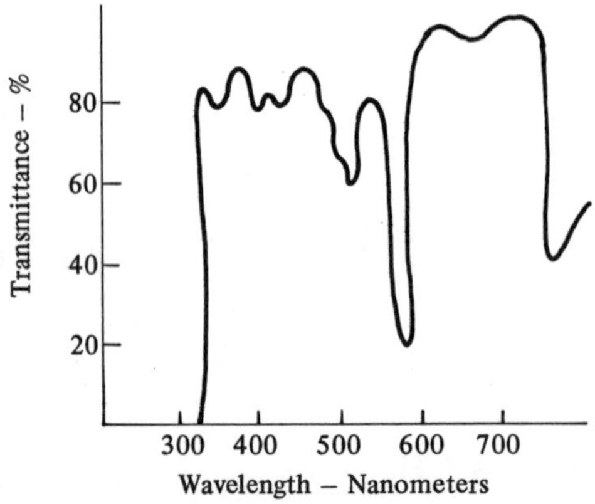

Table R. On 2 Didymium

3.20. Typical Transmission Curves: Tinted Lenses

Table S. Human II

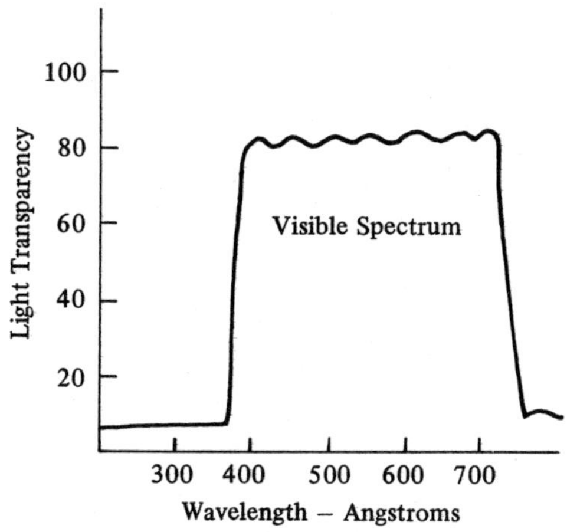

From Spectra-Shield, Inc.

Table T. No IR Model 107

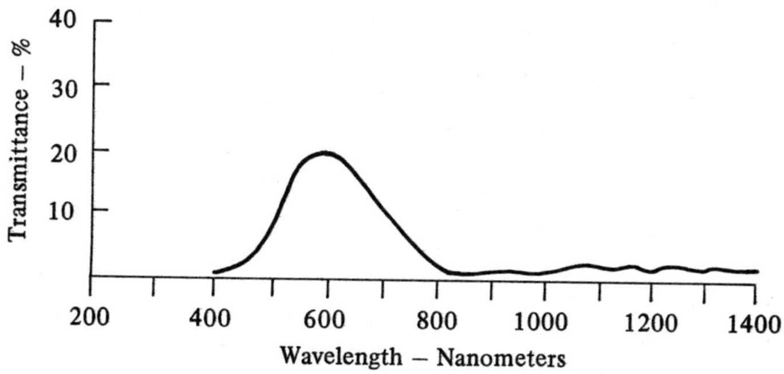

Table U. UV 400

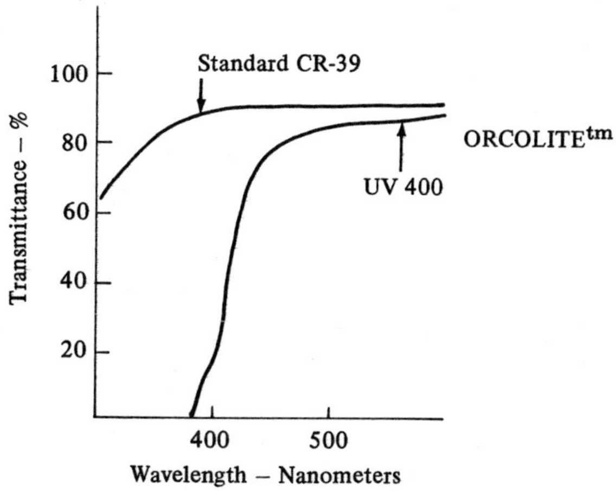

3.20. Typical Transmission Curves: Tinted Lenses

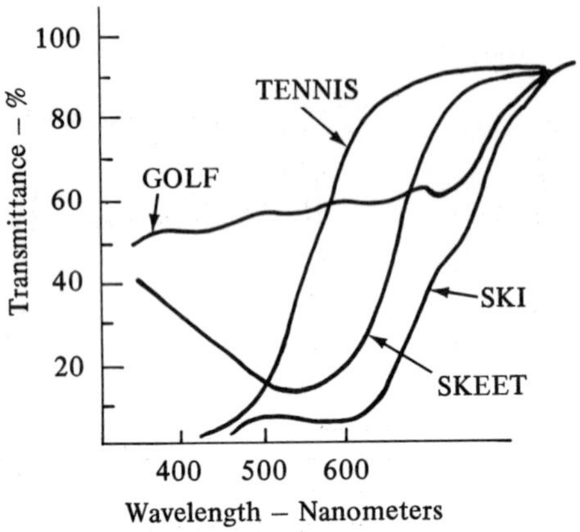

Table V. Sport Tints

BPI[r] and Sport Tints[cm] are registered trademarks of Brain Power Limited.

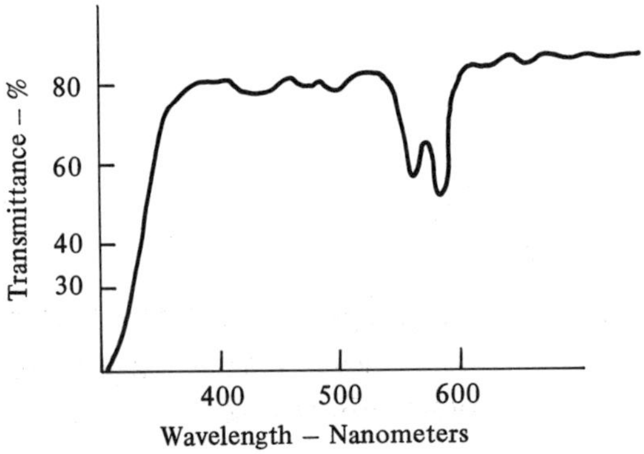

Table W. Coated Neo

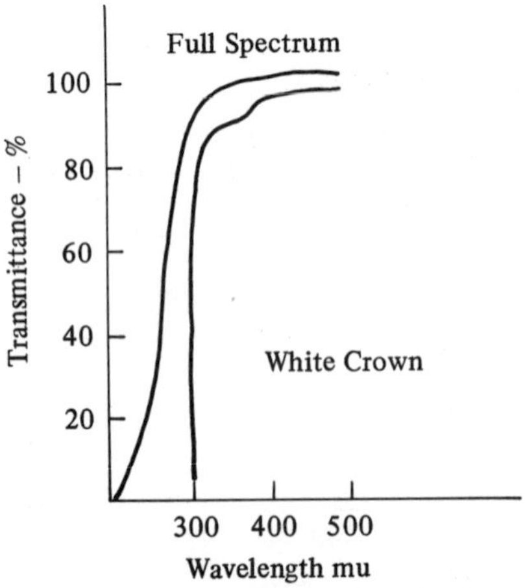

Table X. Full Spectrum

Table Y. Photobrown Extra

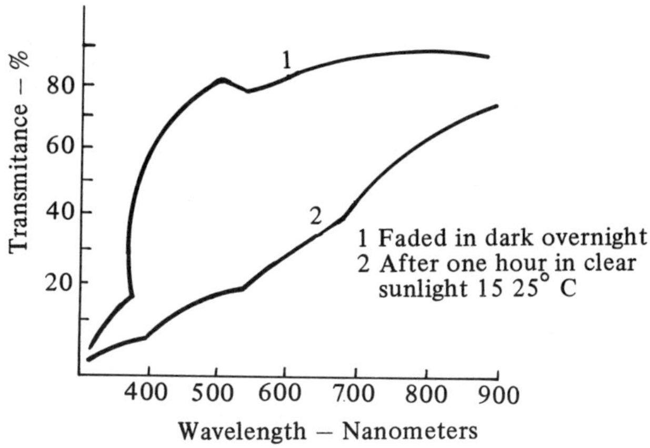

A–F reprinted by permission of the Meyer Optical Company, Kansas City, Missouri.
G reprinted by permission of the Therminon Lens Corporation, Des Moines, Iowa.
H–M reprinted by permission of the Corning Glass Company, Corning, New York.
N reprinted by permission of Bausch and Lomb, Incorporated, Rochester, New York.
O–P reprinted by permission of the American Optical Company, Southbridge, Massachusetts.
Q–R reprinted by permission of BPI Incorporated.
T reprinted by permission of Recreational Innovations, Incorporated.
U reprinted by permission of Optical Radiation, Incorporated.
V is reprinted by permission of BPI, Incorporated.
W is reprinted by permission of Hoya Lens Company.
X is reprinted by permission of Armorlite Incorporated.
Y is reprinted by permission of the Corning Glass Co., New York.

3.21. Absolute Lateral Field of View in Inches Through Segment Widths

Assumptions
Nominal Distance Correction

Power . . . . +2.00 D Lens Addition
Pupil Size . . . . 3 mm. No splitting of Pupil
Center of Rotation . . . . . . 13 mm. From Front of Eye

	Working Distances														
	13 Inches Vertex Distance					*16 Inches Vertex Distance*					*20 Inches Vertex Distance*				
Segment Width	*11 mm.*	*12 mm.*	*13 mm.*	*14 mm.*	*15 mm.*	*11 mm.*	*12 mm.*	*13 mm.*	*14 mm.*	*15 mm.*	*11 mm.*	*12 mm.*	*13 mm.*	*14 mm.*	*15 mm.*
20 mm.	9.4	9.0	8.7	8.4	8.1	11.4	11.0	10.6	10.2	9.8	14.1	13.5	13.0	12.6	12.1
22 mm.	10.5	10.1	9.7	9.4	9.0	12.7	12.3	11.8	11.4	11.0	15.8	15.1	14.6	14.1	13.6
25 mm.	12.1	11.7	11.3	10.9	10.5	14.7	14.2	13.7	13.2	12.7	18.3	17.5	16.9	16.3	15.8
28 mm.	13.8	13.3	12.8	12.3	11.9	16.7	16.1	15.5	15.0	14.5	20.4	19.9	19.2	18.5	17.9
*34 mm.**	17.1	16.5	15.9	15.3	14.8	20.8	20.0	19.2	18.6	18.0	26.0	24.7	23.8	23.0	22.2
*38 mm.**	19.4	18.6	17.9	17.3	16.7	23.5	22.6	21.8	21.0	20.3	29.1	27.9	26.9	25.9	25.0

*Not available — Used for illustration purposes only.

Adapted by permission from Clark, Holmes *et al.*, *Guide to Occupational and Other Visual Needs*, vol. 1. St. Cloud, Minn.: Vision-Ease Corp., 1958.

3.22. Absolute Field of View in Inches Through Various Segment Widths: Cataract Lenses

Segment Width 18 mm.

Vertex Distance	*Total Powers Through Segments* +8.00 D	+10.00 D	+12.00 D
	Field of View at Reading Distance		
8 mm.	12.62″	12.05″	11.49″
9 mm.	11.96″	11.37″	10.79″
10 mm.	11.32″	10.76″	10.19″
11 mm.	10.76″	10.22″	9.62″
12 mm.	10.26″	9.68″	9.12″
13 mm.	9.76″	9.22″	8.65″
14 mm.	9.35″	8.79″	8.20″
15 mm.	8.95″	8.37″	7.81″

Segment Width 20 mm.

Vertex Distance	*Total Powers Through Segments* +8.00 D	+10.00 D	+12.00 D
	Field of View at Reading Distance		
8 mm.	14.02″	13.39″	12.76″
9 mm.	13.28″	12.63″	11.99″
10 mm.	12.58″	11.95″	11.32″
11 mm.	11.95″	11.35″	10.69″
12 mm.	11.39″	10.76″	10.13″
13 mm.	10.85″	10.24″	9.61″
14 mm.	10.39″	9.76″	9.12″
15 mm.	9.94″	9.30″	8.69″

Segment Width 22 mm.

Vertex Distance	*Total Powers Through Segments* +8.00 D	+10.00 D	+12.00 D
	Field of View at Reading Distance		
8 mm.	16.83″	16.06″	15.31″
9 mm.	15.94″	15.16″	14.39″
10 mm.	15.10″	14.34″	13.59″
11 mm.	14.34″	13.63″	12.83″
12 mm.	13.67″	12.87″	12.16″
13 mm.	13.02″	12.29″	11.53″
14 mm.	12.46″	11.72″	10.94″
15 mm.	11.93″	11.16″	10.42″

Reprinted by permission from Univis Lens Co., *Cataract Prescription Handbook*. Courtesy Univis Lens Co., No. Attleboro, Mass.

3.23. Absolute Vertical Field of View in Inches Through Trifocal Intermediates (50% Intermediate)

	Working Distances														
	26 Inches Vertex Distance					*32 Inches Vertex Distance*					*40 Inches Vertex Distance*				
Trifocal Height	*11 mm.*	*12 mm.*	*13 mm.*	*14 mm.*	*15 mm.*	*11 mm.*	*12 mm.*	*13 mm.*	*14 mm.*	*15 mm.*	*11 mm.*	*12 mm.*	*13 mm.*	*14 mm.*	*15 mm.*
6 mm.	3.2	3.1	3.0	2.9	2.8	3.9	3.7	3.6	3.5	3.3	4.9	4.7	4.5	4.3	4.2
7 mm.	4.3	4.1	4.0	3.8	3.7	5.2	5.0	4.8	4.6	4.4	6.5	6.2	6.0	5.8	5.6
8 mm.	5.3	5.1	4.9	4.8	4.6	6.5	6.2	6.0	5.8	5.6	8.1	7.8	7.5	7.2	7.0
10 mm.	7.5	7.2	6.9	6.7	6.4	9.1	8.8	8.4	8.1	7.8	11.3	10.9	10.5	10.1	9.8

Adapted by permission from Clark, Holmes *et al.*, *Guide to Occupational and Other Visual Needs*, vol. 1. St. Cloud, Minn.: Vision-Ease Corp., 1958.

3.24. Available Multifocal Designs

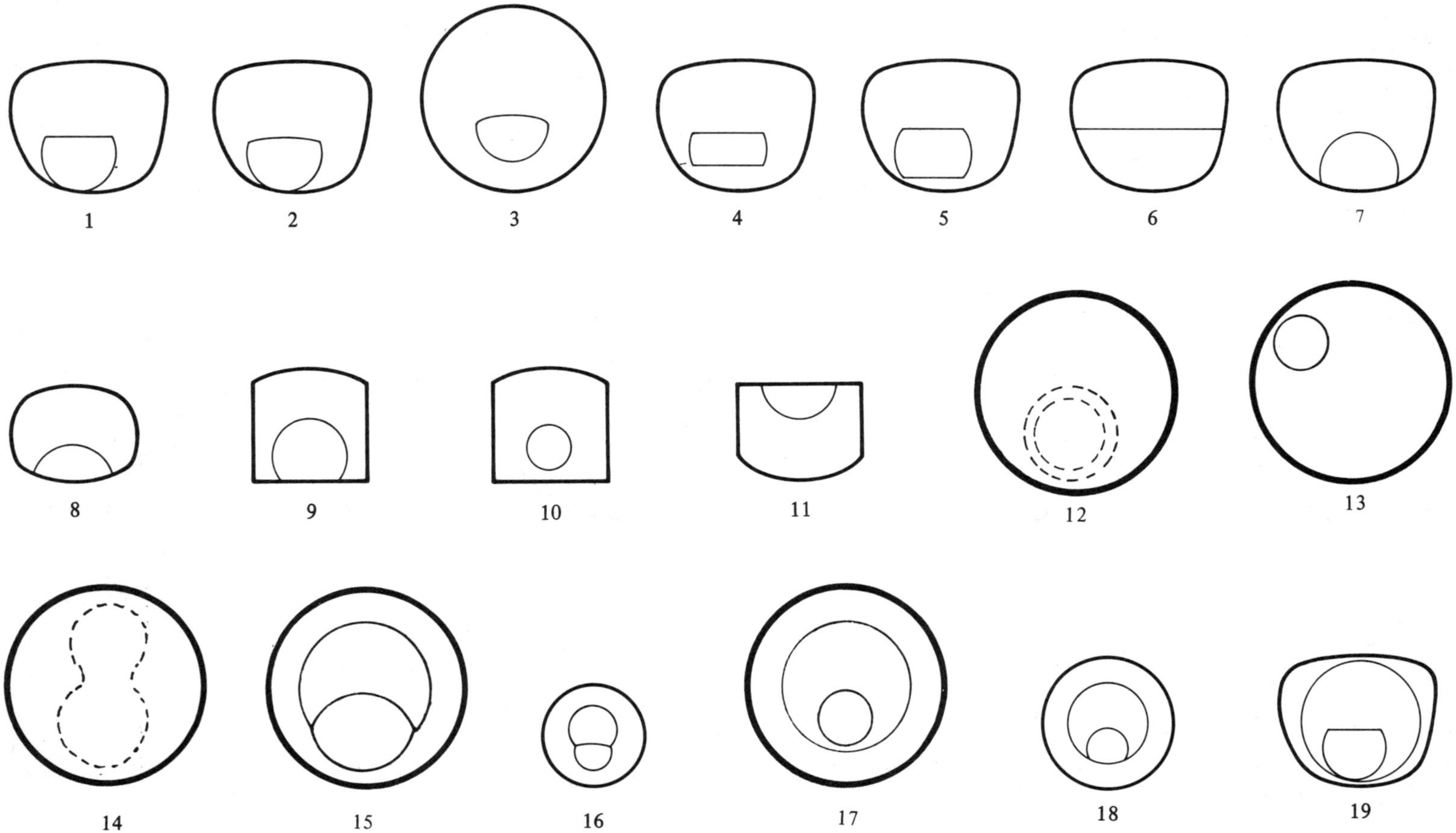

(continued)

3.24. Available Multifocal Designs (continued)

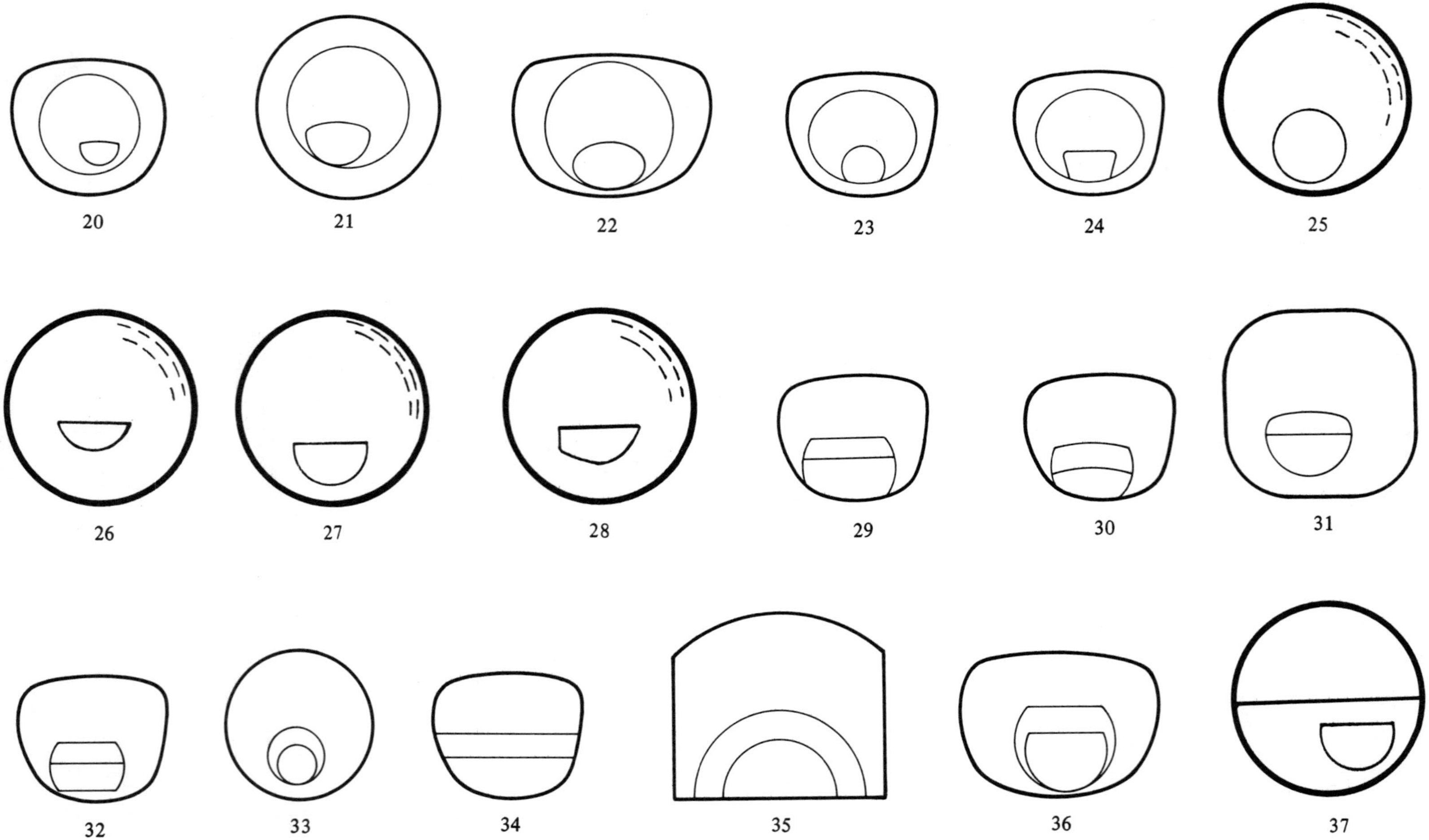

(continued)

3.24. Available Multifocal Designs (continued)

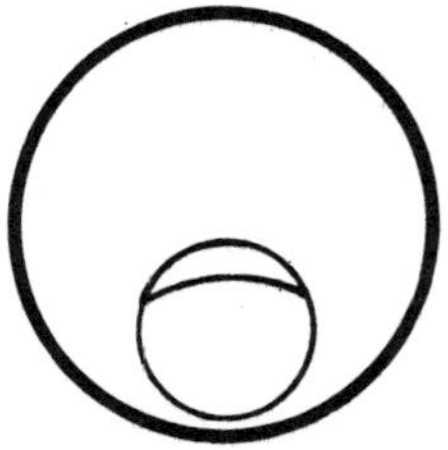
38

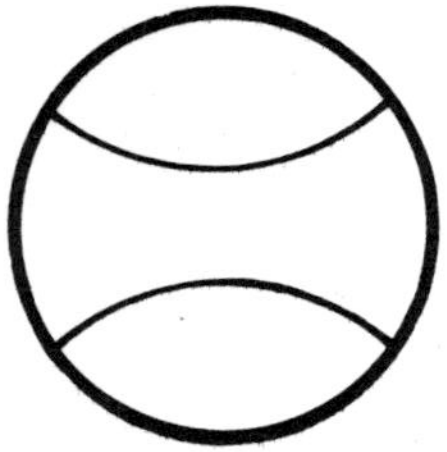
39

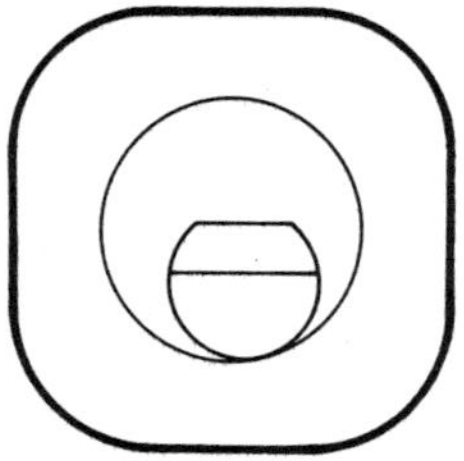
40

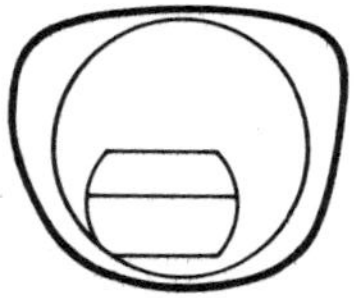
41

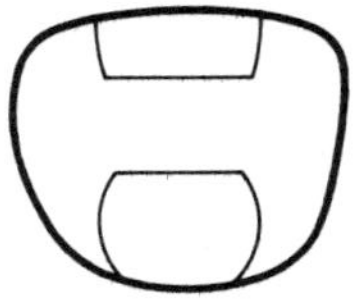
42

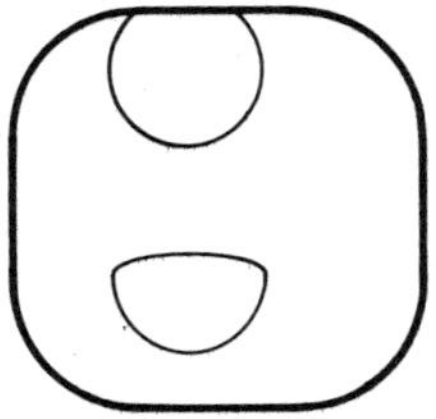
43

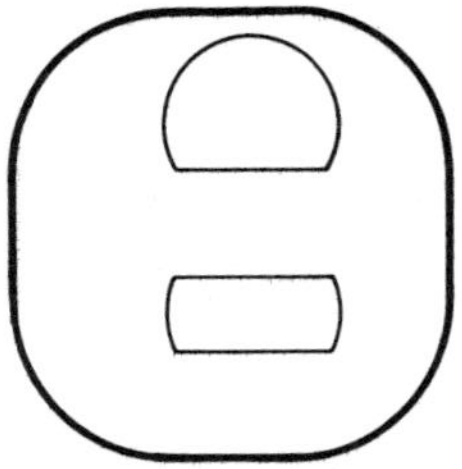
44

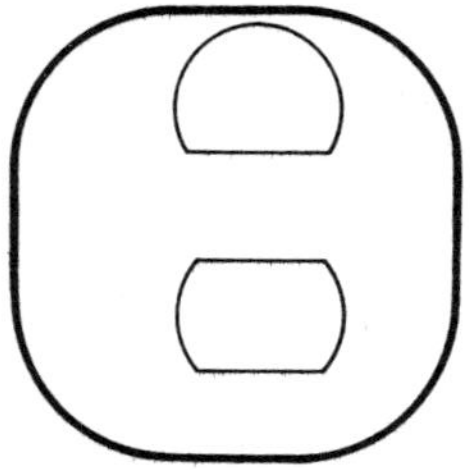
45

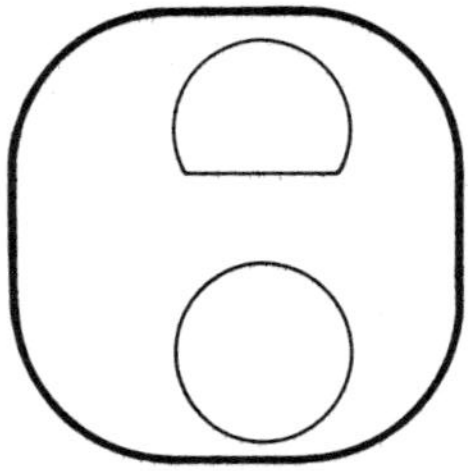
46

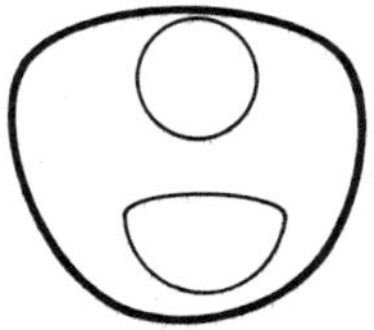
47

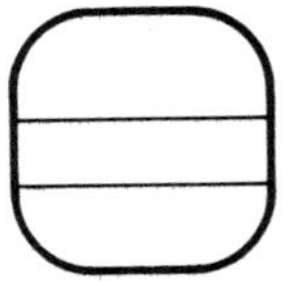
48

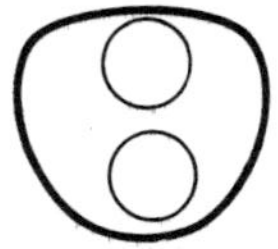
49

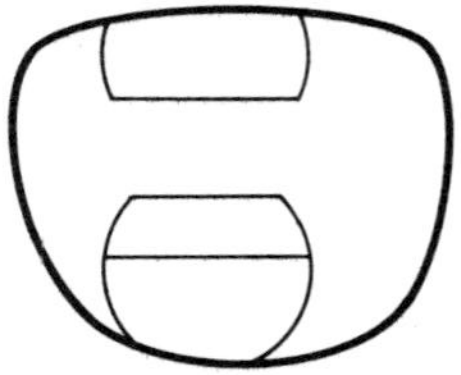
50

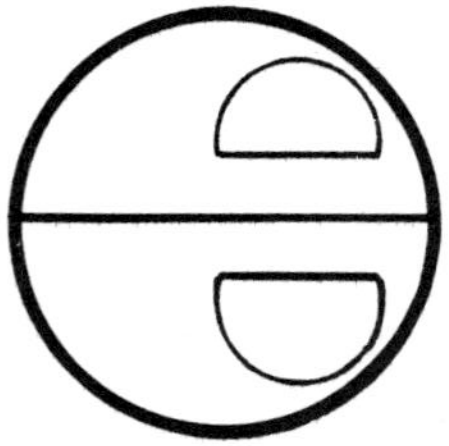
51

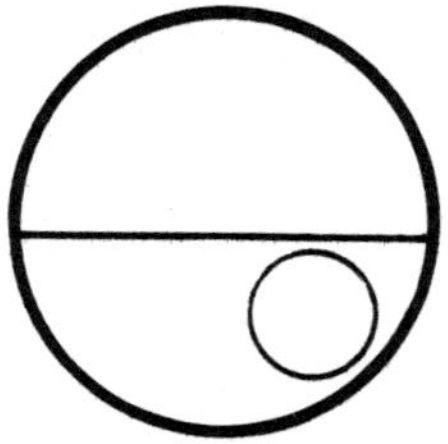
52

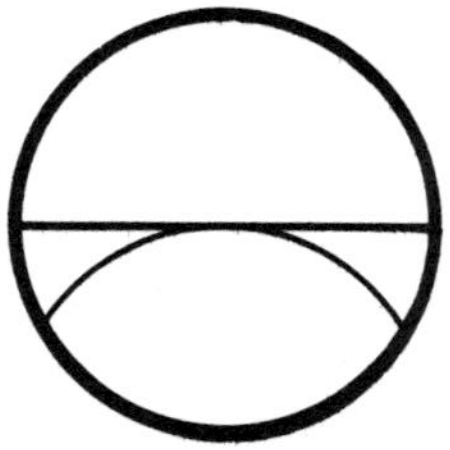
53

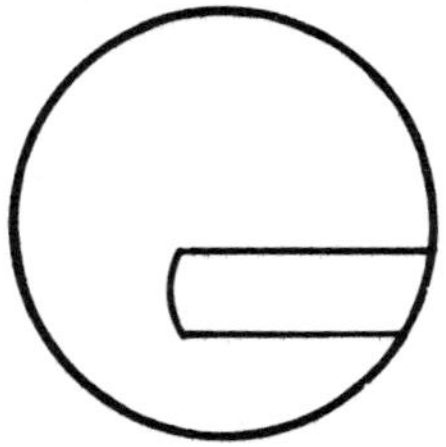
54

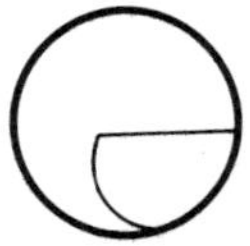
55

(continued)

3.24. Available Multifocal Designs (continued)

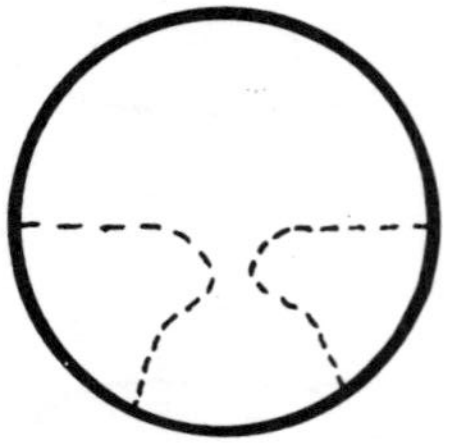

56

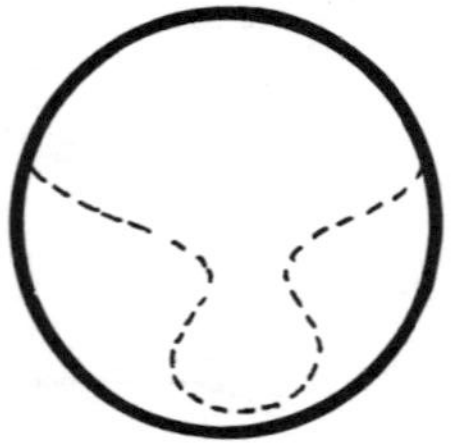

57

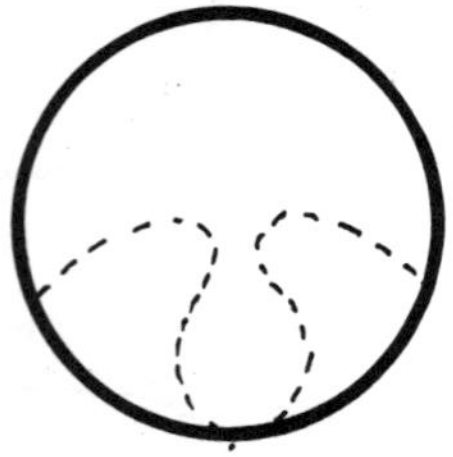

58

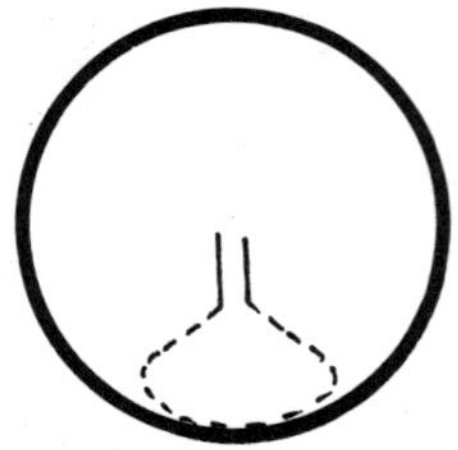

59

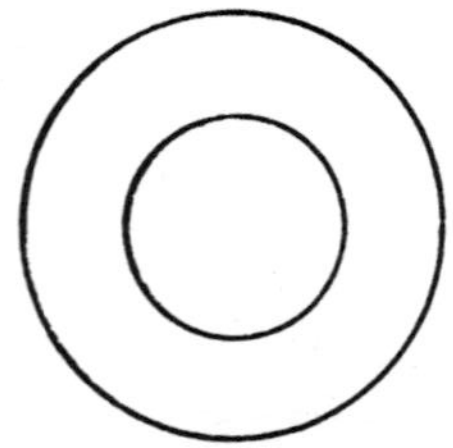

60

3.24. Available Multifocal Designs

Table A. Available Multifocals

Type		*Width of Near Vision Segment*
Bifocals		
1	Flat Top	20, 22, 25, 28, 35, 40[1]
2	Curve Top	22, 25
3	Panoptik (P-Top)	21, 5, 25
4	Ribbon B	9 X 22
5	Ribbon R	14 X (22, 25)
6	Executive	
7	Nochrome	20, 22, 25
7	Kryptok	22, 24, 35, 38
8	Ultex A	38
9	Ultex AL	38
10	Ultex B	20, 22 50[1]
11	Redrite	38, 40
3	Ultex K	
12	Invisible	
13	Button Seg	
14	Myodisc	
Cataract – Regular Lenticulars		
15	Unikat Ultex[2]	35
16	Bifokat[2]	18
17	Unikat Round[2]	
18	Round	22, 30
19	Flat Top	7 X (23, 25)
20	Curve Top	22
21	Panoptik	19.5
Cataract – Aspheric Lenticulars		
22	Round Field – Oval Seg	22
23	Oval Field – Round Seg	22
24	Oval Field – Flat Top Seg	22
Cataract – Aspherics		
25	Welsh Four Drop – Round	22
26	Welsh Four Drop – Flat Top	22
25	Hyperaspheric – Round	22
27	Hyperaspheric – Flat Top	22
28	Frieder	30
1	Full Field – Flat Top	22
7	Full Field – Round	22
Trifocals		
29	Flat Top	6, 7, 8 X (22, 25, 28) 10 X (28, 35)
30	Curve Top	7 X 24
31	Panoptik	7 X 25
32	Ribbon Seg	14 X 22
33	Round	22 X 30
34	Executive	
35	Ultex X	8 X 32
36	Ultra 7	24
37	ED	25
38	Cromwell	
39	Baseball[3]	
Cataract Lenticular		
40	Flat Top	19
41	Ribbon	22

[1] Plastic only
[2] Temporaries
[3] Great Britain

(continued)

Table A. Available Multifocals (continued)

Type		*Width of Near Vision Segment*
Occupational (Dual)		
42	Flat Tops	22, 25, 28
43	Round/Curve Top	21.5
44	Flat Top Ribbon B	22
45	Flat Top/Ribbon R	22
46	Flat Top/Round	22
47	Round/Panoptik	22
48	Executive	
49	Rounds	22
Miscellaneous		
50	Quadri Flat Top	25
51	Quadri Edd	25
52	Reserve Slab-Off	
53	Down Curve Slab-Off	
54	Prism Seg. Ribbon	
55	Prism Seg. Flat Top	
56	Ultra-Vue	25, 40
57	Varilux 2	
58	10/30	30
59	Unison	25
60	All Around	

[1] Plastic only
[2] Temporaries
[3] Great Britain

Refraction and Analysis 4

4.1. Muscle Tonicity

Table A. Normals for Muscle Tonicity (After Morgan)

Tests		*Norms*	*Range*	*Group*
No. 8	Phoria at far	1 exo ± 1	Ortho to 2 exo	(C)
No. 9	Adduction	9 ± 2	7 to 11	(B)
No. 10	Convergence–break	19 ± 4	15 to 23	(B)
	Convergence–recovery	10 ± 2	8 to 12	
No. 11	Abduction–break	7 ± 2	5 to 9	(A)
	Abduction–recovery	4 ± 1	3 to 5	
No. 5	Dynamic Skiametry	+1.37 ± 12	1.25 to 1.50	B
No. 14A	Mon. C.C.	+1.00 ± 25	.75 to 1.25	B
No. 14B	Bin. C.C.	+ .50 ± 25	.25 to .75	B
No. 13B	Phoria at near (Fus. Sup. Conv.) .	3 exo ± 3	Ortho to 6 exo	(C)
No. 16A	Pos. Rel. Conv.	17 ± 3, or No blur	14 to 20, or No blur	B
No. 16B	Pos. Fus. Res.–break	21 ± 3	18 to 24	B
	Pos. Fus. Res.–recovery	11 ± 4	7 to 15	
No. 17A	Neg. Rel. Conv.	13 ± 2, or No blur	11 to 15, or No blur	A
No. 17B	Neg. Fus. Res.–break	21 ± 2	19 to 23	A
	Neg. Fus. Res.–recovery	13 ± 3	10 to 16	
No. 20	Pos. Rel. Acc	−2.37 ± .62	−1.75 to −3.00	A
No. 21	Neg. Rel. Acc	+2.00 ± .25	+1.75 to +2.25	B
	Gradient	4 exo ± 1 Above No. 13B	3 to 5 exo Above No. 13	(C)
No. 19	Amp. Accom.	Age	±2.00 D	A

Table B. O.E.P. Table of Expecteds

Number	*Finding*	*Expected*
3	Habitual phoria at distance	0.5 exophoria
13A	Habitual phoria at near	6 exophoria
4	Distance retinoscopy	Compare with #7
5	Retinoscopy at 20 inches	Compare with #4
6	Retinoscopy at 40 inches	Compare with #4
7	Subjective	Like #4
8	Induced phoria at distance	0.50 exo (compare with #3)
9	Base out to first blur	7 to 9
10	Base out to break/recovery	19/10 minimum
11	Base in to break/recovery	9/5 minimum
12	Vertical phoria and vergences	Ortho (compare to #18)
13B	Induced phoria at near	6 exophoria
14A	Unfused cross cylinder	In ratio with #15A
15A	Induced phoria	In ratio with #14A
14B	Fused cross cylinder	Considered with #15B
15B	Induced phoria	Considered with #14B
16A	Base out to blur out	15 (higher than #17A)
16B	Base out to break/recovery	21/15 minimum
17A	Base in to blur out	14 (lower than 16A)
17B	Base in to break/recovery	22/18 minimum
18	Vertical phoria and vergences	Ortho (compare with #12)
19	Amplitude of accommodation	5.00 D minimum
20	Minus to blur out	−2.25 D to −2.50 D
21	Plus to blur out	+1.75 D to +2.00 D

Table C. Nonembedded and Embedded Syndromes

Nonembedded	*Embedded*
#4 lower than #7	#4 equal to or greater than #7
#9 excessively low (less than one half the mean)	#9 low but not excessively low
#10 recovery excessively low	#10 recovery above the expected
#11 break and recovery excessively low	#11 break and recovery up (recovery above the expected)
#14B net lower than #14A net	#14B net equal to or greater than #14A net
#16B recovery excessively low	#16B break low, but recovery above expected
#19 and #20 excessively low	#19 and #20 not both low (one high, the other low)

Table D. Zone of Comfort

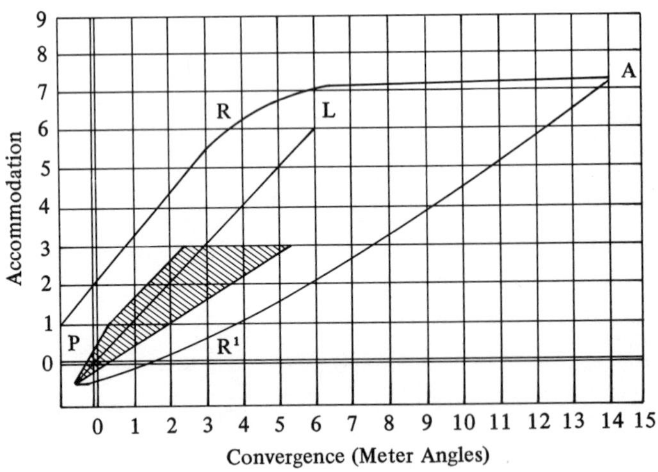

Percival's zone of comfort (after Sheard). Shaded area, zone of comfort; *PRA*, relative positive amplitudes of accommodation; *NR'A*, relative negative amplitudes of accommodation; *A*, near-points of accommodation and convergence; *DL*, line of equal accommodation and convergence.

4.2. System of Dynamic Skiametry (Tait)

Lag of Accommodation

Age	*Lag*	*Age*	*Lag*
38	1.50 D	50	2.28
40	1.67	53	2.37
43	1.75	55	2.50
45	1.87	57	2.75
47	2.00	60	3.00

Modification Factor

Physiologic Exophoria	*Accommodative Convergence*	*Allowance for 1/3 Meter*	*Allowance for 1/5 Meter*
Esophoria or orthophoria or up to 6	12 to 18	1.50	2.00
8	10	1.75	2.50
10	8	2.00	3.00
12	6	2.25	3.50
14	4	2.50	4.00
16	2	2.75	4.50
18	0	3.00	5.00

Reprinted by permission from E.F. Tait, "A quantitive system of dynamic skiametry," *Am. J. Opt.* **30:** (1953).

4.3. Normal Amplitude of Accommodation

Table A. Prince Rule
(U.S. Air Force Standard)

Age	*Normal*	*Age*	*Normal*
17	11.8	32	8.1
18	11.6	33	7.9
19	11.4	34	7.6
20	11.1	35	7.3
21	10.9	36	7.0
22	10.7	37	6.7
23	10.5	38	6.4
24	10.2	39	6.1
25	9.9	40	5.8
26	9.7	41	5.4
27	9.5	42	5.0
28	9.2	43	4.5
29	9.0	44	4.0
30	8.7	45	3.6
31	8.4		

Table B. Donders

Age	*Amp.*	*Age*	*Amp.*	*Age*	*Amp.*
10	14 D	35	5.5 D	60	1.00 D
15	12	40	4.5	65	0.50
20	10	45	3.5	70	0.25
25	8.5	50	2.5	75	0.00
30	7	55	1.75		

Table C. Turner

Age Group	*Mean Value (D)*
Under 13	13
13 – 17	10.6
18 – 22	9.5
23 – 27	7.9
28 – 32	6.6
33 – 37	5.75
38 – 42	4.4
43 – 47	2.5
48 – 52	1.6
53 – 57	1.1
58 – 62	0.7
63 – 67	0.6
Over 67	0.6

Table C reprinted by permission from M.J. Turner, "Observations in the normal subjective amplitude of accommodation," ***Br. J. Physiol. Optics*** **15: 1958.**

4.4. Approximate Adds for 16 Inches by Age

Age	*Total Amp.*	*Usable Amp.*	*P.P.*	*Add*
45	3.50	1.75	11″	0.75
50	2.50	1.25	16	1.25
55	1.75	0.87	22	1.75
60	1.00	0.50	40	2.00
65	0.50	0.25	80	2.25
70	0.25	0.12	160	2.50

4.5. Accommodation Required for Various Ametropias at 16 Inches

Hyperopes		*Myopes*	
Ve	*Acc.*	*Ve*	*Acc.*
0.00	2.45	0.00	2.45
+ 1.00	2.52	− 1.00	2.37
+ 2.00	2.60	− 2.00	2.30
+ 3.00	2.69	− 3.00	2.23
+ 4.00	2.80	− 4.00	2.16
+ 5.00	2.90	− 5.00	2.10
+ 6.00	3.04	− 6.00	2.04
+ 7.00	3.17	− 7.00	1.98
+ 8.00	3.30	− 8.00	1.93
+ 9.00	3.44	− 9.00	1.88
+10.00	3.54	−10.00	1.83
+11.00	3.76	−11.00	1.78
+12.00	3.94	−12.00	1.74
+13.00	4.16	−13.00	1.70
+14.00	4.39	−14.00	1.66
+15.00	4.54	−15.00	1.62
+16.00	4.90	−16.00	1.58
+17.00	5.17	−17.00	1.54
+18.00	5.45	−18.00	1.50
+19.00	5.75	−19.00	1.46
+20.00	6.07	−20.00	1.43

Ve: Effective Vertex Power

Reprinted by permission from the Bureau of Visual Science, *The Effect of the Ametropic Distance Upon the Accommodation and Reading Addition*, Southbridge, Mass.: American Optical Co., 1950.

4.6. Relative Approximate Age for the Onset of Presbyopia

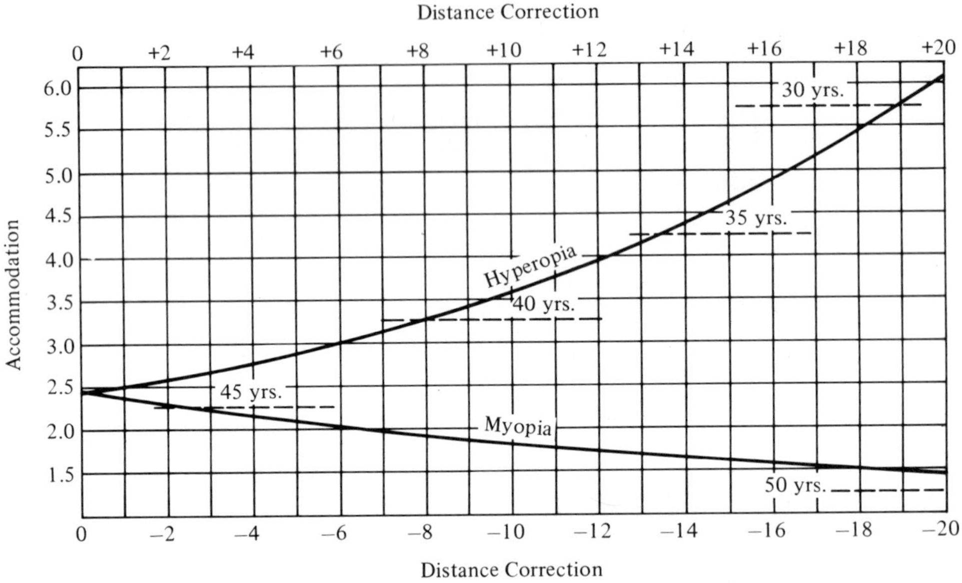

4.7. Convergence Deficiencies

Table A. Relation of Various Types of Convergence Deficiencies

Condition	*Phoria At Far*	*Phoria At Near*	*ACA*	*Tonic*
Convergence Insufficiency	Neg.	Large exo	Low	Normal
Convergence Excess	Neg.	Large eso	High	Normal
Divergence Insufficiency	Eso	Neg.	Low to Normal	High Normal
Divergence Excess	Exo	Neg.	High	Low

Table B. Classification of Binocular Anomalies

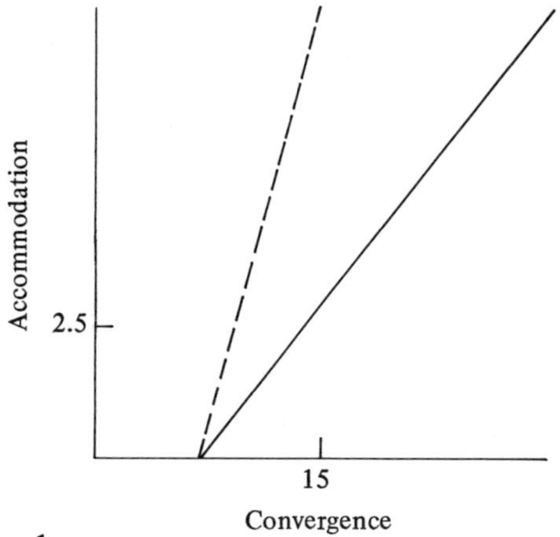

1

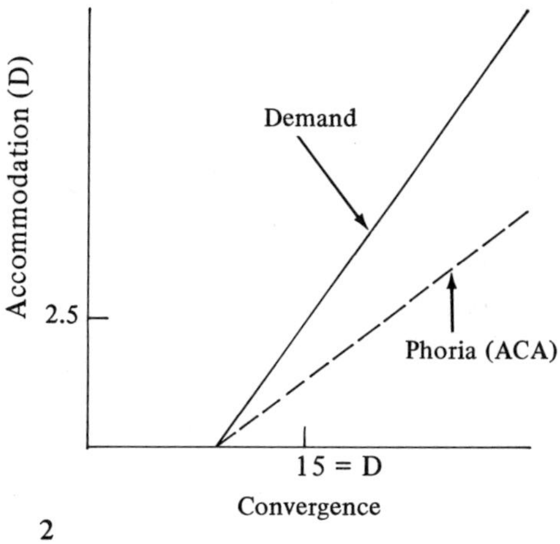

2

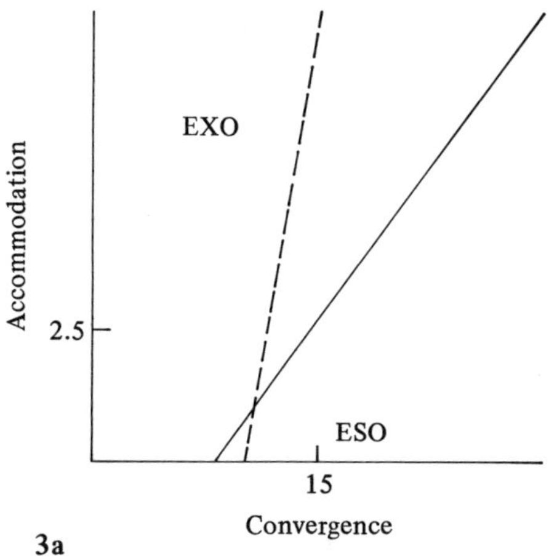

3a

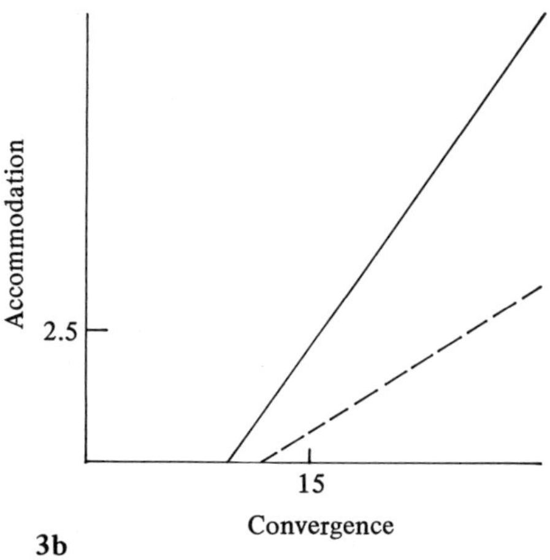

3b

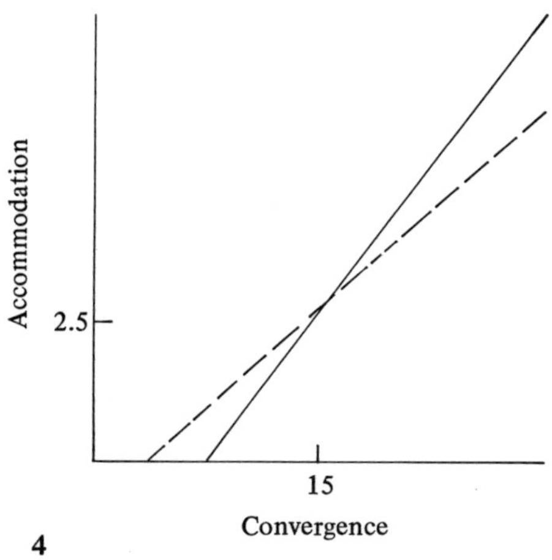

4

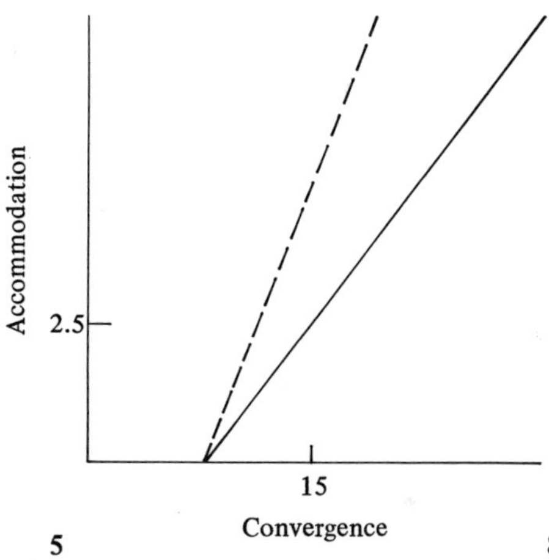

5

4.7. Convergence Deficiencies

Table B. Classification of Binocular Anomalies (continued)

1. *Convergence Insufficiency*
   Orthophoric or near-orthophoric at distance, and has a high exophoria at near, indicating a low AC/A ratio. The graph is of limited extent toward the right, owing to the poor nearpoint of convergence. The graph has a high slope, indicating a low AC/A ratio.
2. *Convergence Excess*
   Orthophoria or near-orthophoria at distance and a high esophoria at near. AC/A ratio is high.
3. *Divergence Insufficiency*
   (a) The patient may have a high esophoria at distance with a lesser esophoria at near, indicating excessive tonic convergence, but normal accomodative convergence; or (b) the patient may have a higher esophoria at near than at distance, indicating that both tonic convergence and accomodative convergence are excessive.
4. *Divergence Excess*
   A high exophoria at distance and near-orthophoria at near. High AC/A ratio.
5. *"False" Convergence Insufficiency*
   The patient has orthophoria or near-orthophoria at distance, and a high exophoria at near, usually accompanied by a low nearpoint of convergence – all of which would be expected in convergence insufficiency. However, it differs from classical convergence insufficiency in that the zone of clear, single binocular vision is normal.

Table C. Guides for Prescribing Prisms

Lateral

Sheard

−2/3 phoria −1/3 compensating duction.
The duction is base out to blur for exophoria and base in to blur for esophoria. A plus result indicates a need for prism.

Percival

Exophoria: Base in to blur −2/3 total fusional reserve (16A+17A)
Esophoria: Base out to blur −2/3 total fusional reserve (16A+17A)

Thorington

Exophoria at near −10Δ (presbyopia)

Vertical

Base down to break – base up to break

A plus result indicates base down prism.
For compound prisms in Rx's see Table 2.2

4.8. The Ocular Muscles

Table A. Actions of the Ocular Muscles

	In Primary Position			*Abducted*			*Abducted*		
Muscle	*Lat.*	*Vert.*	*Tors.*	*Lat.*	*Vert.*	*Tors.*	*Lat.*	*Vert.*	*Tors.*
Int. Rectus	In	0	0	In	0	0	In	0	0
Ext. Rectus	Out	0	0	Out	0	0	Out	0	0
Sup. Rectus	In	Up	Extort	Less	Less	More	Less	More	Less
Inf. Rectus	In	Down	Intort	Less	Less	More	Less	More	Less
Sup. Oblique	Out	Down	Extort	Less	More	Less	Less	Less	More
Inf. Oblique	Out	Up	Intort	Less	More	Less	Less	Less	More

The relationship of the version movement and the muscle under test for each eye is shown in the following table:

Movement	*Right Eye*	*Left Eye*
(a) Levo-Version	Medial Rectus	Lateral Rectus
(b) Dextro-Version	Lateral Rectus	Medial Rectus
(c) Levo-Supra-Version	Inferior Oblique	Superior Rectus
(d) Levo-Infra-Version	Superior Oblique	Inferior Rectus
(e) Dextro-Supra-Version	Superior Rectus	Inferior Oblique
(f) Dextro-Infra-Version	Inferior Rectus	Superior Oblique

"More" or "Less" refers to relationship with primary position.

Table B. Synergists

Muscle	*Primary action*	*Secondary action*	*Synergists*
Lateral rectus (LR)	Abduction	None	SO and IO
Medial rectus (MR)	Adduction	None	SR and IR
Superior rectus (SR)	Elevation	Adduction Incycloduction	IO MR and IR SO
Inferior rectus (IR)	Depression	Adduction Excycloduction	SO MR and SR IO
Superior oblique (SO)	Incycloduction	Depression Abduction	SR IR LR and IO
Inferior oblique (IO)	Excycloduction	Elevation Abduction	IR SR IR and SO

Table C. Antagonists

		Antagonists	
Muscle	*Action*	*Primary*	*Secondary*
Lateral rectus (LR)	Abduction	MR	SR and IR
Medial rectus (MR)	Adduction	LR	SO and IO
Superior rectus (SR)	Elevation Adduction Incycloduction	IR	SO SO, LR, and IO IO and IR
Inferior rectus (IR)	Depression Adduction Excycloduction	SR	IO SO, LR, and IO SO, SR
Superior oblique (SO)	Incycloduction Depression Abduction	IO	IR SR and IO SR, MR, and IR
Inferior oblique (IO)	Excycloduction Elevation Abduction	SO	SR LR and SO SR, MR, and IR

4.9. True Prism Values from the Phoropter Reading

Account is taken of the oblique lines of sight caused by the prism used in the test.

Measured Prism	*Distance R_x* +7	+6	+5	+4	+3	+2	−2	−3	−4	−5	−6	−7
8	10.5	9.5	9.25	9.0	8.75	8.5	8.0	7.50	7.25	7.0	7.0	6.5
7	9.25	8.5	8.0	7.75	7.50	7.25	7.0	6.25	6.0	6.0	6.0	5.5
6	8.0	7.25	7.0	6.75	6.5	6.25	6.0	5.75	5.5	5.0	5.0	5.0
5	6.5	6.0	5.75	5.5	5.5	5.25	5.0	4.75	4.5	4.25	4.25	4.0
4	5.25	5.0	4.5	4.5	4.25	4.0	4.0	3.75	3.5	3.5	3.5	3.25
3	4.0	3.5	3.5	3.25	3.25	3.0	3.0	2.75	2.5	2.5	2.5	2.5
2	2.75	2.5	2.25	2.25	2.0	2.0	2.0	2.0	2.0	2.0	2.0	1.5

True Prismatic Value

For tests at near, deduct 10 percent from the above figures.
There is no factor required between +1 and −1.

4.10. True Cylindrical Components from the Ophthalmometer Reading

Expected Cylindrical Correction at the Spectacle Point for Various Ametropias and Corneal Readings
Distance separating spectacle point and cornea = 12 1/3 mm.

Spherical Component of Correcting Lens Dioptres	*When Keratometer reading of corneal astigmatism in dioptres is* −1	−2	−3	−4	−5	−6	−7	−8
	corresponding cylinder ( ) in dioptres to be prescribed is							
+10	−0.78	−1.57	−2.38	−3.21	−4.06	− 4.93	− 5.82	− 6.73
8	−0.82	1.66	2.52	3.40	4.30	5.22	6.17	− 7.12
6	−0.87	1.75	2.66	3.59	4.55	5.52	6.52	− 7.55
5	−0.89	1.80	2.73	3.69	4.67	5.67	6.71	− 7.76
4	−0.91	1.85	2.81	3.79	4.80	5.83	6.89	− 7.98
3	−0.94	1.90	2.88	3.90	4.93	5.99	7.07	− 8.19
2	−0.96	1.95	2.96	4.00	5.06	6.15	7.27	− 8.42
+ 1	−0.99	2.00	3.04	4.10	5.19	6.31	7.47	− 8.65
0	−1.01	−2.05	−3.11	−4.21	−5.33	− 6.48	− 7.66	− 8.88
− 1	−1.04	2.10	3.19	4.32	5.47	6.65	7.86	9.12
2	−1.06	2.15	3.27	4.42	5.60	6.82	8.07	9.35
3	−1.09	2.21	3.35	4.53	5.74	6.99	8.27	9.58
4	−1.12	2.26	3.43	4.64	5.88	7.16	8.47	9.83
5	−1.14	2.32	3.52	4.76	6.03	7.34	8.69	10.08
6	−1.17	2.37	3.60	4.87	6.18	7.52	8.90	10.32
8	−1.22	2.48	3.78	5.11	6.48	7.89	9.34	10.84
10	−1.28	2.59	3.95	5.34	6.77	8.26	9.78	11.36
12	−1.34	2.71	4.13	5.59	7.09	8.64	10.24	11.89
15	−1.43	2.89	4.41	5.97	7.58	9.24	10.96	12.73
−20	−1.58	−3.20	−4.89	−6.63	−8.42	−10.28	−12.22	−14.18

The physiological astigmia should be added to these values.
Reprinted by permission from H.H. Emsley, *Visual Optics*, 4th ed. London: Hatton Press, 1949.

4.11. Isopters in the Normal Visual Field–Tangent Screen (After Roenne)

Table A. White

Visual Angle	*Object (mm.)*	*Distance (mm.)*	*Out*	*Out Down*	*Down*	*In Down*	*In*	*In Up*	*Up*	*Out Up*
9°	160	1,000	107	102	76	67	62	72	69	95
4.5°	80	1,000	104	99	76	67	62	72	69	91
2.25°	40	1,000	101	96	76	67	62	72	69	91
1.14°	20	1,000	99	96	76	67	62	72	69	88
34.2′	10	1,000	93	89	76	67	62	67	69	79
17.2′	5	1,000	82	72	69	59	60	64	66	75
8.6′	5	2,000	72	62	51	47	50	47	51	50
4.3′	2.5	2,000	33	34	27	25	31	25	24	25
2.1′	2.5	4,000	10	17	13	12	15	15	11	12
1.0′	1.25	4,000	10	9	8	7	6	6	4	6
0.5′	0.63	4,000	About 1°20′							
0.45′	0.63	4,800	Recognizable at the fixation point.							

4.11. Isopters in the Normal Visual Field–Tangent Screen (After Roenne)

Table B. Color

Visual Angle	Object (mm.)	Distance (mm.)	Blue (Degrees)				Red (Degrees)				Green (Degrees)			
			Out	Down	In	Up	Out	Down	In	Up	Out	Down	In	Up
1.7′	1	2,000	4.4	3.5	4.4	3.2	2	1.8	0.2	1.3	1.6	1.4	1.3	1.3
3.4′	2	2,000	7.3	6.4	7.7	5.3	4	2.4	3.7	3.0	3.8	2.5	3.2	2.5
5.1′	3	2,000	11	11	13	8	6	4.5	6.5	4.2	5	3.0	4.6	3.0
8.6′	5	2,000	17	14	18	12	8	5	8	6	7	4.6	7	5.0
17.2′	10	2,000	27	22	25	20	13	9	13	8	9	7.6	9.7	6.6
34.4′	20	2,000	33	28	32	27	20	13	18	13	15	10	14	9.6
1°9′	40	2,000	–	–	–	–	32	20	20	19	22	16	17	14
10.4′	1	330	38	16	23	15	13	7	11	8	6	4	6	4
20.8′	2	330	50	20	26	17	22	11	14	11	13	7	10	6
31.2′	3	330	74	29	30	24	42	13	17	15	17	18	12	9
52.0′	5	330	80	33	35	30	53	21	23	22	28	12	14	12
1°44′	10	330	87	47	43	37	79	35	29	31	49	16	21	18
3°28′	20	330	89	55	46	41	85	46	36	37	65	21	22	21
6°56′	40	330	92	58	48	43	87	52	41	42	70	30	29	29

4.12. Visual Angle Subtended by Various Tangent Screen Targets Presented at Various Viewing Distances.*

Target Size (mm)	*Viewing Distance (mm)* 330	500	1000	1500	2000	3000	4000
0.50	5' 13"	3' 26"	1' 43"	1' 9"	52"	34"	26"
0.63	6' 34"	4' 20"	2' 10"	1' 27"	1' 5"	43"	32"
1.0	10' 25"	6' 53"	3' 26"	2' 18"	1' 43"	1' 9"	52"
1.5	15' 38"	10' 19"	5' 9"	3' 26"	2' 35"	1' 43"	1' 17"
2.0	20' 50"	13' 45"	6' 53"	4' 35"	3' 26"	2' 18"	1' 43"
3.0	31' 15"	20' 38"	10' 19"	6' 53"	5' 9"	3' 26"	2' 35"
4.0	41' 40"	27' 30"	13' 45"	9' 10"	6' 53"	4' 35"	3' 26"
5.0	53' 5"	34' 23"	17' 11"	11' 28"	8' 36"	5' 44"	4' 18"
10.0	1° 44' 10"	1° 8' 45"	34' 23"	22' 55"	17' 11"	11' 28"	8' 36"
20.0	3° 28' 21"	2° 17' 31"	1° 8' 45"	45' 50"	34' 23"	22' 55"	17' 11"
30.0	5° 12'	3° 26' 16"	1° 43' 8"	1° 8' 45"	51' 34"	34' 23"	25' 47"
40.0	6° 56'	4° 34'	2° 17' 31"	1° 31' 40"	1° 8' 45"	45' 50"	34' 23"

*The targets subtending less than about 6 minutes of arc (in the upper right portion of the table, above the descending stepped line) do not form a correspondingly small image on the retina.

Reprinted from *First Interprofessional Standard for Visual Field Testing*, National Academy of Sciences, 1975.

4.13. Estimated Image Size Differences for Various Anisometropias

Anisometropic Difference in Diopters	*Axial Ametropic: % Image Size Difference*	*Refractive Ametropia: % Image Size Difference* +Rx	–Rx
1.00	.28%	1.50%	1.25%
1.50	.42%	2.25%	1.88%
2.00	.55%	3.00%	2.50%
2.50	.69%	3.75%	3.13%
3.00	.83%	4.50%	3.75%
3.50	.96%	5.25%	4.38%
4.00	1.10%	6.00%	5.00%
4.50	1.24%	6.75%	5.63%
5.00	1.38%	7.50%	6.25%
5.50	1.52%	8.25%	6.875%
6.00	1.65%	9.00%	7.50%
6.50	1.79%	9.75%	8.13%
7.00	1.93%	10.50%	8.75%
7.50	2.07%	11.25%	9.38%
8.00	2.20%	12.00%	10.00%
8.50	2.34%	12.75%	10.63%
9.00	2.48%	13.50%	11.25%
9.50	2.61%	14.25%	11.88%
10.00	2.75%	15.00%	12.50%

Assuming 12 mm. vertex distance

4.14. Working Distances in Various Occupations

Occupation	*Inches*
Accountant	10, 21, 28
Air Conditioning Mechanic	19
Appliance Repairman (Small)	18, 20–30
Architect	11–18, 20–30
Arc Welder	14–22
Artist (Fine)	16–22
Artist (Commercial)	13–23
Assembler (Small Parts)	16–20
Automobile Repairman	12–18
Automobile Serviceman	20–34
Banker	16–26
Barber	14–18
Bartender	14–21
Beauty Parlor Operator	10–16
Bicycle Repairman	16–20
Body & Fender Repairman	14
Bookbinder	16–21
Bookkeeper	16, 21, 28
Butcher	24–28
Cabinet Maker	20
Card Player	14, 16–25
Card Sorter (IBM)	18–20
Carpenter	18–20, 36
Carpet Installer	14–20
Cashier	18–22
Chiropractor	13–28
Cinema Photographer	16–18
Clergyman	16, 20–22
Compositor	12–16
Cook	17, 21–32
Cosmetologist	10–18
Dairy Farmer	24
Dentist	14–24
Dental Assistant	20–24
Desk Clerk (Hotel)	22–29

Occupation	*Inches*
Desk Worker	16–18, 30–36
Drattsman	8–12, 16, 22–30
Drill Press Operator	14–20
Electrician	12–14, 16–20
File Clerk	16–24
Film Editor	14–16
Film Splicer	14–16
Florist	16–20
Forming Press Operator	18–20
Gardener	14–16, 20
Gas Station Attendant	18–34
Glazier	18–24
Grain Farmer	23
Grocery Clerk	18–22
Gunsmith	13–16
Hosiery Inspector	12–14
Housewife	16–34
IBM Card Sorter	18–20
Ironer	24–30
Key Punch Operator	18
Knitting Machine Operator	20–25
Laboratory Technician	12–16
Lathe Operator	12–20
Laundry Marker	16–18
Letter Carrier	17–34
Librarian	16, 22–30
Linoleum Layer	14–20
Linotyper	16–24
Locksmith	14–18
Lumber Yard Man	16–20
Machinist	14–20
Manicurist	10–22
Minister	20–22

(continued)

4.14. Working Distances in Various Occupations (continued)

Occupation	*Inches*
Model Maker	14
Nurse	11–20
Offset Stripper	21, 24–30
Organist	19
Painter	18
Paper Hanger	16–24, 18–32
Pharmacist	18–34
Photoengraver	10–12, 20–24
Paper Hanger	16–24, 18–32
Photoengraver	10–12, 20–24
Photolithographer	16–38
Pianist	20–33
Pilot (Commercial)	18
Pilot (Private)	26
Pistol Shooter	17–34
Plasterer	19
Plumber	12–26
Podiatrist	10–18
Precision Grinder	15–20
Presser	16–20
Pressman (Printing)	13–27
Projectionist	16–20
Quality Control Engineer	14, 22–25
Rabbi	20–22
Radio Engineer	12–18
Receptionist	16–24
Recordist (Sound)	18–22
Roofer	20
Sales Clerk	18–24
Saw Mill Operator	16–20
Screw Machine Operator	16–20
Seamer	10–12, 18–22
Secretary	16–24
Sheet Metal Worker	18–35
Shoe Clerk	18–24
Spotter (Cleaners)	16–33
Stenographer	16–24
Stenotyper	16–18
Stripper	10–16
Surgeon	14–24
Surveyor	13–16, 20–27
Tailor	12, 18, 28
Teacher	17, 23, 28
Telephone Operator	20
Teller (Bank)	16–20
Tile Setter	18–24
Tool & Die Maker	12–20
Trout Fisherman	10
TV Repairman	10-20
Typesetter	15–19
Upholsterer	19
Veterinarian	14–23
Violinist	16–20, 30
Watch Repairman	9–18
Welder	18–20
X-Ray Technician	12–30

Reprinted by permission from Clark, Holmes *et al.*, *Guide to Occupational and Other Visual Needs*, St. Cloud, Minn.: Vision-Ease Corp., vol. 1, 1958; vol. 2, 1972.

4.15. Range of Clear Vision Through Various Adds

	Usable Accommodation										
Add	*+225*	*+200*	*+175*	*+150*	*+125*	*+100*	*+75*	*+50*	*+25*	*0*	*Extreme Far Point (Inches)*
+ 50	13	14	16	18	20	23	26	32	40	52	80
+ 75	12	13	14.5	16	18	20	23	26	32	40	53
+100	11.5	12	13.25	14.5	16	18	20	23	26	32	40
+125	10.5	11.5	12.25	13.25	14.5	16	18	20	23	26	32
+150	10	10.5	11.5	12.25	13	14.5	16	18	20	23	26
+175	9.5	10	10.5	11.5	12	13	14.5	16	18	20	23
+200	9	9.5	10	10.5	11.5	12	13	14.5	16	18	20
+225	8.5	9	9.5	10	10.5	11.5	12	13	14.5	16	18
+250	8	8.5	8.75	9.5	10	10.5	11.5	12	13	14.5	16
+275	7.5	8.0	8.5	9	9.5	10	10.5	11.5	12	13	14.5
+300	7.25	7.5	8.0	8.5	9	9.5	10	10.5	11.5	12	13
+325	7	7.25	7.5	8	8.5	9	9.5	10	10.5	11.5	12
+350	6.75	7	7.25	7.5	8	8.5	9	9.5	10	10.5	11.5
+375	6.5	6.75	7	7.25	7.5	8	8.5	9	9.5	10	10.5
+400	6	6.5	6.75	7	7.25	7.5	8	8.5	9	9.5	10
	Near Point For Clear Vision (Inches)										Extreme Far Point (Inches)

For an Add of +200, an accommodation of +100; the range of clear vision would be 12 to 20 inches.

Reprinted by permission from Clark, Holmes *et al.*, *Guide to Occupational and Other Visual Needs*, St. Cloud, Minn.: Vision-Ease Corp., vol. 1, 1958.

4.16. Ratio of Blood Pressure to Intraocular Pressure

Normal ratios: (systemic blood pressure divided by the intraocular pressure)
BP/IOP Systolic = 5.75 or greater
Diastolic = 3.25 or greater

Systemic Blood Pressure Hg (mm)	*Intraocular Pressure Hg (mm)* 16	18	20	22	24	26	28	30	32	34
60	3.8	3.3	3.0	2.7	2.5	2.3	2.1	2.0	1.9	1.8
70	4.4	3.9	3.5	3.2	2.9	2.7	2.5	2.3	2.2	2.1
80	5.0	4.4	4.0	3.6	3.3	3.1	2.9	2.6	2.5	2.4
90	5.6	5.0	4.5	3.9	3.7	3.4	3.2	3.0	2.8	2.6
100	6.3	5.6	5.0	4.5	4.2	3.8	3.6	3.3	3.1	2.9
110	6.9	6.1	5.5	5.0	4.6	4.2	3.9	3.6	3.4	3.2
120	7.5	6.7	6.0	5.5	5.0	4.6	4.3	4.0	3.7	3.5
130	8.1	7.2	6.5	5.9	5.4	5.0	4.7	4.3	4.1	3.8
140	8.8	7.8	7.0	6.4	5.8	5.4	5.0	4.6	4.4	4.1
150	9.4	8.3	7.5	6.8	6.3	5.8	5.4	5.0	4.7	4.4
160	10.0	8.9	8.0	7.3	6.7	6.2	5.7	5.3	5.0	4.7
170	10.6	9.4	8.5	7.7	7.1	6.5	6.1	5.7	5.3	5.0
180	11.2	10.8	9.0	8.2	7.5	6.9	6.4	6.0	5.6	5.3
190	11.9	10.6	9.5	8.6	7.9	7.3	6.7	6.3	5.9	5.6
200	12.5	11.1	10.0	9.1	8.3	7.7	7.1	6.7	6.2	5.9
210	13.1	11.7	10.5	9.5	8.7	8.1	7.5	7.0	6.6	6.2
220	13.8	12.2	11.0	10.0	9.2	8.5	7.9	7.4	6.8	6.5
230	14.4	12.7	11.5	10.4	9.6	8.8	8.2	7.7	7.2	6.8
240	15.0	13.3	12.0	10.9	10.0	9.2	8.6	8.0	7.5	7.1

4.17. Systolic and Diastolic Blood Pressures: Norms

Age	*Systolic*	*Diastolic*	*Age*	*Systolic*	*Diastolic*
0–4 M F	94	61	50–54 M	135	83
			F	137	84
5–9 M F	102	56	55–59 M	138	84
			F	139	84
10–14 M F	113	59	60–64 M	142	85
			F	144	85
15–19 M	121	69	65–69 M	143	83
F	118	67	F	154	85
20–24 M	123	76	70–74 M	145	82
F	116	72	F	159	85
25–29 M	125	78	75–79 M	146	81
F	117	74	F	158	84
30–34 M	126	79	80–84 M	145	82
F	120	75	F	157	83
35–39 M	127	80	85–89 M	145	79
F	124	78	F	154	82
40–44 M	129	81	90–94 M	145	78
F	127	80	F	150	79
45–49 M	130	82	95–106 M	146	78
F	131	82	F	149	81

4.18. Effective Power Change Induced by Altering Vertex Distance of Cataract Lenses

Table A. Away from Eye

Lens Power Before Movement Away From Eye	*Effective Lens Power Required When Movement of Lens Away From Eye Is:*									
	1 mm.	*2 mm.*	*3 mm.*	*4 mm.*	*5 mm.*	*6 mm.*	*7 mm.*	*8 mm.*	*9 mm.*	*10 mm.*
+ 7.00 D	+ 6.95 D	+ 6.90 D	+ 6.86 D	+ 6.81 D	+ 6.76 D	+ 6.72 D	+ 6.67 D	+ 6.63 D	+ 6.59 D	+ 6.54 D
7.25 D	7.20	7.15	7.10	7.05	7.00	6.95	6.90	6.85	6.81	6.76
7.50 D	7.44	7.39	7.33	7.28	7.23	7.18	7.13	7.08	7.03	6.98
7.75 D	7.69	7.63	7.57	7.52	7.46	7.41	7.35	7.30	7.24	7.19
8.00 D	7.94	7.87	7.81	7.75	7.69	7.63	7.58	7.52	7.46	7.41
8.25 D	8.18	8.12	8.05	7.99	7.92	7.86	7.80	7.74	7.68	7.62
8.50 D	8.43	8.36	8.29	8.22	8.15	8.09	8.02	7.96	7.90	7.83
8.75 D	8.67	8.60	8.53	8.45	8.38	8.31	8.24	8.18	8.11	8.05
9.00 D	8.92	8.84	8.76	8.69	8.61	8.54	8.47	8.40	8.33	8.26
9.25 D	9.17	9.08	9.00	8.92	8.84	8.76	8.69	8.61	8.54	8.47
9.50 D	9.41	9.32	9.24	9.15	9.07	8.99	8.91	8.83	8.75	8.68
9.75 D	9.66	9.56	9.47	9.38	9.30	9.21	9.13	9.04	8.96	8.88
10.00 D	9.90	9.80	9.71	9.62	9.52	9.43	9.35	9.26	9.17	9.09
10.25 D	10.15	10.04	9.94	9.85	9.75	9.66	9.56	9.47	9.38	9.30
10.50 D	10.39	10.28	10.18	10.08	9.98	9.88	9.78	9.69	9.59	9.50
10.75 D	10.64	10.52	10.41	10.31	10.20	10.10	10.00	9.90	9.80	9.71
11.00 D	10.88	10.76	10.65	10.54	10.43	10.32	10.21	10.11	10.01	9.91
11.25 D	11.12	11.00	10.88	10.77	10.65	10.54	10.43	10.32	10.22	10.11
11.50 D	11.37	11.24	11.12	10.99	10.87	10.76	10.64	10.53	10.42	10.31
11.75 D	11.61	11.48	11.35	11.22	11.10	10.98	10.86	10.74	10.63	10.51
12.00 D	11.86	11.72	11.58	11.45	11.32	11.19	11.07	10.95	10.83	10.71
12.25 D	12.10	11.96	11.82	11.68	11.54	11.41	11.28	11.16	11.03	10.91
12.50 D	12.35	12.20	12.05	11.90	11.76	11.63	11.49	11.36	11.24	11.11
12.75 D	12.59	12.43	12.28	12.13	11.99	11.84	11.71	11.57	11.44	11.31
13.00 D	12.83	12.67	12.51	12.36	12.21	12.06	11.92	11.78	11.64	11.50
13.25 D	13.08	12.91	12.74	12.58	12.43	12.27	12.13	11.98	11.84	11.70

(continued)

Table A. Away from Eye (continued)

Lens Power Before Movement Away From Eye	*Effective Lens Power Required When Movement of Lens Away From Eye Is:* 1 mm.	2 mm.	3 mm.	4 mm.	5 mm.	6 mm.	7 mm.	8 mm.	9 mm.	10 mm.
+13.50 D	+13.32 D	+13.15 D	+12.97 D	+12.81 D	+12.65 D	+12.49 D	+12.33 D	+12.18 D	+12.04 D	+11.89 D
13.75 D	13.56	13.38	13.21	13.03	12.87	12.70	12.54	12.39	12.24	12.09
14.00 D	13.81	13.62	13.44	13.26	13.08	12.92	12.75	12.59	12.43	12.28
14.25 D	14.05	13.86	13.67	13.48	13.30	13.13	12.96	12.79	12.63	12.47
14.50 D	14.29	14.09	13.90	13.70	13.52	13.34	13.16	12.99	12.83	12.66
14.75 D	14.54	14.33	14.12	13.93	13.74	13.55	13.37	13.19	13.02	12.85
15.00 D	14.78	14.56	14.35	14.15	13.95	13.76	13.57	13.39	13.22	13.04
15.25 D	15.02	14.80	14.58	14.37	14.17	13.97	13.78	13.59	13.41	13.23
15.50 D	15.26	15.03	14.81	14.60	14.39	14.18	13.98	13.79	13.60	13.42
15.75 D	15.51	15.27	15.04	14.82	14.60	14.39	14.19	13.99	13.79	13.61
16.00 D	15.75	15.50	15.27	15.04	14.81	14.60	14.39	14.18	13.99	13.79
16.25 D	15.99	15.74	15.49	15.26	15.03	14.81	14.59	14.38	14.18	13.98
16.50 D	16.23	15.97	15.72	15.48	15.24	15.01	14.79	14.57	14.37	14.16
16.75 D	16.47	16.21	15.95	15.70	15.45	15.22	14.99	14.77	14.56	14.35
17.00 D	16.72	16.44	16.18	15.92	15.67	15.43	15.19	14.96	14.74	14.53
17.25 D	16.96	16.67	16.40	16.14	15.88	15.63	15.39	15.16	14.93	14.71
17.50 D	17.20	16.91	16.63	16.36	16.09	15.84	15.59	15.35	15.12	14.89
17.75 D	17.44	17.14	16.85	16.57	16.30	16.04	15.79	15.54	15.31	15.07
18.00 D	17.68	17.37	17.08	16.79	16.51	16.25	15.99	15.73	15.49	15.25
18.25 D	17.92	17.61	17.30	17.01	16.72	16.45	16.18	15.92	15.68	15.43
18.50 D	18.16	17.84	17.53	17.23	16.93	16.65	16.38	16.11	15.86	15.61
18.75 D	18.40	18.07	17.75	17.44	17.14	16.85	16.57	16.30	16.04	15.79
19.00 D	18.65	18.30	17.98	17.66	17.35	17.06	16.77	16.49	16.23	15.97
19.25 D	18.89	18.54	18.20	17.87	17.56	17.26	16.96	16.68	16.41	16.14
19.50 D	19.13	18.77	18.42	18.09	17.77	17.46	17.16	16.87	16.59	16.32
19.75 D	19.37	19.00	18.65	18.30	17.97	17.66	17.35	17.06	16.77	16.49

(continued)

Table A. Away from Eye (continued)

Lens Power Before Movement Away From Eye	*Effective Lens Power Required When Movement of Lens Away From Eye Is:*									
	1 mm.	*2 mm.*	*3 mm.*	*4 mm.*	*5 mm.*	*6 mm.*	*7 mm.*	*8 mm.*	*9 mm.*	*10 mm.*
+20.00 D	+19.61 D	+19.23 D	+18.87 D	+18.52 D	+18.18 D	+17.86 D	+17.54 D	+17.24 D	+16.95 D	+16.67 D
20.25 D	19.85	19.46	19.09	18.73	18.39	18.06	17.74	17.43	17.13	16.84
20.50 D	20.09	19.69	19.31	18.95	18.59	18.25	17.93	17.61	17.31	17.01
20.75 D	20.33	19.92	19.53	19.16	18.80	18.45	18.12	17.80	17.48	17.18
21.00 D	20.57	20.15	19.76	19.37	19.00	18.65	18.31	17.98	17.66	17.36
21.25 D	20.81	20.38	19.98	19.59	19.21	18.85	18.50	18.16	17.84	17.53
21.50 D	21.05	20.61	20.20	19.80	19.41	19.04	18.69	18.34	18.01	17.70
21.75 D	21.29	20.84	20.42	20.01	19.62	19.24	18.88	18.53	18.19	17.87

Table B. Towards Eye

Lens Power Before Movement Toward Eye	*Effective Lens Power Required When Movement of Lens Toward Eye Is:*									
	1 mm.	*2 mm.*	*3 mm.*	*4 mm.*	*5 mm.*	*6 mm.*	*7 mm.*	*8 mm.*	*9 mm.*	*10 mm.*
+ 7.00 D	+ 7.05 D	+ 7.10 D	+ 7.15 D	+ 7.20 D	+ 7.25 D	+ 7.31 D	+ 7.36 D	+ 7.42 D	+ 7.47 D	+ 7.53 D
7.25 D	7.30	7.36	7.41	7.47	7.52	7.58	7.64	7.70	7.76	7.82
7.50 D	7.56	7.61	7.67	7.73	7.79	7.85	7.92	7.98	8.04	8.11
7.75 D	7.81	7.87	7.93	8.00	8.06	8.13	8.19	8.26	8.33	8.40
8.00 D	8.06	8.13	8.20	8.26	8.33	8.40	8.47	8.55	8.62	8.70
8.25 D	8.32	8.39	8.46	8.53	8.60	8.68	8.76	8.83	8.91	8.99
8.50 D	8.57	8.65	8.72	8.80	8.88	8.96	9.04	9.12	9.20	9.29
8.75 D	8.83	8.91	8.99	9.07	9.15	9.23	9.32	9.41	9.50	9.59
9.00 D	9.08	9.16	9.25	9.34	9.42	9.51	9.61	9.70	9.79	9.89
9.25 D	9.34	9.42	9.51	9.61	9.70	9.79	9.89	9.99	10.09	10.19

(continued)

Table B. Towards Eye (continued)

Lens Power Before Movement Toward Eye	*Effective Lens Power Required When Movement of Lens Toward Eye Is:*									
	1 mm.	*2 mm.*	*3 mm.*	*4 mm.*	*5 mm.*	*6 mm.*	*7 mm.*	*8 mm.*	*9 mm.*	*10 mm.*
+ 9.50 D	+ 9.59 D	+ 9.68 D	+ 9.78 D	+ 9.88 D	+ 9.97 D	+10.07 D	+10.18 D	+10.28 D	+10.39 D	+10.50 D
9.75 D	9.85	9.94	10.04	10.15	10.25	10.36	10.46	10.58	10.69	10.80
10.00 D	10.10	10.20	10.31	10.42	10.53	10.64	10.75	10.87	10.99	11.11
10.25 D	10.36	10.46	10.58	10.69	10.80	10.92	11.04	11.17	11.29	11.42
10.50 D	10.61	10.73	10.84	10.96	11.08	11.21	11.33	11.46	11.60	11.73
10.75 D	10.87	10.99	11.11	11.23	11.36	11.49	11.62	11.76	11.90	12.04
11.00 D	11.12	11.25	11.38	11.51	11.64	11.78	11.92	12.06	12.21	12.36
11.25 D	11.38	11.51	11.64	11.78	11.92	12.06	12.21	12.36	12.52	12.68
11.50 D	11.63	11.77	11.91	12.05	12.20	12.35	12.51	12.67	12.83	12.99
11.75 D	11.89	12.03	12.18	12.33	12.48	12.64	12.80	12.97	13.14	13.31
12.00 D	12.15	12.30	12.45	12.61	12.77	12.93	13.10	13.27	13.45	13.64
12.25 D	12.40	12.56	12.72	12.88	13.05	13.22	13.40	13.58	13.77	13.96
12.50 D	12.66	12.82	12.99	13.16	13.33	13.51	13.70	13.89	14.08	14.29
12.75 D	12.91	13.08	13.26	13.44	13.62	13.81	14.00	14.20	14.40	14.61
13.00 D	13.17	13.35	13.53	13.71	13.90	14.10	14.30	14.51	14.72	14.94
13.25 D	13.43	13.61	13.80	13.99	14.19	14.39	14.60	14.82	15.04	15.27
13.50 D	13.68	13.87	14.07	14.27	14.48	14.69	14.91	15.13	15.37	15.61
13.75 D	13.94	14.14	14.34	14.55	14.77	14.99	15.21	15.45	15.69	15.94
14.00 D	14.20	14.40	14.61	14.83	15.05	15.28	15.52	15.77	16.02	16.28
14.25 D	14.46	14.67	14.89	15.11	15.34	15.58	15.83	16.09	16.35	16.62
14.50 D	14.71	14.93	15.16	15.39	15.63	15.88	16.14	16.41	16.68	16.96
14.75 D	14.97	15.20	15.43	15.67	15.92	16.18	16.45	16.73	17.01	17.30
15.00 D	15.23	15.46	15.71	15.96	16.22	16.48	16.76	17.05	17.34	17.65
15.25 D	15.49	15.73	15.98	16.24	16.51	16.79	17.07	17.37	17.68	18.00
15.50 D	15.74	16.00	16.26	16.52	16.80	17.09	17.39	17.69	18.01	18.35
15.75 D	16.00	16.26	16.53	16.81	17.10	17.39	17.70	18.02	18.35	18.70

(continued)

Table B. Towards Eye (continued)

Lens Power Before Movement Toward Eye	*Effective Lens Power Required When Movement of Lens Toward Eye Is:*									
	1 mm.	*2 mm.*	*3 mm.*	*4 mm.*	*5 mm.*	*6 mm.*	*7 mm.*	*8 mm.*	*9 mm.*	*10 mm.*
+16.00 D	+16.26 D	+16.53 D	+16.81 D	+17.09 D	+17.39 D	+17.70 D	+18.02 D	+18.35 D	+18.69 D	+19.05 D
16.25 D	16.52	16.80	17.08	17.38	17.69	18.01	18.34	18.68	19.03	19.40
16.50 D	16.78	17.06	17.36	17.67	17.98	18.31	18.65	19.01	19.38	19.76
16.75 D	17.04	17.33	17.64	17.95	18.28	18.62	18.97	19.34	19.72	20.12
17.00 D	17.29	17.60	17.91	18.24	18.58	18.93	19.30	19.68	20.07	20.48
17.25 D	17.55	17.87	18.19	18.53	18.88	19.24	19.62	20.01	20.42	20.85
17.50 D	17.81	18.13	18.47	18.82	19.18	19.55	19.94	20.35	20.77	20.21
17.75 D	18.07	18.40	18.75	19.11	19.48	19.86	20.27	20.69	21.12	21.58
18.00 D	18.33	18.67	19.03	19.40	19.78	20.18	20.59	21.03	21.48	21.95
18.25 D	18.59	18.94	19.31	19.69	20.08	20.49	20.92	21.37	21.84	22.32
18.50 D	18.85	19.21	19.59	19.98	20.39	20.81	21.25	21.71	22.20	22.70
18.75 D	19.11	19.48	19.87	20.27	20.69	21.13	21.58	22.06	22.56	23.08
19.00 D	19.37	19.75	20.15	20.56	20.99	21.44	21.91	22.41	22.92	23.46
19.25 D	19.63	20.02	20.43	20.86	21.30	21.76	22.25	22.75	23.28	23.84
19.50 D	19.89	20.29	20.71	21.15	21.61	22.08	22.58	23.10	23.65	24.22
19.75 D	20.15	20.56	20.99	21.44	21.91	22.40	22.92	23.46	24.02	24.61
20.00 D	20.41	20.83	21.28	21.74	22.22	22.73	23.26	23.81	24.39	25.00
20.25 D	20.67	21.10	21.56	22.03	22.53	23.05	23.59	24.16	24.76	
20.50 D	20.93	21.38	21.84	22.33	22.84	23.38	23.93	24.52		
20.75 D	21.19	21.65	22.13	22.63	23.15	23.70	24.28			
21.00 D	21.45	21.92	22.41	22.93	23.46	24.03				
21.25 D	21.71	22.19	22.70	23.22	23.78					
21.50 D	21.97	22.47	22.98	23.52						
21.75 D	22.23	22.74	23.27							

Reprinted by permission from T. H. Calkins, *Essentials of Modern Lens Theory and Practice*. Rochester, NY: Shuron Continental Co.

4.19. Sources for Specialized Frames

Table A. Frames

Baby Specs	Benson (28 Eye)
Bed Specs	Framel, Swift, T Hamblin, Selsi
Colored Metallic Finish	Cal Mart, Pacific Univ, Frame Specialties
Contact Lens Insertion	CosOMedic
Cataract Temporaries	Younger
Custom (colors, designs)	Imperial Ltd.
Detached Retina	Kono
Entropion	Kono
Elevator Pads	Superior
Flat Bridge	Pathway, Goldsmith
Folding	Jan, Tworoger
Folding Half Eye	Clear Vision
Flip Ups	Jan, Rovbart, Tworoger, Frawel, Brooks, Gordon, Rachel
Hemisropsia	Jardon, Benson
Hypoallergenic	*see* Stainless Steel, Opryl
Inverted Half Eye	Jan
Make Up	Cos-medic, Franel, Univis, Fashion, Kono
Moist Chamber	Benson
Off Face	Astro-optics, Optical Devices, Pro-optics, Arox
Oversize ZYL	Clear Vision
Ptosis Crutch	Benson
Rear View Mirror	Ultra Light
Rubber Bridge	Criss
Saftey	Airco, Boic, B & L, Fish-Schurman, U.S. Safety, Willson, Titmus
Side Shields	Bernell, B & L, Titmus
Sports	
Billards	Imperial, London Williamson
Divers Mask (Rx)	Aqua Optics, Younger, Tworoger
Floating	Aqua-Floats
Goggle (Headband)	Lloyd (Rx), Criss, Sport Optics, Franel (Rx), Rainbo (Rx)
Goggles (Rx)	Herslof, Criss, Embassy, Martin Wells, Willson
Mask Over Specs	Rawlings
Sport Band	Embassy, Criss, Lloyd
Swimming Goggle	Opti-Sport (Rx)
Shooting Glasses	U.S. Optical, B & L, Welling
Ski Goggle (Rx)	Zyloware, Uvex
Wrap Around	Eketalon, Embassy, MK
Underwater	Younger, Scubba Spec, Hillsinger, H.S.
Bonding (Rx to Mask)	Custom, Benson, Venice
Stainless Steel	Interoptic
Xeropthalmia	Kono

Table B. Sources

Airco
804 W. Roslyn Rd.
Colonial Hts., VA 23834

American Optical Co.
14 Mechanic St.
Southbridge, MA 01550

A.M. Poriss Co.
8 Crossroads Plaza
West Hartford, CT 06117

Aqua-Floats
Optic-Glass Float Co.
P.O. Box 15457
Tulsa, OK 75115

Aqua Optics
575 West 6th Street
San Pedro, CA 90731

Arox
P.O. Box 24740
Los Angeles, CA

Bausch & Lomb Co.
1400 N. Goodman St.
Rochester, NY 14602

Benson Optical
1812 Park Avenue
Minneapolis, MN 55440

BOIC
175 Rock Road
P.O. Box 401
Glen Rock, NJ 07452

Cal-Mart
607 South Hill Street
Suite 631
Los Angeles, CA 90014

Cos Medic
Suite 106
2824 Franklin Street
Michigan City, IN 46360

Criss Optical Mfg. Co.
P.O. Box 220
Augusta, KS 67010

Custom Ltd.
816 15th St. NW
Washington, DC 20005

Ektelon
7079 Mission Gorge Rd.
San Diego, CA 92120

Embassy Creations
P.O. Box 143
Holmes, PA 19843

Fashion Optics
2685 Culver Ave.
Dayton, OH

Fish-Schurman
70 Port-Mar Road
New Rochelle, NY 10802

Frame Specialties
P.O. Box 663
Oregon City, OR 97045

Franel Optical Supply Co.
P.O. Box 96
Maitland, FL 32751

Futura Optics
139 No. Clark Drive
Beverly Hills, CA 90211

P. Goldsmith Ltd.
18 Station Close
Potters Bar
Hertfordshire, England

Gordon Optical Supply
7751 Burnet Ave.
Van Nuys, CA 91405

Hilsinger Corporation
30 West Bacon St.
Plainville, MA 02762

H. S. Products Co.
900 East 92 St.
Brooklyn, NY 11238

Imperial Optical Co.
P.O. Box 1180
545 W. 18th Street
Hialeah, Florida 33011

Interoptic Eyewear
5 Westchester Plaza
Elmsford, NY 10523

Jan Optical
351 Scally Place
Westbury, NY

Jardon Plastics
17100 W. 12 Mile
Southfield, MI 48076

Lloyd Distributors
23931 Craftsman Circle
Calabasas, CA 91302

London Williamson Ltd.
32A-37 Cowper St.
London, EC2A 4AR, England

(continued)

Table B. Sources (continued)

May Manufacturing
7 Barnabas Rd.
P.O. Box 473
Marion, MA 02735

Martin Wells, Ltd.
88 Bent Street
St. Marys, NSW, Australia

MK Eye Guard
Champion Glove Co.
2200 E. Ovid St.
Des Moines, IA 50313

Optical Devices, Ltd.
12 E Yates Road So.
Memphis, TN 38117

Opti-Craft, Inc.
Box 4344
Portland, OR 97208

Opti-Sport Co.
2460 Williamette St.
Eugene, OR 97505

Pacific Universal
168 Vista Ave.
Pasadena, CA 91107

Pinpoint Prescriptions Inc.
1239 Upper Happy Valley Rd.
Lafayette, CA 94579

Pro Optics
317 Woodwork Lane
Palatine, IL 60067

Pro-tec, Inc.
1108 Northrup Way
Bellevue, WA 98004

Rawlings Sporting Goods
2300 Del Mar St.
St. Louis, MO

Scott USA
P.O. Box 187
Sun Valley, ID 83353

Scuba Spec, Inc.
P.O. Box 22356
Savannah, GA 31403

Shane-Michael Optical Co.
70 Elmira St.
San Francisco, CA 94124

R.P. Smith Co.
P.O. Box 700
Evergreen, CO 80439

Smith Sports Optics
P.O. Box 11
Ketchum, ID 83340

Solari Sports Products
1670 Cordova St.
Los Angeles, CA 90007

Space Age Optics
P.O. Box 8424
Kansas City, MO 64114

Sport Optics
P.O. Box 11
Ketchum, ID 83340

Superior Optical Co.
16 E. 23 Street
New York, NY

Super Sports Spec.
Herslof Optical Co.
1200 W. Carmen Ave.
Milwaukee, WI 53225

Swift Instruments
952 Dorchester Rd.
Boston, MA 02125

John Tworoger
249 W 34 Street
New York, NY 10001

Univis
10 Maguire Road
Lexington, MA 02173

Ultra Light Touring Shop
Box 208
Brinkhaven, OH 93006

U.S. Optical Specialities, Inc.
604 Mission Street
San Francisco, CA 94105

U.S. Safety Service
1535 Walnut
P.O. Box 1237
Kansas City, MO 64141

Uvex Winter Optical
232 West Exchange St.
Providence, RI 02903

Venice Eye Clinic
950 Cooper Street
Venice, CA 33595

Willson Division
ESB Inc.
P.O. Box 622
2nd and Washington Sts.
Reading, PA 19603

Younger Mfg.
3788 So. Broadway Place
Los Angeles, CA 90007

Zyloware
11–15 47 Ave.
Long Island City, NY

4.20. Measurement Standards for Dress Ophthalmic Dress Frames (ANSI)

Physical Dimensions and Measurements

General. The requirements of this section are to be maintained at the frame manufacturing level.

Front Measurements. The method of measuring and marking front sizes shall be in accordance with the boxing system published in *The Optical Journal and Review of Optometry*. Front products released prior to the publication of this standard may continue to be marked in other systems.

Tolerances

Tolerances, General. Ophthalmic frame design specifications shall be based on a uniform 115° included angle lens bevel. Any measurement technique that verifies the tolerance range may be used by manufacturers. All measurements shall be made prior to the initial insertion of the lenses.

DBL Dimension. The DBL tolerance shall be ±0.5 mm (±0.020 in).

Thickness of Eyewires. The vertical thickness difference between right and left lower eyewires of plastic frames shall be 0.5 mm (0.020 in) maximum. The measurement shall be made at the points of maximum vertical distance from the geometric centers of the lenses. This requirement is intended to avoid misinterpreted prescription readings when utilizing conventional focimeters.

Eye Size. Eye sizes shall be marked according to the indicated lens size for each eye size. The tolerance on eye size shall be +0.25 mm (+0.010 in) maximum.

Temple Measurements and Tolerances. Temples shall be measured and marked for overall length in the metric system in multiples and increments of 5 mm, with a tolerance of ±2 mm. Temple products released prior to the publication of this standard may continue to be measured and marked in inches, with a tolerance of ±3/32 in.

4.21. Conversion Table for Temple Lengths; mm/inches

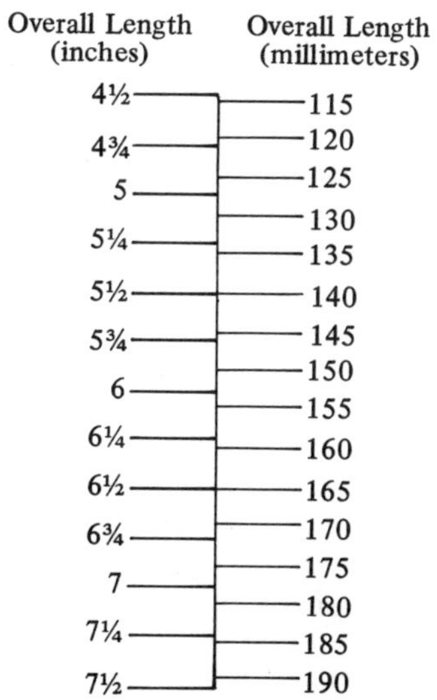

4.22. Distribution of Refractive Errors

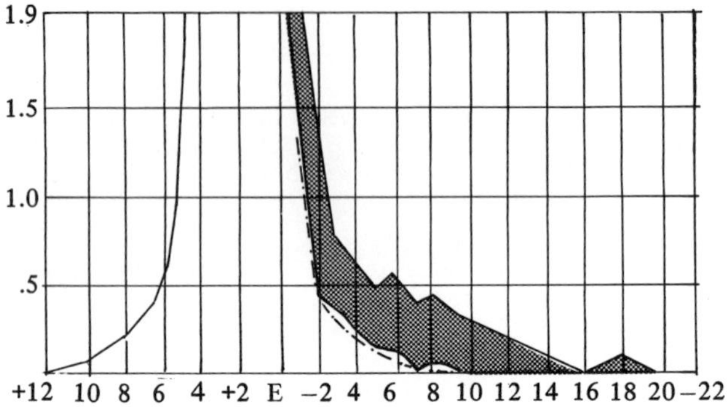

Scheerer's frequency curve of refraction. The shaded area covers the cases of myopia with degenerative fundus changes. The broken line shows the theoretically derived binomial curve on the myopic side.

Reprinted from Duke Elder, *Textbook of Opththalmology*, Vol. IV.

Table A. Distribution of Refractive Changes Between Ages 20 and 40

	Percent
Change of more than +1.00 D	2
Change of +0.62 D to +1.00 D	8
Change of no more than ±0.50 D	76
Change of −0.12 D to −1.00 D	5
Change of more than −1.00 D	10

From T. Grosvener, Longitudinal study of refractive changes between ages 20 and 40, *Opt Weekly*, April, 1977.

Table B. Spherical Ametropia as a Function of Age

	Incidence of Ametropia		
Age	*Hypermetropia*	*Emmetropia*	*Myopia*
45–49	16.3%	77.2%	6.7
50–54	23.5%	70.4%	6.2
55–59	35.4%	59.3%	5.0
60–64	40.1%	52.3%	7.4
65–69	43.9%	43.9%	12.3
70–74	47.7%	43.8%	8.8
Over 75	47.9%	36.9%	15.3

From M.J. Hirsh, Changes in refractive status after the age of 45, *Amer J of Optom*, 35: 229.

Table C. Incidence of Myopia in Children of Various Racial Groups

Racial Group	*Percent of Myopes*
Chinese	17
Korean	13
Japanese	12
Caucasian	12
Spanish	9
Portugese	7
Filipino	7
Puerto Rican	4
Part Hawaiian	4
Hawaiian	3

From Crawford and Hamman

Table D. Astigmatism

By Axis		*By Amount*		
Axis	*%*	*Power*		*%*
180°	24.5	1.50	Against the Rule	.04
45°	2	1.00		.06
90°	17	.50		2.3
135°	3	.50	With the Rule	26.0
		1.00		21.0
		2.00		4.2
		4.00		.4

From W.J. Lyle, Corneal astigmatism and age, *Amer J Optom*, 48:407.

4.23. Typical Expected Results on the Kinetic Cover Test

	K.C.T. Target	
	Moving Closer	*Moving Away*
Vergence Anomalies		
1. Basic exo	exo increase	exo decrease
2. Divergence excess	exo approximately the same	exo approximately the same
3. Convergence insufficiency	exo increase	exo decrease
4. Basic eso	eso decrease	eso increase
5. Divergence insufficiency	eso decrease	eso increase
6. Convergence excess	eso approximately the same	eso approximately the same
Orthophoria	small exo may be induced	ortho or small eso (allowing 5 p.d.) may be induced

Reprinted from Griffin, John: ***Binocular Anomalies, Procedures for Vision Therapy,*** **(p. 44), published by Professional Press, Inc., 101 East Ontario Street, Chicago, Illinois 60611.**

4.24. Recommended Illuminations for the Optometric Exam

Procedure	*Illuminance*
External examination of the eye	100 fc. (1,100 lux) at the examining chair measured in the plane parallel to and 1 m from the floor
Observation of pupillary reflexes, ophthalmoscopy, slit lamp examinations, retinoscopy, keratometry	5 to 10 fc. (55 to 110 lux) measured in the plane parallel to and 1 m from the floor
Distance tests charts	At least 12 to 20 fc. (130 to 215 lux) assuming a 0.8 reflecting factor
Near point cards	Same as distance charts
Binocular cross-cylinder	1 to 2 fc. (10 to 20 lux)
Addition measurements using the cross-cylinder grid target	1 fc. (10 lux)
Tangent screen	7 fc. (75 lux)
Color vision testing	Macbeth or daylight lamp at 80 fc. (860 lux)

Reprinted from Long, W.F.: ***Recommended Light Levels for Clinical Procedures,*** **Optometric Monthly (October, 1979, pp. 89–92) published by the Professional Press, Inc., 101 East Ontario Street, Chicago, Illinois 60611.**

4.25. Heights of 20/200 E for Various Distances

Distance	*Height*
20 ft	87 mm
18 ft	79 mm
16 ft	70 mm
14 ft	61 mm
12 ft	52 mm
10 ft	44 mm

4.26. Tonometry

Table A. Calibration Scale for Schötz Tonometers

	5.5 g	*7.5 g*	*10 g*	*15 g*
Tonometer Reading			*Pressure, mm Hg*	
0.0	41.5	59.1	81.7	127.5
0.5	37.8	54.2	75.1	117.9
1.0	34.5	49.8	69.3	109.3
1.5	31.6	45.8	64.0	101.4
2.0	29.0	42.1	59.1	94.3
2.5	26.6	38.8	54.7	88.0
3.0	24.4	35.8	50.6	81.8
3.5	22.4	33.0	46.9	76.2
4.0	20.6	30.4	43.4	71.0
4.5	18.9	28.0	40.2	66.2
5.0	17.3	25.8	37.2	61.8
5.5	15.9	23.8	34.4	57.6
6.0	14.6	21.9	31.8	53.6
6.5	13.4	20.1	29.4	49.9
7.0	12.2	18.5	27.2	46.5
7.5	11.2	17.0	25.1	43.2
8.0	10.2	15.6	23.1	40.2
8.5	9.4	14.3	21.3	38.1
9.0	8.5	13.1	19.6	34.6
9.5	7.8	12.0	18.0	32.0
10.0	7.1	10.9	16.5	29.6
10.5	6.5	10.0	15.1	27.4
11.0	5.9	9.0	13.8	25.3
11.5	5.3	8.3	12.6	23.3
12.0	4.9	7.5	11.5	21.4

By Schiøtz tonometry the average mean intraocular pressure was found to be 15.5 mm Hg.

A pressure of 21 mm Hg or more may be looked upon with suspicion.

Table B. Applanometry Conversion Scale

Diameter (in mm)	Intraocular Pressure (in mm Hg) 5 grams	7.5 grams	10 grams
3.5	41	58	79
3.6	39	55	74
3.7	37	52	69
3.8	35	49	65
3.9	33	46	61
4.0	32	44	58
4.1	30	42	55
4.2	29	40	52
4.3	27	38	49
4.4	26	36	46
4.5	25	34	43
4.6	24	32	41
4.7	23	30	39
4.8	22	29	37
4.9	21	27	35
5.0	20	26	33.5
5.1	19	25	32
5.2	18	24	30.5
5.3	17	23	29
5.4	16	22	27.5
5.5	15	21	26
5.6	14	20	25
5.7	13.5	19	24
5.8	13	18	23
5.9	12.5	17	22
6.0	12	16	21
6.2	11.5	15	19
6.4	11	14	17
6.6	10.5	13	16
6.8	10	12	15

Posner-Inglima revised conversion table. For use with the Applanometer.

Table C. Relation of MacKay-Marg Measurements to NCT

MacKay-Marg	NCT	MacKay-Marg	NCT	MacKay-Marg	NCT
15	8	30	24	45	40
16	9	31	25	46	41
17	10	32	26	47	42
18	11	33	27	48	43
19	12	34	28	49	44
20	13	35	29	50	45
21	14	36	30	51	46
22	15	37	31	52	47
23	16	38	32	53	48
24	17	39	33	54	49
25	19	40	34	55	50
26	20	41	35	56	51
27	21	42	36	57	52
28	22	43	37	58	53
29	23	44	38	59	54
				60	55

Reprinted from Augsberger, Polasky, and Wolby, Clinical tonometric measurements with the non-contact tonometer, *American Journal of Optometry*, April, 1974.

4.27. Hirshberg Test

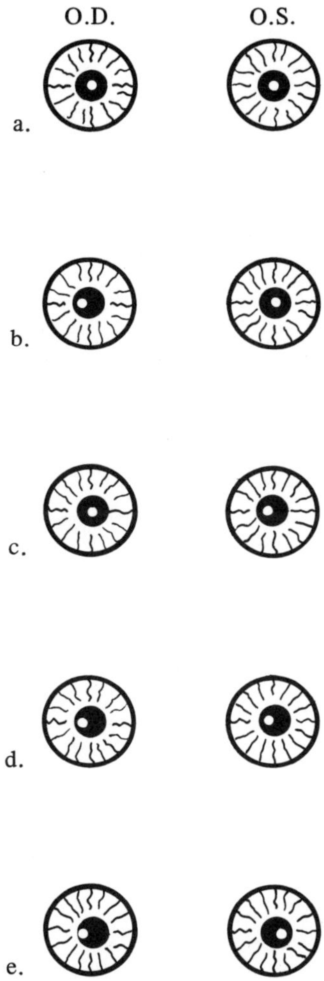

a. Bifoveal fixation, zero angle kappa
b. O.S. fixating, zero angle kappa and 22 p.d. ET of O.D.
c. O.S. fixating, + 1mm angle kappa, and 22 p.d. ET of O.D.
d. O.S. fixating, + 1mm angle kappa, and 44 p.d. ET of O.D.
e. O.S. fixating, — 1mm angle kappa, and 22. p.d. ET of O.D.

Reprinted from Optometric Monthly (p. 15) published by Professional Press, Inc., 101 East Ontario Street, Chicago, Illinois 60611.

Contact Lenses 5

5.1. Minimum Central Thicknesses Recommended for Fused Bifocals

Reading addition (D)	*Minimum central thickness (mm.)*					
	Segment widths (mm.) 5.00	*5.50*	*6.00*	*6.50*	*7.00*	*7.50*
+1.50	0.12	0.14	0.17	0.20	0.23	0.28
+1.75	0.14	0.16	0.19	0.23	0.27	0.32
+2.00	0.16	0.18	0.22	0.26	0.31	0.37
+2.25	0.17	0.20	0.25	0.29	0.35	0.42
+2.50	0.19	0.23	0.27	0.33	0.40	0.47
+2.75	0.21	0.25	0.30	0.36	0.44	0.52
+3.00	0.22	0.27	0.33	0.40	0.48	0.57

Reprinted by permission from J. de Carle, in J. Stone and A. J. Phillips (eds.), *Contact Lenses. A Textbook for Practitioner and Student.* London: Barrie & Jenkins, and Brit. Optical Assn., 1974.

5.2. Recommended Diameter of the Distance Portion in Concentric Bifocals

Pupil diameter (mm.)	*Distance portion diameter (mm.)*	*Pupil diameter (mm.)*	*Distance portion diameter (mm.)*
4.5	3.20	3.2	2.25
4.4	3.10	3.1	2.20
4.3	3.05	3.0	2.10
4.2	2.95	2.9	2.05
4.1	2.90	2.8	2.00
4.0	2.80	2.7	1.90
3.9	2.75	2.6	1.85
3.8	2.70	2.5	1.75
3.7	2.60	2.4	1.70
3.6	2.55	2.3	1.65
3.5	2.45	2.2	1.55
3.4	2.40	2.1	1.50
3.3	2.30	2.0	1.45

Reprinted by permission from J. Stone and A. J. Phillips, *Contact Lenses. A Textbook for Practitioner and Student.* London: Barrie & Jenkins, and Brit. Optical Assn., 1974.

5.3. Minimum Central Thicknesses Recommended for Ballast Bifocals

Positive lenses, 9.00 mm. overall size all 1½ Δ prism ballast		*Negative lenses, 9.00 mm. overall size*		
BVP (D)	*Central thickness (mm.)*	*BVP (D)*	*Central thickness (mm.)*	*Prism (Δ)*
0.00	0.32			
+0.50	0.34	− 0.50	0.31	1½
+1.00	0.35	− 1.00	0.30	1½
+1.50	0.36	− 1.50	0.29	1½
+2.00	0.37	− 2.00	0.27	1½
+2.50	0.39	− 2.50	0.26	1½
+.300	0.40	− 3.00	0.25	1½
+3.50	0.41	− 3.50	0.24	1½
+4.00	0.42	− 4.00	0.25	2
+4.50	0.44	− 4.50	0.25	2
+5.00	0.45	− 5.00	0.24	2
+5.50	0.46	− 5.50	0.23	2
+6.00	0.47	− 6.00	0.22	2
+6.50	0.49	− 6.50	0.25	2½
+7.00	0.50	− 7.00	0.24	2½
+7.50	0.51	− 7.50	0.23	2½
+8.00	0.52	− 8.00	0.22	2½
+8.50	0.54	− 8.50	0.25	3
+9.00	0.55	− 9.00	0.24	3
+9.50	0.56	− 9.50	0.23	3
+10.00	0.57	−10.00	0.22	3
+10.50	0.59	−10.50	0.25	3½
+11.00	0.60	−11.00	0.24	3½
+11.50	0.61	−11.50	0.23	3½
+12.00	0.62	−12.00	0.22	3½
+12.50	0.64	−12.50	0.25	4
+13.00	0.65	−13.00	0.24	4
+13.50	0.66	−13.50	0.23	4
+14.00	0.67	−14.00	0.22	4

Reprinted by permission from J. Stone and A. J. Phillips, *Contact Lenses. A Textbook for Practitioner and Student.* London: Barrie & Jenkins, and Brit. Optical Assn., 1974.

5.4. Conversion of Inches to Millimeters

mm	*inches*	*mm*	*inches*	*mm*	*inches*
.80	.032	.50	.020	.30	.012
.78	.031	.49	.019	.29	.011
.76	.030	.48	.019	.28	.011
.74	.029	.47	.019	.27	.011
.72	.029	.46	.018	.26	.010
.70	.028	.45	.018	.25	.010
.68	.027	.44	.017	.24	.009
.66	.026	.43	.017	.23	.009
.64	.025	.42	.017	.22	.009
.62	.024	.41	.016	.21	.008
.60	.024	.40	.016	.20	.008
.59	.023	.39	.015	.19	.007
.58	.023	.38	.015	.18	.007
.57	.022	.37	.015	.17	.007
.56	.022	.36	.014	.16	.006
.55	.022	.35	.014	.15	.006
.54	.021	.34	.013	.14	.006
.53	.021	.33	.013	.13	.005
.52	.020	.32	.013	.12	.005
.51	.020	.31	.012	.11	.004
				.10	.004

5.5. Recommended Thicknesses for Rigid Contact Lenses

Table A. Recommended Thicknesses for Rigid Contact Lenses (Thin)

	Minus Diameters (mm.)							*Plus Diameters (mm.)*					
	7.0	*7.5*	*8.0*	*8.5*	*9.0*	*9.5*		*7.0*	*7.5*	*8.0*	*8.5*	*9.0*	*9.5*
Plano	.15	.16	.17	.17	.18	.19	+ 1.00	.17	.18	.19	.20	.21	.22
− 1.00	.15	.16	.17	.17	.18	.19	+ 2.00	.17	.18	.19	.20	.21	.22
− 1.50	.14	.15	.16	.16	.17	.18	+ 3.00	.18	.19	.20	.21	.22	.23
− 2.50	.13	.13	.14.	.15	.15	.16	+ 4.00	.19	.20	.21	.22	.23	.24
− 3.00	.12	.12	.13	.14	.14	.15	+ 5.00	.20	.21	.22	.23	.24	.25
− 3.50	.12	.12	.13	.13	.14	.15	+ 6.00	.21	.22	.24	.25	.27	.29
− 4.00	.11	.11	.12	.12	.13	.14	+ 7.00	.22	.23	.25	.27	.29	.33
− 4.50	.10	.10	.11	.11	.12	.13	+ 8.00	.23	.24	.26	.28	.31	.36
− 5.00	.09	.09	.10	.10	.11	.12	+ 9.00	.25	.26	.28	.31	.34	.41
− 5.50	.09	.09	.10	.10	.10	.11	+10.00	.25	.27	.30	.33	.38	.46
− 6.00	.09	.09	.09	.09	.10	.10	+11.00	.26	.29	.31	.34	.42	.50
− 7.00	.09	.09	.09	.09	.10	.10	+12.00	.27	.29	.32	.38	.46	.54
− 7.50	.09	.09	.09	.09	.09	.10	+13.00	.28	.30	.36	.41	.50	.58
− 8.00	.09	.09	.09	.09	.09	.10	+14.00	.30	.33	.40	.46	.55	.63
− 8.50	.09	.09	.09	.09	.09	.10	+15.00	.32	.37	.44	.52	.60	.70
− 9.00	.09	.09	.09	.09	.09	.10	+16.00	.34	.38	.46	.53	.62	.72
−10.00	.09	.09	.09	.09	.09	.10	+17.00	.36	.40	.48	.55	.64	.74
−11.00	.09	.09	.09	.09	.09	.09	+18.00	.37	.42	.50	.57	.67	.77
−12.00	.09	.09	.09	.09	.09	.09	+19.00	.40	.44	.53	.60	.70	.80
−13.00	.09	.09	.09	.09	.09	.09	+20.00	.42	.47	.55	.63	.73	.83

Reprinted by permission from Young Contact Lens Co., Boston, Mass.

5.5. Recommended Thicknesses for Rigid Contact Lenses

Table B. Recommended Thicknesses for Rigid Lenses (Regular)

	Minus Diameters (mm.)								Plus Diameters (mm.)						
	7.5	*8.0*	*8.5*	*9.0*	*9.5*	*10.00*	*10.5*		*7.5*	*8.0*	*8.5*	*9.0*	*9.5*	*10.00*	*10.5*
Plano	.21	.21	.22	.24	.24	.26	.26	+ 1.00	.23	.23	.24	.25	.27	.28	.28
– 1.00	.19	.19	.20	.22	.23	.24	.24	+ 2.00	.25	.25	.26	.27	.29	.31	.31
– 2.00	.18	.18	.19	.19	.20	.21	.21	+ 3.00	.26	.27	.28	.30	.31	.33	.33
– 3.00	.17	.17	.18	.18	.18	.19	.19	+ 4.00	.28	.29	.30	.31	.33	.34	.35
– 4.00	.16	.16	.17	.17	.17	.18	.18	+ 5.00	.30	.31	.32	.33	.35	.37	.40
– 5.00	.15	.15	.16	.16	.16	.17	.17	+ 6.00	.31	.32	.34	.36	.39	.41	.44
– 6.00	.14	.14	.15	.15	.15	.16	.16	+ 7.00	.33	.35	.37	.39	.42	.45	.48
– 7.00	.13	.13	.14	.14	.14	.15	.15	+ 8.00	.35	.37	.40	.42	.45	.49	.52
– 8.00	.12	.12	.13	.13	.13	.14	.14	+ 9.00	.37	.39	.42	.45	.48	.52	.56
– 9.00	.11	.11	.12	.12	.12	.13	.13	+10.00	.38	.41	.44	.48	.52	.56	.60
–10.00	.11	.11	.11	.12	.12	.13	.13	+11.00	.39	.43	.47	.51	.55	.59	.64
–11.00	.10	.11	.11	.11	.11	.12	.12	+12.00	.41	.45	.49	.53	.58	.63	.69
–12.00	.10	.10	.11	.11	.11	.12	.12	+13.00	.42	.46	.51	.56	.60	.67	.73
–13.00	.09	.10	.10	.11	.11	.12	.12	+14.00	.44	.49	.54	.59	.64	.71	.78
–14.00	.09	.09	.10	.10	.11	.12	.12	+15.00	.46	.51	.56	.61	.68	.75	.82
–15.00	.09	.09	.09	.10	.10	.11	.12	+16.00	.48	.53	.58	.63	.71	.79	.86
–16.00	.08	.09	.09	.10	.10	.11	.11	+17.00	.50	.55	.60	.65	.74	.82	.90
–17.00	.08	.08	.09	.10	.10	.11	.11	+18.00	.52	.57	.62	.67	.76	.85	.94
–18.00	.07	.08	.09	.10	.10	.11	.11	+19.00	.54	.59	.65	.69	.79	.89	.98
–19.00	.07	.08	.08	.09	.10	.10	.11	+20.00	.57	.62	.68	.75	.83	.92	1.02

Reprinted by permission from Young Contact Lens Co., Boston, Mass.

Table C. Supplementary Thickness to be Added to a Contact Lens Incorporating Prism
Center Thickness Prism Factor Chart

	– Diopters of Prism –													
Lens Diameter (mm.)	*¾*	*1*	*1¼*	*1½*	*1¾*	2	*2¼*	*2½*	*2¾*	*3*	*3¼*	*3½*	*3¾*	*4*
7.75	0.06	0.08	0.10	0.12	0.14	0.16	0.18	0.20	0.22	0.24	0.26	0.28	0.30	0.32
8.00	0.06	0.08	0.10	0.12	0.14	0.16	0.18	0.20	0.22	0.25	0.27	0.29	0.31	0.33
8.25	0.06	0.08	0.11	0.13	0.15	0.17	0.19	0.21	0.23	0.25	0.27	0.29	0.32	0.34
8.50	0.07	0.09	0.11	0.13	0.15	0.17	0.20	0.22	0.24	0.26	0.28	0.30	0.33	0.35
8.75	0.07	0.09	0.11	0.13	0.16	0.18	0.20	0.22	0.25	0.27	0.29	0.31	0.34	0.36
9.00	0.07	0.09	0.11	0.14	0.16	0.18	0.21	0.23	0.25	0.28	0.30	0.32	0.35	0.37
9.25	0.07	0.09	0.12	0.14	0.17	0.19	0.21	0.24	0.26	0.28	0.31	0.33	0.35	0.38
9.50	0.07	0.10	0.12	0.15	0.17	0.19	0.22	0.24	0.27	0.29	0.32	0.34	0.36	0.39
9.75	0.07	0.10	0.13	0.15	0.17	0.20	0.22	0.25	0.27	0.30	0.32	0.35	0.37	0.40
10.00	0.08	0.10	0.13	0.15	0.18	0.20	0.23	0.26	0.28	0.31	0.33	0.36	0.38	0.41
10.25	0.08	0.11	0.13	0.16	0.18	0.21	0.24	0.26	0.29	0.31	0.34	0.37	0.39	0.42
10.50	0.08	0.11	0.13	0.16	0.19	0.21	0.24	0.26	0.29	0.32	0.35	0.38	0.40	0.43
10.75	0.08	0.11	0.14	0.16	0.19	0.22	0.25	0.27	0.30	0.33	0.36	0.38	0.41	0.44
11.00	0.08	0.11	0.14	0.17	0.20	0.22	0.25	0.28	0.31	0.34	0.37	0.39	0.42	0.45
11.25	0.09	0.12	0.14	0.17	0.20	0.23	0.26	0.29	0.32	0.34	0.37	0.40	0.43	0.46
11.50	0.09	0.12	0.15	0.18	0.21	0.23	0.26	0.29	0.32	0.35	0.38	0.41	0.44	0.47
11.75	0.09	0.12	0.15	0.18	0.21	0.24	0.27	0.30	0.33	0.36	0.39	0.42	0.45	0.48
12.00	0.09	0.12	0.15	0.18	0.21	0.25	0.28	0.31	0.34	0.37	0.40	0.43	0.46	0.49
12.25	0.09	0.13	0.16	0.19	0.22	0.25	0.28	0.31	0.34	0.38	0.41	0.44	0.47	0.50
12.50	0.09	0.13	0.16	0.19	0.22	0.26	0.29	0.32	0.35	0.38	0.41	0.45	0.48	0.51

Add the Above Thickness to Regular Center Thickness

Reprinted by permission from Neefe Optical Laboratory, Big Spring, Texas.

5.6. Prescription Requirements for First-Quality Contact Lenses

Table A. Prescription Requirements for Corneal Lenses (All measurements are made in air with lenses in an air-dried state.)

Parameter		*Tolerance*
Diameter		± 0.05 mm
Posterior optic zone diameter	Light blend	± 0.1 mm
	Medium or heavy blend	± 0.2 mm
Posterior central curve (base curve) radius		± 0.025 mm
Posterior secondary, intermediate, or peripheral curve width		
	Light blend	± 0.05 mm
	Medium or heavy blend	± 0.10 mm
Posterior secondary, intermediate, or peripheral curve radius		± 0.1 mm
Refractive power	+10.00 D to –10.00 D	± 0.12 D (Notes 1, 2, 3)
	More than ± 10.00 D	± 0.25 D
Prism power (measured from the geometric center)		
If lens power is:	+10.00 D to –10.00 D	± 0.25Δ
	More than ± 10.00 D	± 0.50 Δ
Cylinder power	less than 2.00 D	± 0.25 D
	2.00 D to 4.00 D	± 0.37 D
	greater than 4.00 D	± 0.50 D
Cylinder axis		± 5°
Toric base curve radii	Δ r 0 to 0.20 mm	± 0.02 mm (Note 3)
	Δ r 0.21 to 0.40 mm	± 0.03 mm
	Δ r 0.41 to 0.60 mm	± 0.05 mm
	Δ r > 0.60 mm	± 0.07 mm
Bifocal refractive power addition		± 0.25 D (Note 2)
Bifocal segment height		–0.1 mm to +0.2 mm
Center thickness		less than ± 0.02 mm (Note 4)
Edges		As specified
Anterior peripheral curve radius		± 0.2 mm
Anterior optic zone diameter		± 0.1 mm
Optical quality and surface quality		No bubbles, striae, waves, inhomogenieties, crazing, pits, scratches, chips, lathe marks, or stone marks
Color		Pigment inert and uniformly distributed

NOTE 1: If the lens base curve and power errors are cumulative (that is, base curve and lens power errors both add plus power or both add minus power to the refractive correction) the cumulative error shall not exceed 0.25 D.
NOTE 2: The cumulative errors in power between the right and left lenses shall not exceed 0.25 D.
NOTE 3: Symbols used are as follows:
D — diopters
Δ — prism diopters
Δr — difference between radii of principal meridians
NOTE 4: The algebraic differences in thickness error between right and left lenses shall not exceed 0.02 mm.

Table B. Prescription Requirements for Scleral Lenses (All measurements are made in air with lenses in an air-dried state.)

Parameter		*Tolerance*
Outside diameter (size)		± 0.5 mm
Posterior central curve (base curve) radius		± 0.03 mm
Refractive power	+10.00 D to −10.00 D	± 0.12 D (Notes 1 and 2)
	More than ± 10.00 D	± 0.25 D (Notes 1 and 2)
Prism power (measured from the geometric center)		± 0.25 Δ
Cylinder axis		± 5°
Center thickness		± 0.03 mm
Edges		Well rounded and polished
Anterior central curve radius		± 0.01 mm
Surface quality		Free of cutting rings, scratches, polishing rings, etc.
Transition		As specified
Fenestration		As specified
Clearance		As specified ± 0.02 mm

NOTE 1: If the lens base curve and power errors are cumulative (that is, base curve and lens power errors both add plus power or both add minus power to the refractive correction) the cumulative error shall not exceed 0.25 D.

NOTE 2: The cumulative errors in power between the right and left lenses shall not exceed 0.25 D.

5.7. Keratometer Conversion Chart

Table A. Power to Radii (Convex and Concave)

Keratometer Power Reading	*Convex Radius*	*Concave Radius*	*Keratometer Power Reading*	*Convex Radius*	*Concave Radius*
36.00	9.38	9.42	47.75	7.07	7.09
36.25	9.31	9.35	48.00	7.03	7.05
36.50	9.25	9.29	48.25	6.99	7.02
36.75	9.18	9.22	48.50	6.96	6.98
37.00	9.12	9.16	48.75	6.92	6.95
37.25	9.06	9.10	49.00	6.89	6.91
37.50	9.00	9.04	49.25	6.85	6.88
37.75	8.94	8.98	49.50	6.82	6.84
38.00	8.88	8.92	49.75	6.78	6.81
38.25	8.82	8.86	50.00	6.75	6.77
38.50	8.77	8.80	50.25	6.72	6.74
38.75	8.71	8.75	50.50	6.68	6.70
39.00	8.65	8.69	50.75	6.65	6.67
39.25	8.60	8.63	51.00	6.62	6.64
39.50	8.54	8.58	51.25	6.59	6.61
39.75	8.49	8.52	51.50	6.55	6.57
40.00	8.44	8.47	51.75	6.52	6.54
40.25	8.33	8.37	52.00	6.49	6.51
40.50	8.39	8.42	52.25	6.46	6.48
40.75	8.28	8.31	52.50	6.43	6.45
41.00	8.23	8.26	52.75	6.40	6.42
41.25	8.18	8.21	53.00	6.37	6.39
41.50	8.13	8.16	53.25	6.34	6.36
41.75	8.08	8.11	53.50	6.31	6.33
42.00	8.04	8.07	55.75	6.05	6.08
42.25	7.99	8.02	56.00	6.03	6.05
42.50	7.94	7.97	56.25	6.00	6.02
42.75	7.89	7.92	56.50	5.97	6.00
43.00	7.85	7.88	56.75	5.95	5.97
43.25	7.80	7.83	57.00	5.92	5.94
43.50	7.76	7.79	57.25	5.90	5.92
43.75	7.71	7.74	57.50	5.87	5.89
44.00	7.67	7.70	57.75	5.84	5.87
44.25	7.63	7.65	58.00	5.82	5.84
44.50	7.58	7.61	58.25	5.79	5.82
44.75	7.54	7.57	58.50	5.77	5.79
45.00	7.50	7.53	58.75	5.75	5.77
45.25	7.46	7.49	59.00	5.72	5.74
45.50	7.42	7.44	59.25	5.70	5.72
45.75	7.38	7.40	59.50	5.67	5.69
46.00	7.34	7.36	59.75	5.65	5.67
46.25	7.30	7.32	60.00	5.63	5.65
46.50	7.26	7.28	60.25	5.60	5.62
46.75	7.22	7.24	60.50	5.58	5.60
47.00	7.18	7.21	60.75	5.56	5.58
47.25	7.14	7.17	61.00	5.53	5.55
47.50	7.11	7.13			

(continued)

5.7. Keratometer Conversion Chart

Table B. Concave Surfaces

Diopters	*Radii*	*Diopters*	*Radii*	*Diopters*	*Radii*	*Diopters*	*Radii*	*Diopters*	*Radii*
60.00	5.65	53.87	6.29	47.87	7.07	41.87	8.09	35.87	9.44
59.87	5.66	53.75	6.30	47.75	7.09	41.75	8.11	35.75	9.48
59.75	5.67	53.62	6.32	47.62	7.11	41.62	8.14	35.62	9.51
59.62	5.68	53.50	6.33	47.50	7.13	41.50	8.16	35.50	9.54
59.50	5.69	53.37	6.35	47.37	7.15	41.37	8.19	35.37	9.58
59.37	5.71	53.25	6.36	47.25	7.17	41.25	8.21	35.25	9.61
59.25	5.72	53.12	6.38	47.12	7.19	41.12	8.24	35.12	9.64
59.12	5.73	53.00	6.39	47.00	7.21	41.00	8.27	35.00	9.68
59.00	5.74	52.87	6.41	46.87	7.23	40.87	8.29	34.87	9.71
58.87	5.75	52.75	6.42	46.75	7.25	40.75	8.32	34.75	9.75
58.75	5.77	52.62	6.44	46.62	7.27	40.62	8.34	34.62	9.78
58.62	5.78	52.50	6.45	46.50	7.29	40.50	8.37	34.50	9.82
58.50	5.79	52.37	6.47	46.37	7.31	40.37	8.40	34.37	9.86
58.37	5.80	52.25	6.48	46.25	7.33	40.25	8.42	34.25	9.89
58.25	5.82	52.12	6.50	46.12	7.35	40.12	8.45	34.12	9.93
58.12	5.83	52.00	6.51	46.00	7.37	40.00	8.47	34.00	9.96
58.00	5.84	51.87	6.53	45.87	7.39	39.87	8.50	33.87	10.00
57.87	5.85	51.75	6.54	45.75	7.40	39.75	8.53	33.75	10.04
57.75	5.87	51.62	6.56	45.62	7.42	39.62	8.55	33.62	10.08
57.62	5.88	51.50	6.57	45.50	7.44	39.50	8.58	33.50	10.11
57.50	5.89	51.37	6.59	45.37	7.46	39.37	8.61	33.37	10.15
57.37	5.90	51.25	6.61	45.25	7.49	39.25	8.64	33.25	10.19
57.25	5.92	51.12	6.62	45.12	7.51	39.12	8.66	33.12	10.23
57.12	5.93	51.00	6.64	45.00	7.53	39.00	8.69	33.00	10.27
57.00	5.94	50.87	6.65	44.87	7.55	38.87	8.72	32.87	10.30
56.87	5.96	50.75	6.67	44.75	7.57	38.75	8.75	32.75	10.34
56.75	5.97	50.62	6.69	44.62	7.59	38.62	8.77	32.62	10.38
56.62	5.98	50.50	6.70	44.50	7.61	38.50	8.80	32.50	10.42
56.50	6.00	50.37	6.72	44.37	7.64	38.37	8.84	32.37	10.46
56.37	6.01	50.25	6.74	44.25	7.65	38.25	8.86	32.25	10.50
56.25	6.02	50.12	6.75	44.12	7.68	38.12	8.89	32.12	10.55
56.12	6.04	50.00	6.77	44.00	7.70	38.00	8.92	32.00	10.59
56.00	6.05	49.87	6.79	43.87	7.72	37.87	8.95	31.87	10.63
55.87	6.06	49.75	6.80	43.75	7.75	37.75	8.98	31.75	10.67
55.75	6.08	49.62	6.82	43.62	7.77	37.62	9.01	31.62	10.71
55.62	6.09	49.50	6.84	43.50	7.79	37.50	9.04	31.50	10.75
55.50	6.10	49.37	6.86	43.37	7.81	37.37	9.07	31.37	10.80
55.37	6.12	49.25	6.87	43.25	7.83	37.25	9.10	31.25	10.84
55.25	6.13	49.12	6.89	43.12	7.86	37.12	9.13	31.12	10.88
55.12	6.15	49.00	6.91	43.00	7.88	37.00	9.16	31.00	10.93
55.00	6.16	48.87	6.93	42.87	7.90	36.87	9.19	30.87	10.97
54.87	6.17	48.75	6.94	42.75	7.93	36.75	9.22	30.75	11.02
54.75	6.19	48.62	6.96	42.62	7.95	36.62	9.26	30.62	11.06
54.62	6.20	48.50	6.98	42.50	7.97	36.50	9.29	30.50	11.11
54.50	6.22	48.37	7.00	42.37	8.00	36.37	9.32	30.37	11.15
54.37	6.23	48.25	7.02	42.25	8.02	36.25	9.35	30.25	11.20
54.25	6.24	48.12	7.03	42.12	8.04	36.12	9.38	30.12	11.25
54.12	6.26	48.00	7.05	42.00	8.07	36.00	9.41	30.00	11.29
54.00	6.27								

Reprinted by permission from Bausch and Lomb, Rochester, N. Y.

Table C. Extended Range (+1.25 Orthogon)

Drum Reading	*Corneal Power in Diopters*	*Radius in mm Cx*	*CC*
43.000	50.134	6.732	6.759
43.125	50.279	6.712	6.739
43.250	50.425	6.693	6.720
43.375	50.571	6.674	6.701
43.500	50.717	6.655	6.681
43.625	50.862	6.636	6.662
43.750	51.008	6.617	6.643
43.875	51.154	6.598	6.624
44.000	51.299	6.579	6.605
44.125	51.445	6.560	6.587
44.250	51.591	6.542	6.568
44.375	51.737	6.523	6.550
44.500	51.882	6.505	6.531
44.625	52.028	6.487	6.513
44.750	52.174	6.469	6.495
44.875	52.320	6.451	6.477
45.000	52.465	6.433	6.459
45.125	52.611	6.415	6.441
45.250	52.757	6.397	6.423
45.375	52.903	6.380	6.405
45.500	53.048	6.362	6.388
45.625	53.194	6.345	6.370
45.750	53.340	6.327	6.353
45.875	53.486	6.310	6.335
46.000	53.631	6.293	6.318
46.125	53.777	6.276	6.301
46.250	53.923	6.259	6.284
46.375	54.069	6.242	6.267
46.500	54.214	6.225	6.250
46.625	54.360	6.209	6.233
46.750	54.506	6.192	6.217
46.875	54.651	6.175	6.200
47.000	54.797	6.159	6.184
47.125	54.943	6.143	6.167
47.250	55.089	6.126	6.151
47.375	55.234	6.110	6.135
47.500	55.380	6.094	6.119
47.625	55.526	6.078	6.103
47.750	55.672	6.062	6.087
47.875	55.817	6.046	6.071
48.000	55.963	6.031	6.055
48.125	56.109	6.015	6.039
48.250	56.255	5.999	6.024
48.375	56.400	5.984	6.008
48.500	56.546	5.969	5.993
48.625	56.692	5.953	5.977
48.750	56.838	5.938	5.962
48.875	56.983	5.923	5.947
49.000	57.129	5.908	5.931
49.125	57.275	5.893	5.916
49.250	57.421	5.878	5.901
49.375	57.566	5.863	5.886
49.500	57.712	5.848	5.871
49.625	57.858	5.833	5.857
49.750	58.003	5.819	5.842
49.875	58.149	5.804	5.827
50.000	58.295	5.789	5.813
50.125	58.441	5.775	5.798
50.250	58.586	5.761	5.784
50.375	58.732	5.746	5.769
50.500	58.878	5.732	5.755
50.625	59.024	5.718	5.741
50.750	59.169	5.704	5.727
50.875	59.315	5.690	5.713
51.000	59.461	5.676	5.699
51.125	59.607	5.662	5.685
51.250	59.752	5.648	5.671
51.375	59.898	5.935	5.657
51.500	60.044	5.621	5.643
51.625	60.190	5.607	5.630
51.750	60.335	5.594	5.616
51.875	60.481	5.580	5.603
52.000	60.627	5.567	5.589

If the supplementary lens is a Tillyer deduct approximately .05 mm. from the result.

5.7. Keratometer Conversion Chart

Table D. Extended Range (–1.00 Orthogon)

Drum Reading	Corneal Power in Diopters	Radius in mm Cx	CC	Drum Reading	Corneal Power in Diopters	Radius in mm Cx	CC
36.000	30.874	10.931	10.964	39.000	33.447	10.090	10.121
36.125	30.981	10.893	10.926	39.125	33.554	10.058	10.088
36.250	31.089	10.856	10.889	39.250	33.662	10.026	10.056
36.375	31.196	10.819	10.851	39.375	33.769	9.994	10.024
36.500	31.303	10.782	10.814	39.500	33.876	9.963	9.993
36.625	31.410	10.745	10.777	39.625	33.983	9.931	9.961
36.750	31.518	10.708	10.740	39.750	34.090	9.900	9.930
36.875	31.625	10.672	10.704	39.875	34.198	9.869	9.899
37.000	31.732	10.636	10.668	40.000	34.305	9.838	9.868
37.125	31.839	10.600	10.632	40.125	34.412	9.807	9.837
37.250	31.946	10.564	10.596	40.250	34.519	9.777	9.806
37.375	32.054	10.529	10.561	40.375	34.626	9.747	9.776
37.500	32.161	10.494	10.526	40.500	34.734	9.717	9.746
37.625	32.268	10.459	10.491	40.625	34.841	9.687	9.716
37.750	32.375	10.425	10.456	40.750	34.948	9.657	9.686
37.875	32.482	10.390	10.421	40.875	35.055	9.628	9.656
38.000	32.590	10.356	10.387	41.000	35.162	9.598	9.627
38.125	32.697	10.322	10.353	41.125	35.270	9.569	9.598
38.250	32.804	10.288	10.319	41.250	35.377	9.540	9.569
38.375	32.911	10.255	10.286	41.375	35.484	9.511	9.540
38.500	33.018	10.221	10.252	41.500	35.591	9.483	9.511
38.625	33.126	10.188	10.219	41.625	35.698	9.454	9.483
38.750	33.233	10.155	10.186	41.750	35.806	9.426	9.454
38.875	33.340	10.123	10.153	41.875	35.913	9.398	9.426
				42.000	36.020	9.370	9.398

If the supplementary lens is a Tillyer, deduct approximately .05 mm. from the result.

5.7. Keratometer Conversion Chart

Table E. Extended Range (+2.25 Orthogon)

Drum	*Corneal Power*	*CX Radius*	*Drum*	*Corneal Power*	*CX Radius*
38.0	49.74	6.79	45.0	59.02	5.72
25	50.67	6.74	25	59.35	5.69
50	50.40	6.70	50	59.68	5.66
75	50.73	6.65	75	60.01	5.62
39.0	51.06	6.61	46.0	60.34	5.59
25	51.39	6.57	25	60.67	5.56
50	51.73	6.52	50	61.00	5.53
75	52.06	6.48	75	61.33	5.50
40.0	52.39	6.44	47.0	61.66	5.47
25	52.72	6.40	25	61.99	5.44
50	53.05	6.36	50	62.32	5.41
75	53.38	6.32	75	62.65	5.39
41.0	53.71	6.28	48.0	62.99	5.36
25	54.04	6.24	25	63.32	5.33
50	54.38	6.21	50	63.65	5.29
75	54.71	6.17	75	63.99	5.26
42.0	55.04	6.13	49.0	64.32	5.24
25	55.37	6.10	25	64.65	5.21
50	55.70	6.06	50	64.98	5.19
75	56.03	6.02	75	65.31	5.17
43.0	56.36	5.99	50.0	65.64	5.14
25	56.69	5.95	25	65.97	5.11
50	57.02	6.92	50	66.30	5.09
75	57.35	5.88	75	66.63	5.06
44.0	57.69	5.85	51.0	66.97	5.04
25	58.02	5.81	25	67.30	5.01
50	58.35	5.78	50	67.62	4.99
75	58.68	5.75	75	67.96	4.96
			52.0	68.29	4.94

If the additional lens is a Tillyer, deduct approximately .08 mm from the result.

For concave surfaces add an additional .05 mm.

5.8. Guide to Slit Lamp Photography of the Cornea

Table A. Electronic Flash and Diaphragm Settings For Black and White Photographs of Cornea (Nikon)

FILM: TRI-X ASA 400

Light on Cornea	*Magnification Settings* 7× *Flash*	7× *Stop*	10× *Flash*	10× *Stop*	16× *Flash*	16× *Stop*	25× *Flash*	25× *Stop*	35× *Flash*	35× *Stop*
SLIT Very Narrow < 1 mm.	1	1.5	1	.5						
	1.4	2	1.4	1.5	1.4	5				
	2	2.5	2	2	2	1.5	2	0		
	2.8	3	2.8	2.5	2.8	2	2.8	1		
	4	3.5	4	3	4	2.5	4	1.5	4	0
Diffusing Filter	1.4	0								
	2	1	2	0						
	2.8	2	2.8	1	2.8	0				
	4	3	4	2	4	1	4	0	4	0
SLIT Wide 1-2 mm.	1	4	1	3	1	2	1	1	1	0
	1.4	5	1.4	4	1.4	3	1.4	2	1.4	1
	2	6	2	5	2	4	2	2.5	2	2
			2.8	6	2.8	4.5	2.8	3	2.8	2.5
					4	5	4	3.5	4	3
Diffusing filter	1	0								
	1.4	2	1.4	0						
	2	3	2	2	2	0				
	2.8	4	2.8	3	2.8	2	2.8	0		
	4	5	4	4	4	3	4	2	4	1
WIDE OPEN	1	4.5	1	3.5	1	2.5	1	1.5	1	1
	1.4	5	1.4	4	1.4	3.5	1.4	2	1.4	1.5
	2	5.5	2	4.5	2	4	2	2.5	2	2
	2.8	6	2.8	5	2.8	4.5	2.8	3	2.8	2.5
			4	5.5	4	5	4	3.5	4	3
Diffusing Filter	1	3	1	2	1	1	1	.5		
	1.4	3.5	1.4	2.5	1.4	2	1.4	1.5		
	2	4	2	3	2	2.5	2	2.0	2	1.5
	2.8	4.5	2.8	3.5	2.8	3	2.8	2.5	2.8	2.0
	4	5	4	4	4	3.5	4	3.0	4	2.5
GREEN FILTER	1	3	1	2	1	1	1	0		
	1.4	4	1.4	2.5	1.4	1.5	1.4	.5		
	2	4.5	2	3	2	2	2	1	2	0
	2.8	5	2.8	3.5	2.8	2.5	2.8	1.5	2.8	.5
	4	5.5	4	4	4	3	4	2	4	1
BLUE FILTER (Fluorescein) Yellow Filter over Objective	1.4	0								
	2	1	2	0						
	2.8	2	2.8	1	2.8	0				
	4	3	4	2	4	1	4	0	4	0

Table B. Electronic Flash and Diaphragm Settings For Color Photographs of Cornea (Nikon)

FILM: HIGH SPEED EKTACHROME, 160 (DAYLIGHT, FOR COLOR SLIDES)

	Magnification Settings 7×		10×		16×		25×		35×	
Light on Cornea	*Flash*	*Stop*	*Flash*	*Stop*	*Flash*	*Stop*	*Flash*	*Stop*	*Flash*	*Stop*
SLIT	2	0								
Very Narrow	2.8	1	2.8	0						
1 mm	4	2	4	1	4	0	4	0	4	0
Diffusing Filter	2.8	0								
	4	1	4	0	4	0	4	0	4	0
	1	2	1	1.5	1	1				
SLIT	1.4	2.5	1.4	2	1.4	1.5				
WIDE	2	3	2	2.5	2	2				
1-2 mm	2.8	3.5	2.8	3	2.8	2.5	2.8	0		
	4	4	4	3.5	4	3	4	1	4	0
	2	0								
Diffusing Filter	2.8	1	2.8	0						
	4	2	4	1	4	0	4	0	4	0
	1	4	1	3.5	1	3	1	2	1	1
	1.4	4.5	1.4	4	1.4	3.5	1.4	3	1.4	2
WIDE OPEN	2	5	2	4.5	2	4	2	3.5	2	2.5
	2.8	5.5	2.8	5	2.8	4.5	2.8	4	2.8	3
	4	6	4	5.5	4	5	4	4.5	4	3.5
	1	3	1	2.5	1	2	1	1	1	0
	1.4	3.5	1.4	3	1.4	2.5	1.4	2	1.4	1
Diffusing Filter	2	4	2	3.5	2	3	2	2.5	2	2
	2.8	4.5	2.8	4	2.8	3.5	2.8	3	2.8	2.5
	4	5	4	4.5	4	4	4	3.5	4	3
	2	0								
GREEN FILTER	2.8	1	2.8	0						
	4	2	4	1	4	0	4	0	4	0
BLUE FILTER	4	0	4	0	4	0	4	0	4	0
(Fluorescein)										
Yellow Filter										
over Objective										

Reprinted by permission from R. I. Rengstorff and C. C. Krausse, "Guide for slit lamp photography of the cornea," *J. Am. Opt. Assoc.* 42: 1971.

Table C. Accessory Fill-in Flash for the Nikon Photo Slit Lamp

Suggested aperture size for proper exposure at various magnifications with two commonly available film speeds*

	Aperture Size	
Magnification	*ASA 200 film*	*ASA 400 film*
35X	5.5, 7.0, 8.0, 9.5	5.0, 5.5, 7.0, 8.0
25X	5.5, 7.0	5.0, 5.5
16X	5.0, 5.5	4.0, 5.0
10X	4.0, 5.0	4.0

***Recommended film for color transparencies is Kodak High-Speed Ektrachrome (ASA 200), and for black and white photographs is Kodak Tri-X (ASA 400). A smaller aperture size will allow underexposure of fill-in flash. Selective underexposure is desirable at high magnification (35X) because of flare produced by the microscope optics.**

Reprinted from Cummings, Clompus, and Ellis, An accessory fill-in flash for the Nikon photo slit lamp, *American Journal of Optometry*, February, 1979.

Table D. Electronic Flash Intensity Settings for the Nikon Photo Slit Lamp

		Magnification			
ASA 64		*7-10*	*11-16*	*17-25*	*26-35*
Conjunctiva		(.54)	*1.09*	*2.18*	(4.37)
Iris		(.78)	*1.56*	*3.125*	(6.25)
Fundus		*3.125*	(6.25)	(12.5)	(25.0)
Cornea	Wide Slit	*2.34*	(4.68)	(9.375)	(18.75)
	Narrow Slit	*3.125*	(6.25)	(12.5)	(25.0)
Crystalline	Wide Slit	*3.125*	(6.25)	(12.5)	(25.0)
lens	Narrow Slit	(6.25	(12.5)	(25.0)	(50.0)
ASA 200					
Conjunctiva		(.175)	(.35)	(.7)	*1.4*
Iris		(.25)	(.50)	*1.0*	*2.0*
Fundus		*1.0*	*2.0*	*4.0*	(8.0)
Cornea	Wide Slit	(.75)	*1.5*	*3.0*	(6.0)
	Narrow Slit	*1.0*	*2.0*	*4.0*	(8.0)
Crystalline	Wide Slit	*1.0*	*2.0*	*4.0*	(8.0)
lens	Narrow Slit	*2.0*	*4.0*	(8.0)	(16.0)
ASA 400					
Conjunctiva		(.0875)	(.175)	.35	*(.7)*
Iris		(.125)	(.25)	.50	*1.0*
Fundus		(.50)	*1.0*	2.0	*4.0*
Cornea	Wide Slit	(.375)	(.75)	1.5	*3.0*
	Narrow Slit	(.50)	*1.0*	2.0	*4.0*
Crystalline	Wide Slit	(.50)	*1.0*	2.0	*4.0*
lens	Narrow Slit	*1.0*	*2.0*	4.0	(8.0)

Electronic flash units have intensivity settings of 1.0, 1.4, 2.0, 2.8 and 4.0. Sometimes, the intensity settings indicated in these tables don't match these exactly—for example, a suggested intensity may turn out to be 1.09 or 1.56. In these cases, the photographer must set the electronic flash to the intensity which most closely approximates the indicated setting. Then, he must either increase the brightness control or stop down the aperture diaphragm and recalculate the correct intensity setting. For example, when a setting of 1.56 is indicated, the intensity should be set at 1.4, the aperture diaphragm should be opened wide, and the brightness should be increased to seven or eight volts. When a setting of 1.09 is indicated, the intensity should be rounded off at 1.0.

The intensities given in italic can be used without unnecessary worry about over- or underexposure.

Reprinted from T.W. Spivak, Photography through the Nikon slit lamp biomicroscope, *Review of Optometry*, November, 1977.

Table E. Exposures Table for Nikon-Contact Endothelium Camera

Film: Kodachrome ASA 64

Lens	*Eye Structure*	*Slit Width*	*Slit Direction*	*Flash Output*	*Diaphragm Opening*	*Notes*
2X	Cornea-Lens	3 mm	20°–30°	4	5.6	
	Cornea-Lens	5 mm	20°–30°	3	8	
	Cornea-Lens	1 mm	20°–30°	5	5.6	
	Conjunctiva	Full open	20°	3	11	#3
	Conjunctiva with green filter	Full open	25°	4	4.8	#1
	Iris	5 mm	30°	4	11	
	Entire eye with diffusion filter	Full open	20°	4	4.8	#2
5X	Cornea-Lens	0.5 mm	20°–30°	5	2.6	
	Cornea-Lens	2 mm	20°–30°	5	2.6	#6
	Cornea-Lens	5 mm	20°–30°	5	5.6	#6
	Cornea-Flourescein and Cobalt Filter	10 mm	20°–30°	5	4	
	Cornea-Flourescein and Cobalt Filter	10 mm	20°–30°	5	4	#4, #9
	Cornea-Flourescein and Cobalt Filter	10 mm	20°–30°	5	4	#5, #10
	Conjunctiva	Full open	30°–40°	3	11	#3
	Conjunctiva-green filter	Full open	30°–40°	3	5.6	
	Iris	5 mm	20°–30°	5	11	

(continued)

Table E. Exposures table for Nikon-Contact Endothelium Camera (continued)

Film: Kidachrome ASA 64

Lens	*Eye Structure*	*Slit Width*	*Slit Direction*	*Flash Output*	*Diaphragm Opening*	*Notes*
10X	Cornea	0.5 mm	20°–30°	5	1.4	
	Cornea	1 mm	20°–30°	5	2.0	#6
	Cornea	3 mm	20°–30°	5	2.8	#6
	Cornea	5 mm	20°–30°	5	4.0	#6
	Conjunctiva	3 mm	20°–30°	4	8	#3
	Conjunctiva-green filter	3 mm	20°–30°	4	4.0	#1
	Iris	3 mm	30°	5	5.6	
	Corneal Endothelium	1 mm	50°–65°	5	1.4	

[1] Green filter (in filter drawer of light tower) is used when primary point of interest is the conjunctival or limbal blood vessels. They will stand out as black structures against a green background.

[2] Diffusion filter is made by using two thicknesses of wax paper placed over the exit lens on the light tower.

[3] Caution must be exercised in aligning the light source to minimize reflected glare or highlight that might obscure a desired detail.

[4] A Wratten #12 filter (produced by Kodak and obtainable from photographic suppliers) is deep yellow—it increases the contrast value in the shades of green from one area to the next.

[5] A Wratten #13 is deep green and does the same as the #12 filter (see #4 above) but to a greater extent and eliminates completely the blue cast frequency seen in flourescein photography.

[6] The same exposure settings can be used to photograph corneal structures utilizing retroillumination.

[7] Where exposure is critical in order to reveal optimum detail it is advised to bracket the exposures one stop more or less than indicated herein.

[8] When using H.S. Ektachrome ASA 200 film step down the diaphragm by 2 full stops from the charts indicated exposures for ASA 64 film—for ASA 100 film close down by 1 stop—keep Note #7 in mind.

[9] Also #12 filter.

[10] Also #13 filter.

Compiled by, and reprinted with the permission of, Sanford E. Kaps, O.D.F.A.A.O., Tenafly, N.J., U.S.A. 07670

Table F. Ocular Features: Settings for Nikon Photo Slit Lamp

No.	*Subject*	*Mag.*	*Illumination Diaphragm*	*Slit Width*	*Other Details*
1.	Whole eye	0.7	min	max	Diffuser filter
2.	Whole eye	1.0	min–med	max	Diffuser filter
3.	Whole eye	1.6	med	max	Diffuser filter
4.	Whole eye	0.7	max	3 mm	Sclerotic scatter (offset illumination)
5.	Whole eye	1.0	max	3 mm	Sclerotic scatter (offset illumination)
6.	Temporal bulbar conjunctiva	1.0	min	max	Diffuser filter
7.	Temporal bulbar conjunctiva	1.6	min–med	max	Diffuser filter
8.	Temporal bulbar conjunctiva	2.5	med	max	Diffuser filter
9.	Iris	1.0	min	max	Diffuser filter
10.	Iris	1.6	min–med	max	Diffuser filter
11.	Iris	2.5	med	max	Diffuser filter
12.	Iris crypts	1.6	med	5 mm	Oblique illumination
13.	Iris crypts	2.5	med	5 mm	Oblique illumination
14.	Iris crypts	3.5	med–max	5 mm	Oblique illumination
15.	Iris pigment frill	3.5	med–max	5 mm	Focal illumination
16.	Central cornea nerve fibres	1.0	med	2 mm	Focal parallelopiped
17.	Central cornea nerve fibres	1.6	med–max	2 mm	Focal parallelopiped
18.	Central cornea nerve fibres	2.5	max	2 mm	Focal parallelopiped
19.	Central cornea nerve fibres	3.5	max	2 mm	Focal parallelopiped
20.	Central cornea	1.0	max	0.2 mm	Optic section
21.	Central cornea	1.6	max	0.2 mm	Optic section
22.	Central cornea	2.5	max	0.2 mm	Optic section
23.	Crystalline lens	1.0	max	0.2 mm	Optic section
24.	Crystalline lens	1.6	max	0.2 mm	Optic section
25.	Crystalline lens	1.6	med	2 mm	Shagreen in specular reflex
26.	Crystalline lens	2.5	med	2 mm	Shagreen in specular reflex

(continued)

Table F. Ocular Features: Settings for Nikon Photo Slit Lamp (continued)

No.	*Subject*	*Mag.*	*Illumination Diaphragm*	*Slit Width*	*Other Details*
27.	Blood vessels at nasal limbus	1.6	min	1 mm	Retroillumination off iris
28.	Blood vessels at nasal limbus	2.5	med	1 mm	Retroillumination off iris
29.	Blood vessels at nasal limbus	3.5	med	1 mm	Retroillumination off iris
30.	Everted lid	1.0	min	max	Diffuser filter
31.	Everted lid	1.6	med	max	Diffuser filter
32.	Everted lid	2.5	med	max	Diffuser filter
33.	Hard lens fluorescein fit	0.7	max	max	Cobalt blue and yellow barrier filters
34.	Hard lens fluorescein fit	1.0	max	max	Cobalt blue and yellow barrier filters
35.	Hard lens fluorescein fit	1.6	max	max	Cobalt blue and yellow barrier filters
36.	Hard lens fluorescein fit	2.5	max	max	Cobalt blue and yellow barrier filters

Recommended list of ocular features for photography by varied techniques with a trial roll of film. Ektachrome 200 ASA film should be used. The camera shutter speed should be set to flash synchro (1/80 sec) and the flash intensity control to maximum (200 ws). Magnification, diaphragm, slit width, and filters should be set as listed in columns 2–5 of the table. A thin piece of tissue paper over the illumination system can be substituted for a diffusion filter.

Reprinted from S. Zanos, B. Holden, and D. Pye, A guide to ocular photography with the Nikon photo slit lamp, *Australian J. Opt.*, March, 1980.

5.9. Conversion Table for Aesthesiometry

Length of the nylon thread (cm)		*6*	*5*	*4*	*3*	*2*	*1*
Recorded pressure (mg/s) as a function of the angle of bend	5°	11	13	22	34	71	153
	8°	15	16	33	43	97	212
	12°	19	20	45	55	120	284
	17°	23	24	55	64	143	365
Mean values of the pressures supplied with the instrument		11	13	21	36	75	145

5.10. Technique for Peripheral Keratometry

Table A. Distance from Apex

Distance of Fixation Point From Center of Mire		11.3	15.1	19.0	23.0	27.1	29.3	31.2	35.5
Ocular Rotation In Degrees		7.5	10	12.5	15.0	17.5	19.4	20.0	22.5
Corneal Power In Diopters	38	2.9	3.3	3.7	4.2	4.6	4.8	5.0	5.4
	39	2.9	3.3	3.7	4.1	4.5	4.7	4.9	5.3
	40	2.8	3.2	3.6	4.0	4.4	4.6	4.8	5.2
	41	2.8	3.2	3.5	3.9	4.3	4.5	4.7	5.1
	42	2.7	3.1	3.4	3.8	4.2	4.4	4.6	4.9
	43	2.6	3.0	3.4	3.7	4.1	4.3	4.5	4.8
	44	2.6	2.9	3.3	3.6	4.0	4.2	4.4	4.7
	45	2.5	2.9	3.2	3.6	3.9	4.1	4.3	4.6
	46	2.5	2.8	3.1	3.5	3.8	4.0	4.2	4.5

Table B. Correction Factor

Difference in mm. between Central & Peripheral K Reading	0 – .5	.5 – 1	1 – 2	2 – 3	3 – 4	4 and up
Correction Factor	0	1	1.5	2	2.5	3

A more accurate assessment of the corneal periphery measured by eccentric fixation can be made with a correction factor. This value, obtained from Table B, is added to the value 2 Fp – Fc where: Fp = the peripheral reading
Fc = the cap reading

For example: Fc = 42.00 Fp = 36.00 2 × 36 – 42 = 30.00
If the reading is taken at 4.00 mm. (Table A) 30 + 3 = 33.00 D

Reprinted by permission from R.M. Mandell, "Methods to measure the peripheral corneal curvature," *J. Am. Opt. Assoc.* 33: 1962.

5.11. Relative Transmission of Tinted Contact Lenses

Table A. Relative Percentages

Tint	*% Transmittancy*	*Tint*	*%Transmittancy*
Clear	95	Green	
Gray		no. 10	75
no. 0	88	no. 1	77
no. 10	82	no. 2	69
no. 1	78	no. 3	70
no. 2	68	Brown	
no. 3	23	no. 1	63
Blue		no. 2	58
no. 10	80	no. 3	54
no. 1	85	Pink	
no. 5	78	no. 1	89
no. 2	64	no. 2	74
no. 3	48	no. 3	70
Lavender	82		

Reprinted by permission from W. Miller and G. Lumpkin, "Light transmission of tinted contact lenses," *Contact Lens Soc. Amer. J.* 6:1972.

5.11. Relative Transmission of Tinted Contact Lenses

Table B. Transmission Charts

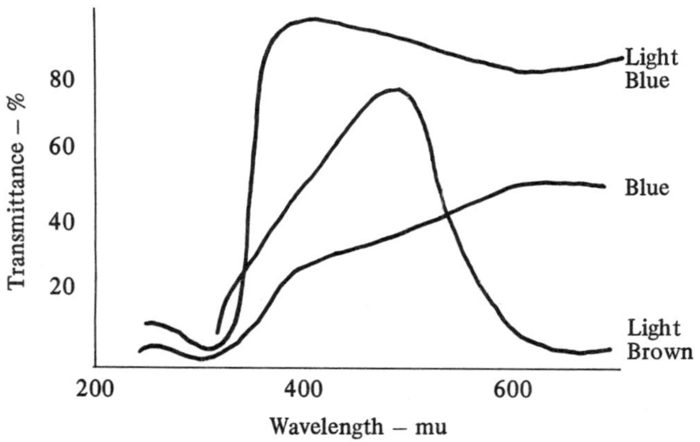

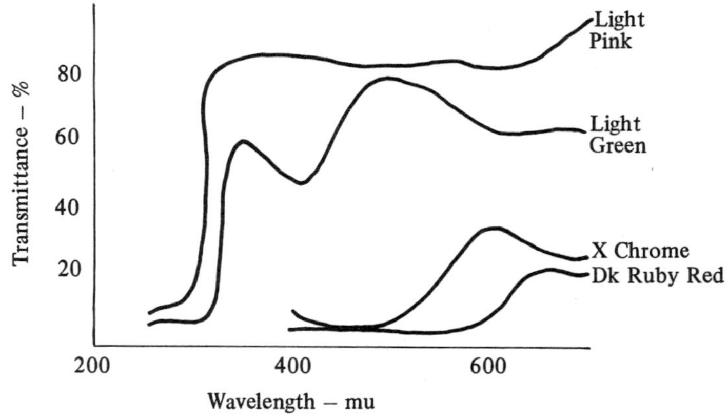

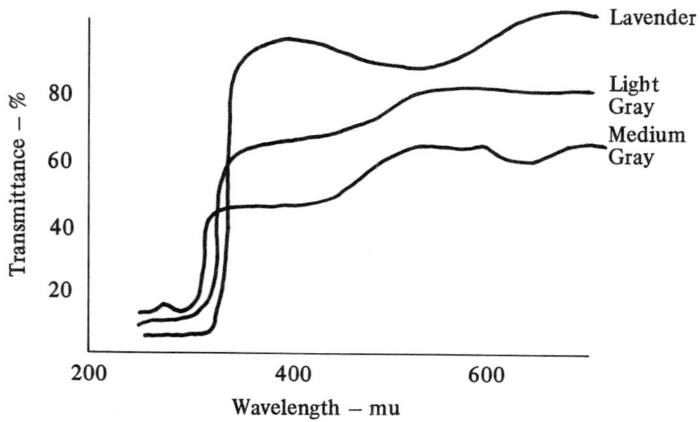

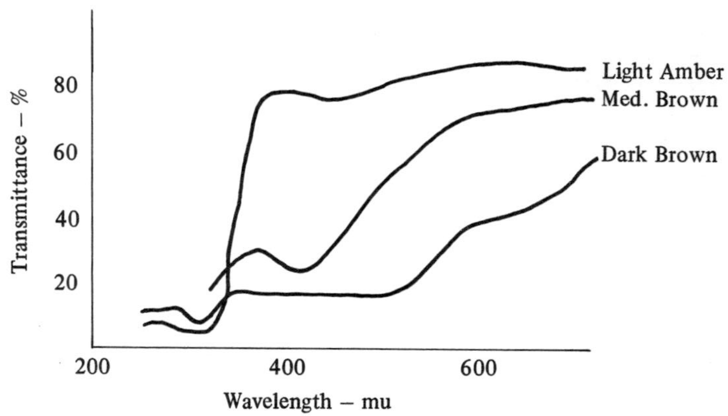

Curves are for Glasflex material with the exception of X Chrome

5.12. Design of Contact Lens-Spectacle Telescopes

Table A. Contact-Spectacle Telescope Constructions

Dioptric Power of Contact Lens	*Dioptric Power of Spectacles*	*Vertex Distance in mm.*	*Mag.*	*Monocular* Field of View in Degrees*
−40	26.3	13	1.52	79
	23.8	17	1.69	61
	22.2	20	1.80	51
	21.1	23	1.91	43
−30	21.8	13	1.35	87
	20.0	17	1.50	68
	18.8	20	1.60	58
	17.7	23	1.68	50
−20	15.9	13	1.26	92
	14.9	17	1.33	76
	14.3	20	1.40	65
	13.7	23	1.46	58

*Assuming 44 mm. eye size.

Table B. Recommended Front Optical Zone Diameters for High Minus Lenticular Contact Lenses. Total Diameter 9.5 mm.

Power	*Front Optical Zone Diameter*
−10 D.	8.0
−20 D.	7.4
−30 D.	7.0
−40 D.	6.6
(P1 front)	3.8

5.13. Corrected Image Size in Anisometropia

Table A. Axial Errors

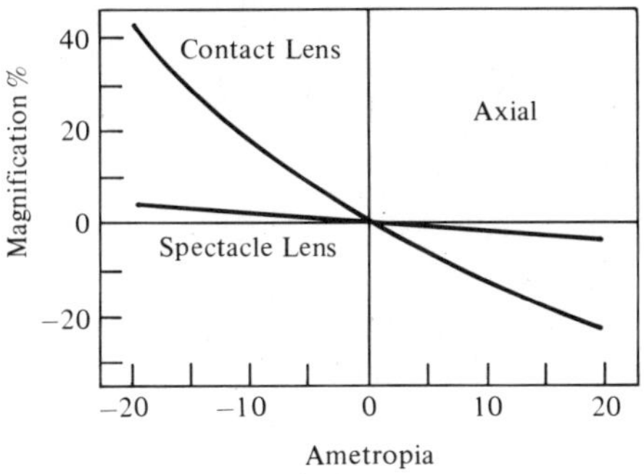

Table B. Refractive Errors

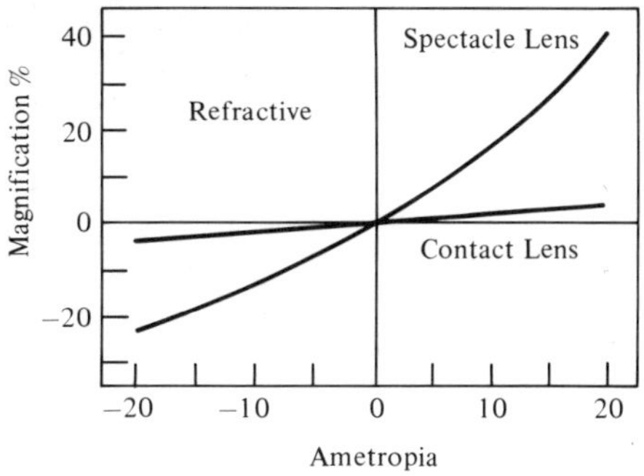

Corrected Ametropic Eye's Image Size Relative to Emmetropic Eye's Image Size.

5.14. Percentage Increase in the Retinal Image Size in the Aphakic Eye Corrected

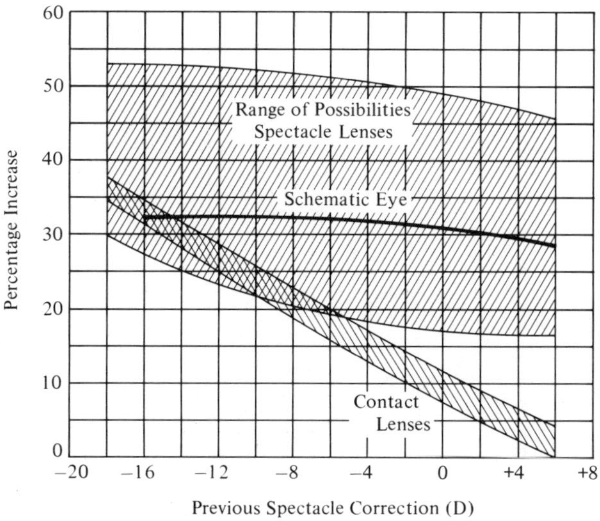

Percentage increase in the retinal image size in the aphakic eye corrected by spectacle and contact lenses. The graph indicates the possible spread of values.

Reprinted by permission from A. G. Bennett, "Percentage increases in the retinal image size in the aphakic use correct spectacles and contact lenses," ***The Contact Lens.*** **4: 1973.**

5.15. Back Vertex Power from Front Vertex Power of Positive Contact Lenses

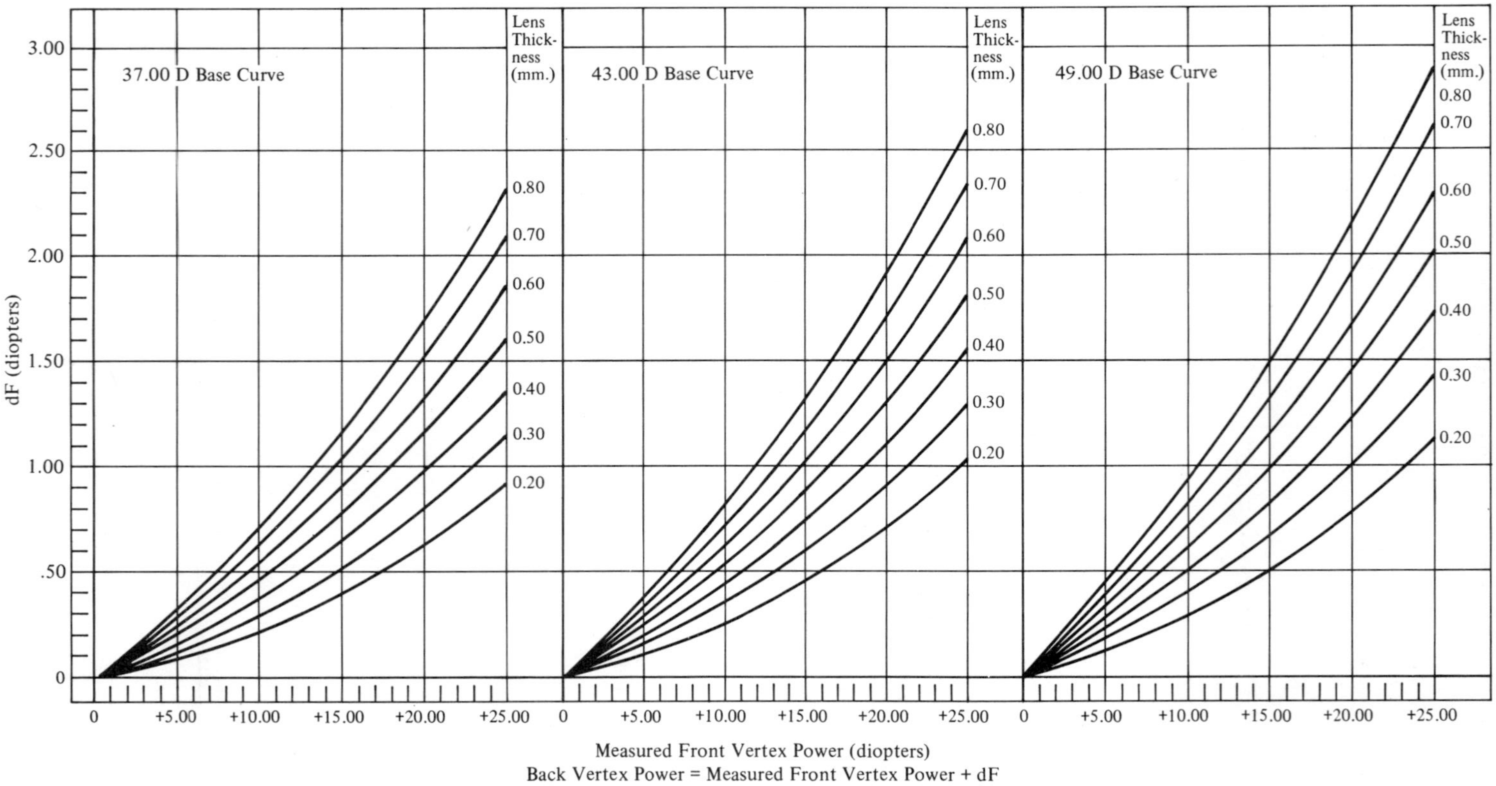

Reprinted by permission from *Encyclopedia of Contact Lens Practice*, Int. Optics Publ. Co., vol. 3, chapter 32. Courtesy of the Bernell Corp., South Bend, Ind.

5.16. Characteristics of the Bausch & Lomb Soflens

Table A. Posterior Apical Radius (Standard Minus Lenses)

	Diameter 12.5				*Diameter 13.6*			
Power	*B Series*	*F Series*	*J Series*	*N Series*	*B3 Series*	*F3 Series*	*J3 Series*	*C Series*
– 0.25	9.00	8.65	8.35	8.05	9.55	9.25	8.95	
– 0.50	8.95	8.60	8.30	8.00	9.50	9.20	8.90	
– 0.75	8.90	8.55	8.30	8.00	9.45	9.15	8.85	
– 1.00	8.85	8.50	8.25	7.95	9.40	9.10	8.80	8.00
– 1.25	8.80	8.50	8.20	7.90	9.35	9.05	8.75	8.00
– 1.50	8.75	8.45	8.15	7.85	9.30	9.00	8.70	7.95
– 1.75	8.70	8.40	8.10	7.85	9.25	8.95	8.65	7.90
– 2.00	8.70	8.35	8.10	7.80	9.20	8.90	8.60	7.85
– 2.25	8.65	8.30	8.05	7.75	9.15	8.85	8.55	7.85
– 2.50	8.60	8.25	8.00	7.75	9.10	8.80	8.50	7.80
– 2.75	8.55	8.25	8.00	7.70	9.05	8.75	8.45	7.75
– 3.00	8.50	8.20	7.95	7.65	9.05	8.75	8.45	7.75
– 3.25	8.45	8.15	7.90	7.65	9.00	8.70	8.40	7.70
– 3.50	8.40	8.10	7.85	7.60	8.95	8.65	8.35	7.65
– 3.75	8.40	8.10	7.85	7.55	8.90	8.60	8.30	7.65
– 4.00	8.35	8.05	7.80	7.55	8.85	8.55	8.25	7.60
– 4.25	8.30	8.00	7.75	7.50	8.80	8.50	8.20	7.55
– 4.50	8.25	7.95	7.75	7.45	8.80	8.50	8.20	7.55
– 4.75	8.25	7.95	7.70	7.45	8.75	8.45	8.15	7.50
– 5.00	8.20	7.90	7.65	7.40	8.70	8.40	8.10	7.45
– 5.50	8.10	7.85	7.60	7.35	8.60	8.30	8.00	7.40
– 6.00	8.05	7.75	7.55	7.25	8.50	8.25	7.95	7.35
– 6.50	7.95	7.70	7.45		8.40	8.15		7.30
– 7.00	7.90	7.60	7.40		8.35	8.10		7.25
– 7.50	7.80	7.55	7.35		8.25	8.00		7.15
– 8.00	7.75	7.50			8.20	7.95		7.10
– 8.50	7.70	7.45			8.10	7.85		7.05
– 9.00	7.60	7.35			8.05	7.80		7.00
– 9.50		7.30			7.95	7.75		6.95
– 10.00					7.90	7.65		6.90
– 10.50					7.80	7.60		6.85
– 11.00					7.75	7.55		6.80
– 11.50					7.70	7.45		6.75
– 12.00					7.60	7.40		6.70
– 12.50					9.55[1]	9.20[1]		6.65
– 13.00					9.45	9.10		6.60
– 13.50					9.35	9.00		6.55
– 14.00					9.25	8.90		6.50
– 14.50					9.15	8.85		6.45
– 15.00					9.05	8.75		6.40
– 15.50					8.95	8.65		6.35
– 16.00					8.85	8.55		6.30
– 16.50					8.75	8.50		6.25
– 17.00					8.70	8.40		6.20
– 17.50					8.60	8.30		6.15
– 18.00					8.50	8.25		6.10
– 18.50					8.45	8.15		6.10
– 19.00					8.35	8.10		6.05
– 19.50					8.25	8.00		6.00
– 20.00					8.20	7.95		5.95
Center Thickness	.11	.14	.11	.14	.11	.14	.15	.07 to .29

[1] **Lenticular from this point**

Table B. Posterior Apical Radius (Plus Lenses)

Power	*N*	*B3*	*F3*	*J3*	*B4*
	12.5-13.5	*13.5*	*13.5*	*13.5*	*14.5*
+ 0.25	8.15	8.75	8.25		9.50
+ 0.50	8.15	8.80	8.30		9.55
+ 0.75	8.20	8.80	8.35		9.60
+ 1.00	8.25	8.85	8.40		9.65
+ 1.25	8.25	8.90	8.45		9.70
+ 1.50	8.30	8.95	8.45		9.75
+ 1.75	8.35	9.00	8.50		9.80
+ 2.00	8.40	9.05	8.55		9.85
+ 2.25	8.40	9.10	8.60		9.90
+ 2.50	8.45	9.15	8.65		9.95
+ 2.75	8.50	9.20	8.70		10.00
+ 3.00	8.55	9.20	8.70		10.05
+ 3.25	8.55	9.25	8.75		10.10
+ 3.50	8.60	9.30	8.80		10.15
+ 3.75	8.65	9.35	8.85		10.20
+ 4.00	8.70	9.40	8.90		10.30
+ 4.25	8.75	9.45	8.95		10.35
+ 4.50	8.75	9.50	9.00		10.40
+ 4.75	8.80	9.55	9.05		10.45
+ 5.00	8.85	9.60	9.10		10.50
+ 5.50	8.95	9.70	9.20		10.65
+ 6.00	9.05	9.80	9.30		10.75
+ 6.50	7.00[2]		8.25		
+ 7.00	7.05		8.35		
+ 7.50	7.10		8.45		
+ 8.00	7.15		8.50		
+ 8.50	7.20		8.60		
+ 9.00	7.25		8.70		
+ 9.50	7.30		8.75		
+10.00	7.35		8.85		
+10.50	7.40		8.95		
+11.00	7.45	7.70	7.40	7.15	
+11.50	7.50	7.75	7.50	7.20	
+12.00	7.55	7.80	7.55	7.25	
+12.50	7.60	7.90	7.60	7.35	
+13.00	7.65	7.95	7.70	7.40	
+13.50	7.70	8.05	7.75	7.45	
+14.00	7.75	8.10	7.80	7.50	
+14.50	7.80	8.20	7.90	7.60	
+15.00	7.90	8.25	7.95	7.65	
+15.50	7.95	8.35	8.05	7.70	
+16.00	8.00	8.45	8.10	7.80	
+16.50	8.05	8.50	8.20	7.85	
+17.00	8.10	8.60	8.25	7.95	
+17.50	8.15	8.70	8.35	8.00	
+18.00		8.75	8.40	8.10	
+18.50		8.85	8.50	8.15	
+19.00		8.95	8.60	8.25	
+19.50		9.05	8.65	8.30	
+20.00		9.15	8.75	8.40	
Center Thickness					
to + 6.00	.19 to .47	.12 to .30	.30		
+ 6.50 to + 10.50	.40 to .57		.42		.12 to .30
+ 11.00 up	.53 to .75	.57	.57	.57	

[2] **Series becomes lenticular at this point and diameter becomes 13.5 mm.**

Table C. Posterior Apical Radius (H_3, HH)

Power	+H3	+H4
+ 6.50	7.35	8.05
+ 7.00	7.40	8.15
+ 7.50	7.50	8.20
+ 8.00	7.55	8.30
+ 8.50	7.60	8.35
+ 9.00	7.70	8.45
+ 9.50	7.75	8.50
+ 10.00	7.80	8.60
+ 10.50	7.90	8.70
+ 11.00	7.95	8.75
+ 11.50	8.00	8.85
+ 12.00	8.10	8.95
+ 12.50	8.15	9.05
+ 13.00	8.25	9.15
+ 13.50	8.30	9.25
+ 14.00	8.40	9.30
+ 14.50	8.50	9.40
+ 15.00	8.55	9.55
+ 15.50	8.65	9.65
+ 16.00	8.75	9.75
+ 16.50	8.80	9.85
+ 17.00	8.90	9.95
+ 17.50	9.00	10.05
+ 18.00	9.10	10.20
+ 18.50	9.20	10.30
+ 19.00	9.25	10.40
+ 19.50	9.35	10.55
+ 20.00	9.45	10.65
Center Thickness	.49 to .60	.46 to .55

Table D. Posterior Apical Radius (Ultra Thin Minus, B_4)

Power	12.5 U	13.5 U3	14.5 U4	14.5 B4	13.5 O_3	14.5 O_4
− 0.25	8.53	9.09	8.99	9.99		
− 0.50	8.49	9.04	8.95	9.93		
− 0.75	8.44	8.99	8.90	9.87		
− 1.00	8.40	8.94	8.86	9.82		
− 1.25	8.36	8.90	8.81	9.76		
− 1.50	8.32	8.85	8.77	9.71	9.25[3]	9.60
− 1.75	8.28	8.81	8.72	9.65	9.20[3]	9.50
− 2.00	8.24	8.76	8.68	9.60	9.15	8.55
− 2.25	8.21	8.72	8.64	9.55	9.10	8.50
− 2.50	8.17	8.68	8.60	9.50	9.05	8.45
− 2.75	8.13	8.63	8.55	9.44	9.00	8.45
− 3.00	8.09	8.59	8.51	9.39	8.95	8.40
− 3.25	8.05	8.55	8.47	9.34	8.90	8.35
− 3.50	8.02	8.51	8.43	9.29	8.85	8.30
− 3.75	7.98	8.47	8.39	9.24	8.80	8.25
− 4.00	7.94	8.43	8.35	9.20	8.75	8.25
− 4.25	7.91	8.38	8.31	9.15	8.70	8.20
− 4.50	7.87	8.34	8.27	9.10	8.70	8.15
− 4.75	7.84	8.30	8.23	9.05	8.65	8.10
− 5.00	7.80	8.27	8.19	9.01	8.60	8.10
− 5.50	7.73	8.19	8.11	8.91	8.50	8.00
− 6.00	7.66	8.11	8.04	8.82	8.40	7.95
− 6.50	7.60	8.04	7.97	8.73	8.35	7.85
− 7.00	7.53	7.96	7.89	8.65	8.25	7.80
− 7.50	7.47	7.89	7.82	8.56	8.20	7.70
− 8.00	7.40	7.82	7.75	8.48	8.10	7.65
− 8.50	7.34	7.75	7.69	8.40	8.05	7.60
− 9.00	7.28	7.68	7.62	8.32	7.95	7.50
Center Thickness	.07	.07	.07 to .08	.12	.035	.035

[3] Made in U_4 molds

5.17. True Lens Thickness from Optical Thickness Measured by a Radiuscope (Flexible Lenses)

(N = 1.43)

Measured Thickness	*True Thickness*	*Measured Thickness*	*True Thickness*
10	14.3	28	40.0
11	15.7	29	41.5
12	17.2	30	42.9
13	18.6	31	44.3
14	20.0	32	45.8
15	21.5	33	47.2
16	22.9	34	48.6
17	24.3	35	50.1
18	25.5	36	51.5
19	27.2	37	52.9
20	28.6	38	54.3
21	30.0	39	55.8
22	31.2	40	57.2
23	32.3	41	58.6
24	34.3	42	60.1
25	35.6	43	61.5
26	37.2	44	62.9
27	38.6	45	64.4
		46	65.8

5.18. Oxygen Permeability of Contact Lens Materials

Lens or material name	Manufacturer or distributor	Oxygen permeability (cn^{-1}/sec) (ml O_2/ml .mm Hg)	Temperature C
AO Thin	American Opt.	9.2	22
Aquaflex (Thin)	Union Corp.	10.8	22
CAB (hard)	Wöhlk	4.3 10^{-11}	RT*
		5.9	RT
CAB (hard)	Eastman Kodak	13.8	35
Calcon	Calcon	7.3	RT
		13.6	25
CLP2A (hard)	Dupont	20.9	37
Duragel 75		40.0	22
Dura Soft	Wesley/Jessen	5.2	
Geleflex 60		40	22
Gelflex 75	Contact Lens Mfg.	16.6	20
Hoya Soft	Hoya	7.0	
Hydrocurve II (55)	Hydrocurve		22
Hydrocurve II 45	Hydrocurve	15.5	22
Hydron 0.6	American	8.1	
Igel 78	Optiflex	27.7	23
Kelvin Canada	Kelvin Canada	22.0	25
		25.0	27
Opticare (hard)	Opticare	2.0	RT
Permalens	Global Vision	34.3	RT
		42.0	36
Plano T	Bausch & Lomb	7.6	RT
Polycon		5.0	RT
Sauflon 70	Contact Lens Mfg.	30.5	RT
		39.2	35
Sauflon 85	Contact Lens Mfg.	48.6	RT
Scanlens	Scanlens	31.0	37
		35.7	37
Silsoft	Dow Corning	3.40	
Smith & Nephew No. 407	Smith Nephew	45.0	RT
Softon		16.0	
Soflens U_4	Bausch & Lomb	7.8	22
Soflens O_4	Brusch & Lomb	14.3	22
Welcon 38%	Titmus-Eurocon	7.3	RT

*RT = Room Termperature

5.19. Relationship Between Center Thickness and Oxygen Performance for Some Gas-Permeable Materials

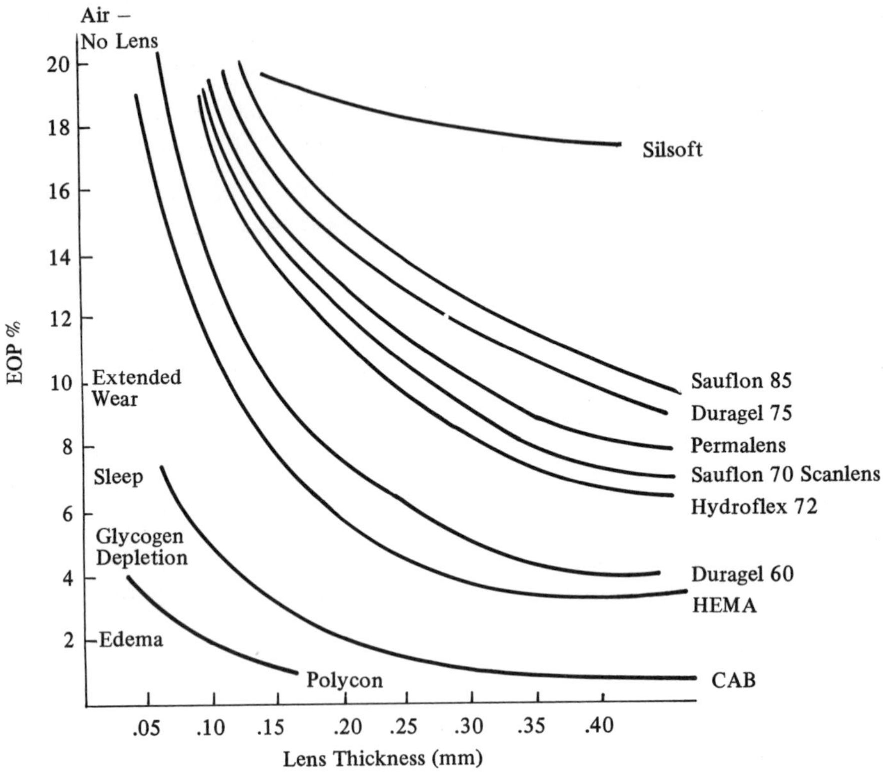

5.20. Availability of Specialty Contact Lenses

Table A. Sources

Rigid	
Aphakia tint	Wesley/Jesson
Aspheric anteriors (for residual astigmatism)	Conforma, Neefe, Prec-cosmet
Aspheric Multifocals	Contour comfort, Breger, Conlensco, W/J Prec-Cosmet, Palco
Cosmetic (add color)	Neefe, Prec-cosmet
Cosmetic (Black pupil)	Neefe
Fenestrated	Medi-cornea, Lombart, Continuous curve, Capitol
Graduated Adds (anterior)	Kendall, Morrison, Sohnges
Half-Tint	Pres-cosmet
Keratoconus	Pre-corneal Contact Lens Co.
Korb technique	Guaranteed
Near vision lens	May
Nissel tints	Lombard
Nystagmus	W/J
Orthokeratology lens	Neefe, W/J
Occluder lens	Neefe
Opaque occluder (black pupil)	Neefe
Periballest	Neefe, Guaranteed
Pupil lens (clear pupil)	Neefe
Sclerals	Prec-cosmet, W/J, Daniker, Omni, Neefe
Trifocal	Neefe
Ultraviolet cut off	Marvel
Vented	Gordon, Morrison
Wet treated (coating)	Morgan, Neefe
X chrome	Lombart, Young
Soft	
Cosmetic	Weicon, Narcissus Medical Foundation, Kelvin
Keratoconus	Flexlens
Piggy Back	Flexlens
Tinted	Weicon, Kelvin
Ventilated	BG Contact Lens Co., LTD.

Table B. Addresses of Sources

Accusoft Contact Lens Lab 116A Vandalia Street Collinsville, IL 62234	Conlensco 34-09 24 Street Long Island City, NY 11016
Alcon Optics Div. of Alcon Labs, Inc. 6201 So. Freeway Forth Worth, TX 76101	Continuous Curve Contact Lenses, Inc. P.O. Box 17157 San Diego, CA 92117
Alden Optical Labs, Inc. 13295 Broadway Alden, NY 14004	Contour Comfort Contact Lens Co. P.O. Box 1612 Waco, TX 76703
Americal Hydron 210 Crossways Park Drive Woodbury, NY 11797	Danker 393 Front Street Hempstead, NY 11550
American Optical Corporation Soft Contact Lens Division 51 New York Avenue Framingham, MA 01701	Dominion Contact Lens Labs, Ltd. P.O. Box 250, Station N Toronto, Ontario M8V3T7
Bausch & Lomb, Soflens Div. 1400 North Goodman Street Rochester, NY 14602	Dow Corning Ophthalmics 4700 Colley Avenue Norfolk, VA 23501
Breger-Mueller Welt Co. 6922 Hollywood Boulevard Los Angeles, CA 90028	Flexlens, Inc. 5625 North High Street Columbus, OH 43085
Burton, Parsons & Co., Inc. 120 Westhampton Ave. Washington, DC 20027	Frontier Contact Lenses, Inc. 1417 San Marco Boulevard Jacksonville, FL 32207
Calcon Laboratories 3556 Lexington Ave. El Monte, CA 91734	Gordon Contact Lenses, Inc. 180 St. Paul Street Rochester, NY 14604
Capitol Contact Lenses, Inc. 4218 Howard Avenue Kensington, MD 20795	Guaranteed Contact Lens Co. 2139 East Indian School Road Phoenix, AZ 85016
Cooper Laboratories, Inc. 5 Palo Alto Square Palo Alto, CA 94304	Kelvin Lenses, LTD. Kelvin House Denton, Manchester, M342AH England
Conforma Laboratories P.O. Box 624 Norfolk, VA 23501	Kendall Optics 221 Fairmont Avenue Fairmont, WV 26554

(continued)

Table B. Addresses of Sources (continued)

Lombart Lenses, Ltd.
Box 1693
Norfolk, VA 23501

Medicornea
P.O. Box 588
Lebanon, IN 46052

Milton Roy Co.
P.O. Box 1899
Sarasota, FL 33578

Morgan Optics
P.O. Box 806
Dallas, TX 75221

Morrison Laboratories
Green & Division Streets
Harrisburg, PA 17105

Narcissus Medical Foundation
1800 Sullivan Avenue
Daly City, CA 94015

Neele Optical Lab.
811 Scurry Street
Big Springs, TX

Omega Optical Co.
P.O. Box 222233
Dallas, TX 75222

Paris Contact Lens Laboratory
4928 Le Jeune Road
Coral Gables, FL 33146

Plastic Contact Lens Co.
21 Dundas Square
Suite 504
Toronto, Ontario

Precision-Cosmet Co., Inc.
11140 Bren Road West
Minnetonka, MN 55343

Pre-Corneal Lens Co.
P.O. Box 22703
Houston, Texas

Research Services Corporation
5280 Trail Lake Drive
Fort Worth, TX 76133

Rynco Scientific Corporation
31 Stewart Street
Floral Park, NY 11001

Salvatori Ophthalmics, Inc.
P.O. Box 4255
Sarasota, FL 33578

Sauflon International, Inc.
(Heyer-Schulte)
1402 E. Elton Ave
Irvine, CA 92714

Wm. Sohnges
7 Brienner Strasse
Munich, Germany

Soft Lenses, Inc.
8006 Engineer Road
San Diego, CA 92111

Syntex Ophthalmics, Inc.
P.O. Box 10476
Phoenix, AZ 85064

UCO Optics, Inc.
Aquaflex Division
3000 Winton Road, South
Rochester, NY 14623

Wesley-Jessen, Inc.
37 South Wabash Avenue
Chicago, IL 60603

Weicon
P.O. Box 54
Aschaffenburg, Germany

Young Contact Lens Co.
475 Commonwealth Avenue
Boston, Mass 02215

5.21. Vertex Distance Conversion Chart

Minus Lenses 11	12	13	14	15	*Spectacle Lens Correction*	*Plus Lenses* 11	12	13	14	15
4.75	4.75	4.75	4.62	4.62	5.00	5.25	5.25	5.37	5.37	5.37
5.12	5.12	5.12	5.12	5.12	5.50	5.87	5.87	5.87	6.00	6.00
5.62	5.62	5.50	5.50	5.50	6.00	6.37	6.50	6.50	6.50	6.62
6.00	6.00	6.00	6.00	5,87	6.50	7.00	7.00	7.12	7.12	7.25
6.50	6.50	6.37	6.37	6.37	7.00	7.62	7.62	7.75	7.75	7.75
6.87	6.87	6.87	6.75	6.75	7.50	8.12	8.25	8.25	8.37	8.50
7.37	7.25	7.25	7.25	7.25	8.00	8.75	8.87	8.87	9.00	9.12
7.75	7.75	7.62	7.62	7.50	8.50	9.37	9.50	9.50	9.62	9.75
8.25	8.12	8.00	8.00	8.00	9.00	10.00	10.12	10.25	10.37	10.37
8.62	8.50	8.50	8.37	8.37	9.50	10.62	10.75	10.87	11.00	11.12
9.00	8.87	8.87	8.75	8.75	10.00	11.25	11.37	11.50	11.62	11.75
9.37	9.37	9.25	9.12	9.12	10.50	11.87	12.00	12.12	12.25	12.50
9.75	9.75	9.62	9.50	9.50	11.00	12.50	12.75	12.87	13.00	13.12
10.25	10.12	10.00	9.87	9.87	11.50	13.12	13.37	13.50	13.75	13.87
10.62	10.50	10.37	10.25	10.12	12.00	13.87	14.00	14.25	14.50	14.62
11.00	10.87	10.75	10.62	10.50	12.50	14.50	14.75	15.00	15.25	15.37
11.37	11.25	11.12	11.00	10.87	13.00	15.25	15.50	15.62	16.00	16.12
11.75	11.62	11.50	11.37	11.25	13.50	15.87	16.12	16.37	16.62	16.87
12.12	12.00	11.87	11.75	11.50	14.00	16.50	16.75	17.12	17.50	17.75
12.50	12.37	12.25	12.00	11.87	14.50	17.25	17.50	17.87	18.25	18.50
12.87	12.75	12.50	12.37	12.25	15.00	18.00	18.25	18.62	19.00	19.37
13.25	13.00	12.87	12.75	12.62	15.50	18.75	19.00	19.37	19.75	20.25
13.62	13.50	13.25	13.00	12.87	16.00	19.37	19.75	20.25	20.50	21.00
14.00	13.75	13.62	13.50	13.25	16.50	20.25	20.50	21.00	21.50	21.87
14.25	14.12	14.00	13.75	13.50	17.00	21.00	21.50	22.00	22.25	22.87
14.75	14.50	14.25	14.00	13.87	17.50	21.75	22.25	22.75	23.25	23.75
15.00	14.75	14.62	14.37	14.12	18.00	22.50	23.00	23.50	24.00	24.62
15.37	15.12	14.87	14.75	14.50	18.50	23.25	23.75	24.50	25.00	25.62
15.75	15.50	15.25	15.00	14.75	19.00	24.00	24.75	25.25	26.00	26.50
16.37	16.12	15.87	15.37	15.67	20.00	25.62	26.37	27.00	27.75	28.50
17.00	16.75	1.650	16.25	16.00	21.00					
17.75	17.37	17.12	16.75	16.50	22.00					
18.37	18.00	17.75	17.37	17.12	23.00					
19.00	18.62	18.25	18.00	17.62	24.00					
19.62	19.25	18.87	18.50	18.12	25.00					

5.22. Design of Standard Contour Lenses

Table A. Base Curve

Corneal Astigmatism	*Initial Base Curve*
Spherical	On K or 0.25 D flatter
.025 to 1.00	On K or 0.25 D steeper
1.00 to 2.00	0.25 to 0.50 D steeper
> 2.00	1/3 the toricity

Table B. Diameter

Base Curve	*Diameter*
40.0 D	98
41.0 D	96
42.0 D	94
43.0 D	92
44.0 D	90
45.0 D	88
46.0 D	86
47.0 D	85

Add .05 for aperatures over 11.00 mm. Subtract for aperatures under 9.00 mm.

Table C. Optic Zone

Base curve radius minus .7
For pupils over 6.00 mm, add .4 mm.
For pupils under 4.00 mm, subtract .2 mm.

Table D. Intermediate Curve

Optic Zone	*Flatter than Base Curve by (mm)*
7.8	1.6
7.6	1.5
7.4	1.4
7.2	1.4
7.0	1.3
6.8	1.3
6.6	1.2
6.5	1.1

Peripheral curve is 1.2 mm flatter than the intermediate.

5.23. Flourescein Fitting Patterns

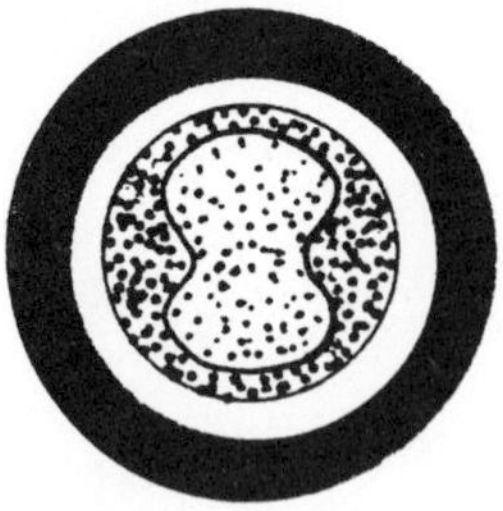

Spherical cornea. Monocurve lens fitted steep.

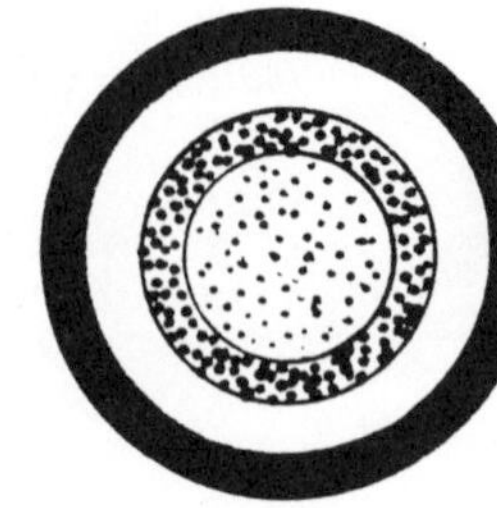

Sperhical cornea. Monocurve lens fitted flat.

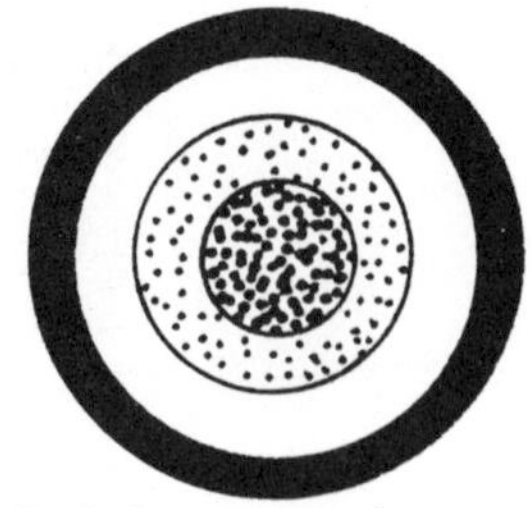

Spherical cornea. Monocurve lens fitted flat. High riding position.

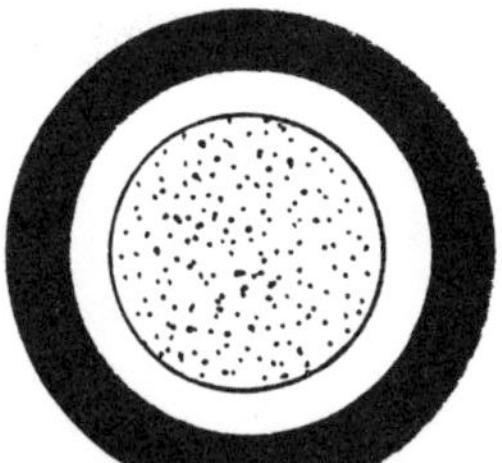

Spherical cornea. Monocurve lens fitted flat. Nasal ridding position.

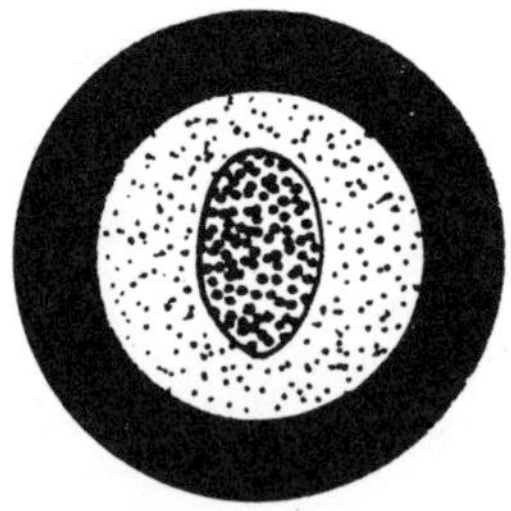

With-the-rule corneal toricity. Monocurve lens fitted slightly steeper than horizontal corneal meridian.

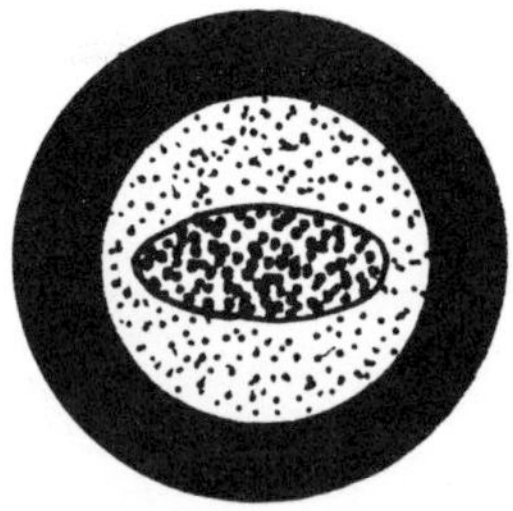

With-the-rule corneal toricity. Monocurve lens fitted slightly flatter than horizontal corneal meridian.

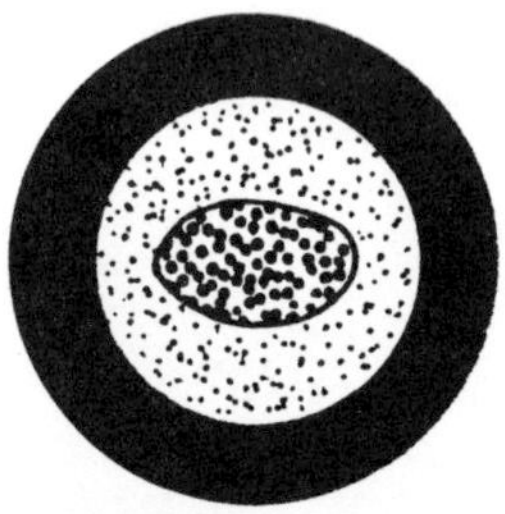

With-the-rule corneal toricity. Monocurve lens fitted much flatter than horizontal corneal meridian.

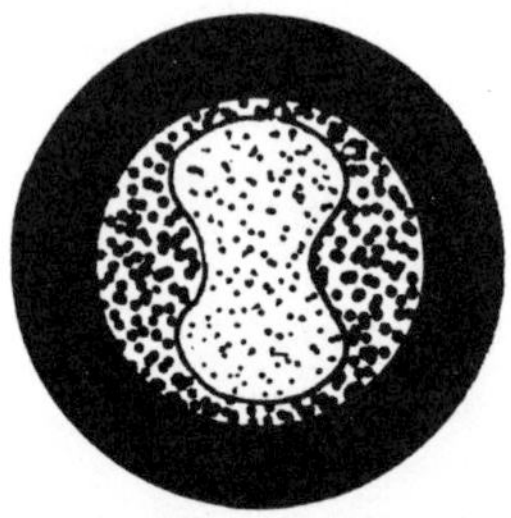

Against-the-rule corneal toricity. Monocurve lens fitted slightly flatter than vertical corneal meridian.

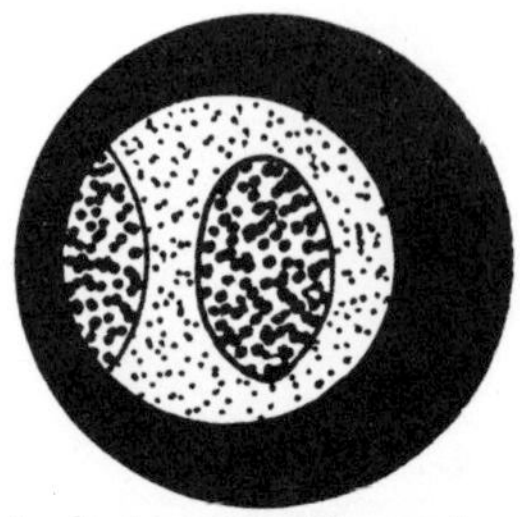

Spherical cornea. Bicurve lens with O.Z. parallel to cornea and P.C. clearance.

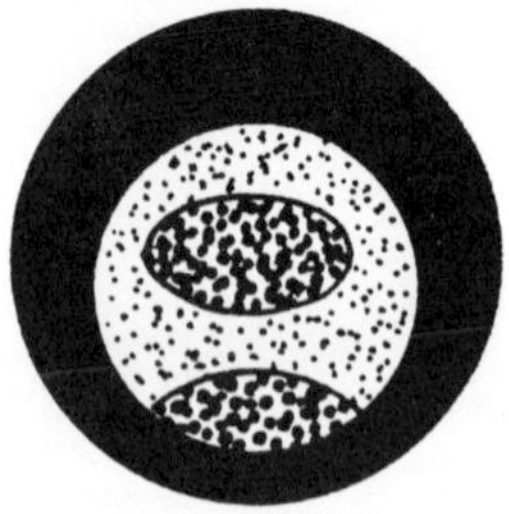

Spherical cornea. Bicurve lens with O.Z. fitted flatter than central cornea.

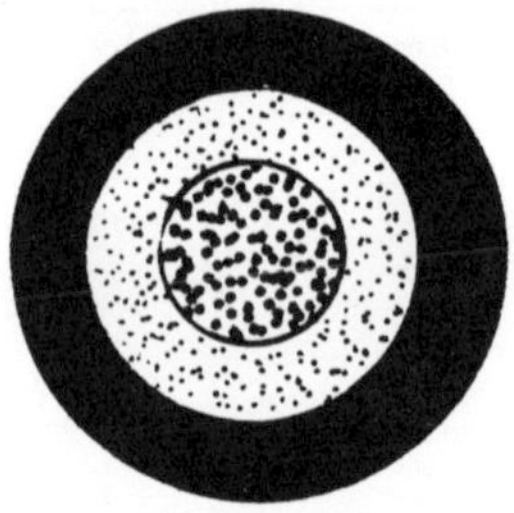

Spherical cornea. Bicurve lens with O.Z. fitted steeper than central cornea.

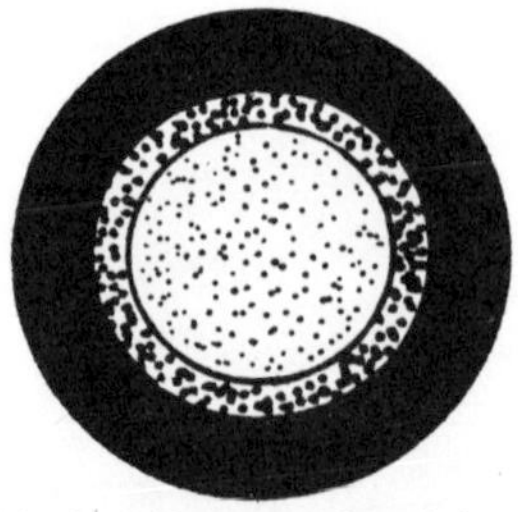

With-the-rule corneal toricity. Bicurve lens with O.Z. fitted slightly steeper than flattest corneal meridian.

Reprinted from Robert Mandell, *Contact Lens Practice*, 2nd Ed. Springfield, Ill.: Chas. C. Thomas, 1974.

5.24. Design of a Minus Carrier Contact Lens

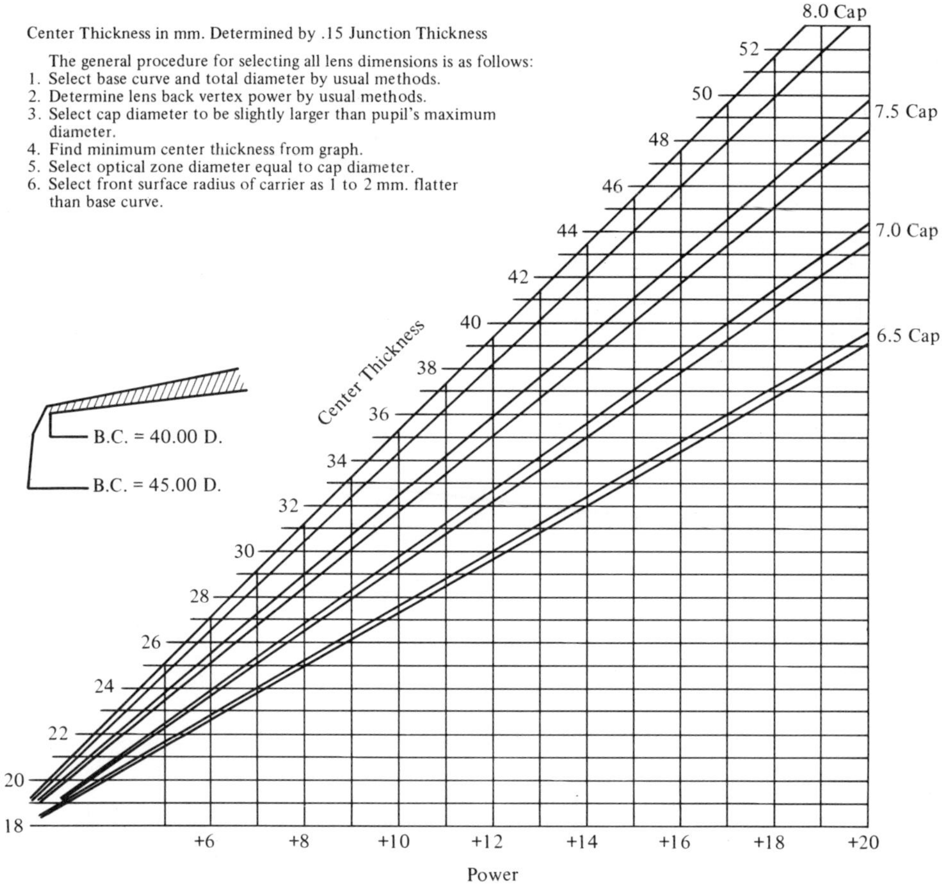

Reprinted by permission from R. B. Mandell, "A method to determine the dimensions of a minus carrier contact lens," *J. Am. Opt. Assoc.* 39: 1968.

5.25. Design of an Inverted Contact Lens Telescope for Unilateral Aphakia

Specifications for the Inverted Telescope

Aphakic minification (percent)	*VD (millimeters)*	*F(+)* (D.S.)*	*F(-)† (D.S.)*
12.3	15.4	8.00	9.12
11.8	15.7	7.50	8.50
11.1	15.8	7.00	7.87
11.2	13.9	8.00	9.00
10.3	15.9	6.50	7.25
10.0	11.1	9.00	10.00
9.7	13.8	7.00	7.75
9.4	15.8	6.00	6.62
8.7	13.4	6.50	7.12
8.7	16.6	5.25	5.75
8.6	10.7	8.00	8.75
8.3	15.1	5.50	6.00
8.1	11.7	7.00	7.62
8.0	13.9	5.75	6.25
7.9	10.9	7.25	7.87
7.7	12.9	6.00	6.50
7.6	16.2	4.62	5.00
7.4	11.9	6.25	6.75
7.2	15.4	4.75	5.12
7.2	14.6	4.87	5.25
7.1	11.0	6.50	7.00
6.9	14.0	5.00	5.37
6.9	10.2	6.75	7.25
6.6	12.7	5.25	5.62
6.7	9.5	7.00	7.50
6.3	11.6	5.50	5.87
6.1	15.7	3.87	4.12
6.0	10.6	5.75	6.12
5.9	14.7	4.00	4.25
5.8	9.8	6.00	6.37
5.7	13.8	4.12	4.37
5.6	9.1	6.25	6.62
5.6	13.1	4.25	4.50

***F(+) is added to the aphakic contact lens correction.**
†F(-) is placed in the spectacle frame.

Reprinted by permission from J. M. Enoch, "A spectacle-contact lens combination used as a reverse galilean telescope in unilateral aphakia," *Am. J. Opt.* 45:1968.

Use of Table

A magnification reduction of 6-8% placed before a unilateral aphakic eye corrected with a contact lens will usually produce fusion.

Assume the patient is refracted at 12 mm and requires +12.50 D. When fit on K with a contact lens, the power needed will be +14.75 D. If one chooses to correct, for example, 6.9% of the residual image size error and the frame is to be worn at 14 mm., the table will give the negative lens necessary to produce this amount of minification.

In the above example, +5.00 is added to the contact lens (+5.00 + 14.75) making a total of +19.75. A −5.37 is incorporated into the spectacle plane.

A rocking pad front and cable (or stiff riding bow) temple are advisable.

5.26. Specialized Fitting Techniques (Korb)

Initial Lens Selection
Base Curve: .15 to .2 mm. flatter than flattest K (single cut)
Diameter: According to corneal size between 8.6 and 9.4 mm.

Table A. Lenticular Flange

Radii Values for the Lenticular Flange Expressed in mm. of Curvature Flatter than the Base Curve of the Lens

L-2 Korb Technique (Lenticular Designs) (Plano to −3.00)

	Plano (.11 CT.)			*−1.00 (.10 CT.)*			*−2.00 (.09 CT.)*			*−3.00 (.08 CT.)*		
	8.2D	*8.6D*	*9.0D*	*8.2D*	*8.6D*	*9.0D*	*8.2D*	*8.6D*	*9.0D*	*8.2D*	*8.6D*	*9.0D*
Base	*7.4L*	*7.8L*	*8.0L*	*7.4L*	*7.8L*	*8.0L*	*7.4L*	*7.8L*	*8.0L*	*7.4L*	*7.8L*	*8.0L*
7.40	3.2	2.6	2.7	2.6	2.2	2.6	2.4	1.7	2.0	2.1	1.5	1.7
7.50	3.1	2.6	2.7	2.6	2.2	2.5	2.4	1.7	2.0	2.0	1.4	1.6
7.60	3.0	2.5	2.6	2.5	2.1	2.4	2.3	1.6	1.9	2.0	1.4	1.6
7.70	2.9	2.4	2.5	2.5	2.0	2.3	2.2	1.5	1.8	1.9	1.3	1.5
7.80	2.8	2.4	2.4	2.4	1.9	2.2	2.2	1.5	1.8	1.8	1.2	1.4
7.90	2.7	2.3	2.3	2.4	1.9	2.0	2.1	1.4	1.7	1.7	1.2	1.3
8.00	2.6	2.2	2.2	2.3	1.8	1.9	2.0	1.4	1.6	1.7	1.2	1.3
8.10	2.6	2.1	2.2	2.3	1.8	1.8	2.0	1.4	1.6	1.7	1.2	1.3
8.20	2.5	2.0	2.1	2.2	1.7	1.7	1.9	1.3	1.5	1.6	1.2	1.2
8.30	2.4	1.9	2.0	2.1	1.6	1.5	1.8	1.2	1.4	1.5	1.2	1.2
8.40	2.4	1.8	1.9	2.0	1.5	1.4	1.8	1.2	1.3	1.5	1.2	1.2
8.50	2.3	1.7	1.8	1.9	1.4	1.3	1.7	1.2	1.2	1.4	1.2	1.2
8.60	2.2	1.6	1.7	1.8	1.3	1.2	1.6	1.2	1.2	1.3	1.2	1.2
8.70	2.1	1.5	1.6	1.8	1.2	1.0	1.5	1.2	1.2	1.2	1.2	1.2

The D refers to diameter, the L to lenticular diameter: i.e. 8.6D = 8.6 mm. diameter, 7.8L = 7.8 lenticular zone.

All lenses have been designed and calculated for an edge thickness of .075 with a maximum deviation of .005 mm. except the following lenses:

8.6 diameters, −2.00 power, 8.50, 8.60, 8.70 bases
8.6 diameters, − 3.00 power, 8.20, 8.30, 8.40, 8.50, 8.60, 8.70 bases
9.0 diameters, −3.00 power, 8.40, 8.50, 8.60, 8.70 bases

The latter lenses have a maximum edge thickness of .09 mm. rather than the preferable .075 mm. This was necessitated by designing an adequate lenticular flange which would support the lens high on the cornea.

Prism tolerance – no prism tolerance is allowed to −2.00 diopters. Over −2.25 diopters to −4.00 diopters, 1/8th of a prism diopter tolerance is permitted. Above −4.00 diopters of power, some flexibility and tolerance is permitted up to an absolute maximum of 1/4th of a diopter of prism.

Over −3.00 in power, flatten the lenticular radius .15 mm. for each additional diopter of minus power.

Table B. Lenticular Thickness

Thicknesses:		*Lenticular*					*Plus*		
Plus Lens Power		*Outside Lenticular Optical Zone* 6.8	*7.0*	*7.2*	*7.4*	*7.6*	*7.8*	*8.0*	*8.2*
+ .75 – 1.87		14	14	14	14	15	16	16	16
2.00 – 2.37		14	14	14	14	15	17	17	17
2.50 – 2.87		14	14	15	15	16	17	17	17
3.00 – 3.37		15	15	16	16	17	17	18	18
3.50 – 3.87		16	16	17	17	18	18	19	19
4.00 – 4.87		17	17	18	19	20	20	20	21
5.00 – 5.37	I	18	19	19	20	21	21	22	22
5.50 – 5.87		18	19	19	21	22	23	23	23
6.00 – 6.37		19	20	20	22	23	23	24	25
6.50 – 6.87		20	20	21	23	24	24	25	26
7.00 – 7.37		21	21	23	24	25	25	26	27
7.50 – 7.87		21	22	24	25	25	26	27	28
8.00 – 8.37		22	24	25	26	26	27	28	30
8.50 – 8.87		23	24	25	26	27	28	29	31
9.00 – 9.37		24	25	26	27	28	29	30	32
9.50 – 9.87		25	26	27	28	29	30	31	33
10.00 – 10.37	II	26	27	28	29	30	32	33	35
10.50 – 10.87		26	27	28	29	31	33	34	36
11.00 – 11.37		27	28	29	30	32	34	36	37
11.50 – 11.87		28	29	30	31	33	35	36	38
12.00 – 12.37		29	30	31	32	35	36	37	39
12.50 – 12.87		30	31	32	33	36	37	38	40
13.00 – 13.37		31	32	34	35	37	38	40	41
13.50 – 13.87		31	33	34	36	37	39	41	42
14.00 – 14.37		32	34	35	37	38	40	42	44
14.50 – 14.87		33	34	36	38	39	41	43	45
15.00 – 15.37		34	35	37	39	40	42	44	46
15.50 – 15.87		34	36	38	40	41	43	45	47
16.00 – 16.37	III	35	37	39	41	42	44	46	49
16.50 – 16.87		35	37	39	41	43	45	47	50
17.00 – 17.37		36	38	40	42	44	46	48	51
17.50 – 17.87		37	39	41	43	45	47	49	52
18.00 – 18.37		38	40	42	44	46	48	50	53
18.50 – 18.87		38	40	42	44	46	49	51	54
19.00 – 19.37		39	41	43	45	47	50	52	54
19.50 – 19.87		40	41	44	46	48	51	53	56
20.00 – 20.50		40	42	45	47	49	52	54	58

Lenses in Group I are calculated for a .12 carrier thickness.
Lenses in Group II are calculated for a .13 carrier thickness.
Lenses in Group III are calculated for a .14 carrier thickness.

Table C. Lenticular Designs

	Diam.	O.Z.	R2	Blend	Edge	Plano to −2.50 D	C	−2.75 to −6.00 D	C	+.25 to +4.00 D	C	+4.25 to +7.00 D	C	+7.25 up D	C
	9.8	8.2	1.4	.7	4/12	8.2	1.5	8.6	1.5	8.2	2.0	8.2	2.0	8.2	2.2
	9.6	8.0	1.4	.7	4/12	8.2	1.5	8.4	1.5	8.2	2.0	8.2	2.0	8.2	2.2
	9.4	7.8	1.4	.7	3/12	8.0	1.6	8.2	1.5	8.0	2.0	7.8	2.0	7.8	2.2
	9.2	7.6	1.4	.7	3/12	8.0	1.6	8.2	1.5	8.0	2.0	7.8	2.0	7.8	2.2
I	9.0	7.5	1.4	.7	3/12	7.8	1.7	8.0	1.5	7.6	1.8	7.5	1.8	7.5	2.0
	8.8	7.4	1.4	.7	2/12	7.8	1.7	7.8	1.5	7.6	1.8	7.5	1.8	7.5	2.0
II	8.6	7.2	1.5	.8	2/12	7.6	1.7	7.6	1.5	7.4	1.8	7.3	2.0	7.2	2.2
	8.4	7.0	1.9	.9	2/12	7.4	1.9	7.4	1.5	7.2	2.0	7.1	2.0	7.0	2.2
III	8.2	6.8	2.3	1.0	1/12	7.2	2.0	7.2	1.7	7.0	2.0	6.9	2.0	6.9	2.5
	8.0	6.7	2.4	1.0	1/12	7.0	2.0	7.2	1.7	7.0	2.0	6.9	2.0	6.9	2.5
	7.8	6.5	2.4	1.0	1/12	6.8	2.0	6.8	1.7	6.8	2.2	6.6	2.5	6.5	2.5
	7.6	6.3	2.4	1.0	1/12	6.6	2.0	6.6	1.7	6.6	2.2	6.4	2.5	6.3	2.5

R2 = posterior peripheral curve.
C = anterior carrier radius above curves and blend expressed as mm. flatter than base curve.

Table D. Single Cut Thicknesses

Single Cut Plus Lens

Plus Power (Back Vertex)	6.5 mm.	7.0 mm.	7.5 mm.	8.0 mm.	8.5 mm.	9.0 mm.	9.5 mm.
+20.00 to +20.75	.40	.45	.51	.58	.65	.72	.84
+19.00 to +19.75	.38	.43	.50	.56	.63	.70	.81
+18.00 to +18.75	.37	.42	.48	.54	.60	.68	.78
+17.00 to +17.75	.36	.41	.46	.52	.58	.65	.75
+16.00 to +16.75	.35	.40	.45	.50	.56	.63	.72
+15.00 to +15.75	.34	.38	.43	.48	.53	.60	.68
+14.00 to +14.75	.32	.36	.41	.46	.51	.57	.64
+13.00 to +13.75	.31	.35	.39	.44	.49	.55	.61
+12.00 to +12.75	.30	.34	.38	.42	.47	.52	.58
+11.00 to +11.75	.28	.32	.36	.40	.44	.49	.55
+10.00 to +10.75	.27	.31	.35	.38	.42	.46	.52
+ 9.00 to + 9.75	.26	.29	.33	.36	.39	.44	.49
+ 8.00 to + 8.75	.25	.28	.31	.34	.37	.41	.46
+ 7.00 to + 7.75	.24	.27	.30	.32	.35	.39	.43
+ 6.00 to + 6.75	.23	.25	.28	.30	.33	.36	.39
+ 5.00 to + 5.75	.21	.24	.26	.28	.30	.33	.37
+ 4.00 to + 4.75	.20	.22	.24	.26	.28	.31	.34
+ 3.00 to + 3.75	.18	.20	.22	.24	.26	.28	.31
+ 2.00 to + 2.75	.17	.19	.21	.22	.24	.26	.28
+ 1.00 to + 1.75	.16	.17	.19	.20	.22	.23	.25
0 to + .75	.16	.16	.17	.18	.19	.21	.22

Table E. S-2 Korb Technique (Single Cut Designs)
Plano to –6.00 Minus Thickness

	Plano				*–1.00*				*–2.00*			
Base	*8.2*	*8.6*	*9.0*	*9.4*	*8.2*	*8.6*	*9.0*	*9.4*	*8.2*	*8.6*	*9.0*	*9.4*
7.40 . . .	–17	–18	–19	–21	–15	–14	–17	–18	–13	–13	–14	–15
7.50 . . .	–17	–18	–19	–20	–15	–14	–17	–18	–13	–13	–14	–15
7.60 . . .	–17	–17	–18	–19	–14	–14	–16	–17	–12	–12	–13	–14
7.70 . . .	–16	–17	–17	–18	–14	–14	–16	–17	–12	–12	–13	–14
7.80 . . .	–16	–16	–17	–18	–14	–14	–16	–17	–12	12	–13	–14
7.90 . . .	–15	–16	–16	–17	–13	–14	–15	–16	–11	12	–12	14
8.00 . . .	–15	–16	–16	–16	–13	–13	–15	–16	–11	12	–12	13
8.10 . . .	–15	–16	–16	–16	–13	–13	–14	–15	–11	11	–12	13
8.20 . . .	–15	–16	–16	–16	–13	–13	–13	–15	11	11	12	12
8.30 . . .	–14	–16	–16	–16	–12	–12	–13	–14	11	11	12	12
8.40 . . .	–14	–15	–15	–15	–12	–12	–12	–13	11	10	11	11
8.50 . . .	–13	–15	–15	–15	–11	–11	–12	–12	10	10	11	11
8.60 . . .	–13	–14	–14	–15	–11	–11	–11	–11	10	10+	10	10
8.70 . . .	–13	–14	–14	–15	–11	–11	–11	–11	10	10+	10	10

	–3.00				*–4.00*			
	8.2	*8.6*	*9.0*	*9.4*	*8.2*	*8.6*	*9.0*	*9.4*
7.40 . . .	–11	–12	–12	–13	–08	–08	–09	–09
7.50 . . .	–11	–11	–12	–13	–08	–08	–08	–09
7.60 . . .	–11	–10	–11	–12	–08	08	–08	–09
7.70 . . .	–10	–09	–10	12	08	08+	08	–08
7.80 . . .	–10	–09	–10	12	08	08+	08	08
7.90 . . .	–10	09	10	11	08	08+	08	08
8.00 . . .	10	09	10	10	08	08+	08+	08
8.10 . . .	10	09	10	10	08	08+	08+	08
8.20 . . .	10	09	09	10	08	08+	08+	08
8.30 . . .	09	08	09	09	07	07+	07+	07+
8.40 . . .	09	08	09	09	07	07+	07+	07+
8.50 . . .	09	08	08	09	07	07+	07+	07+
8.60 . . .	09+	08+	08	09	07	07+	07++	07++
8.70 . . .	09+	08+	08	09	07	07+	07++	07++

	–5.00				*–6.00*			
	8.2	*8.6*	*9.0*	*9.4*	*8.2*	*8.6*	*9.0*	*9.4*
7.40 . . .	–07	–07	–07	–07	06	06	06	06+
7.50 . . .	–07	07	07	07	06	06+	06+	06+
7.60 . . .	07	07+	07	07	06	06+	06++	06++
7.70 . . .	07+	07++	07+	06+	06+	06++	06++	06++
7.80 . . .	07+	07++	07++	07++	06+	06++	06++	06++
7.90 . . .	07+	07++	07++	07++	06+	06++	06++	06++
8.00 . . .	07+	07++	07++	07++	06+	06++	06++	06++
8.10 . . .	07+	07++	07++	07++	06+	06++	L	L
8.20 . . .	07+	07++	07++	07++	06++	06++	L	L
8.30 . . .	07++	07++	07++	06++	06++	06++	L	L
8.40 . . .	07++	07++	06++	06++	L	L	L	L
8.50 . . .	07++	07++	06++	06++	L	L	L	L
8.60 . . .	07++	07++	06++	L++	L	L	L	L
8.70 . . .	07++	07++	06++	L++	L	L	L	L

l.c.: —11 = .05 edge plus or minus .005 mm.
l.c.: 11 = .06 edge plus or minus .005 mm.
l.c.: 11+ = .07 edge plus or minus .005 mm.
l.c.: 11++ = .08 edge plus or minus .005 mm.
l.c.: L = lenticular required.

Courtesy Dr. D. R. Korb, Boston, Mass.

5.27. Specialized Fitting Techniques (Bayshore)

Diameter = .2 smaller than the palpebral aperture.

Base Curve:

Optical Zone	*Base Curve is steeper than K by*
5.6	.65 mm.
5.8	.5
6.0	.4
6.2	.35
6.4	.3
6.5	.3
6.6	.25
	For toric corneas deduct an additional 1/3 the difference between meridians.

Intermediate curves are from 1.0 mm. to 1.5 mm. flatter than the base curve. Peripheral curve is about .2 mm. wide with a radius of 17 mm.

5.28. Specialized Fitting Techniques (Ultrathin)

Table A.

Keratometry/Astigmatism	*Base Curve*
0 to 0.50 ΔK	on K
0.75D to 1.00D ΔK	0.25 D. steeper than K
1.25D to 2.00D ΔK	0.50 D. steeper than K
Greater than 2.00D ΔK	1/3 ΔK

Table B.

Base Curve	*Diameter*	*Peripheral Width*	*Curve O.Z.*
Steeper than 45.00 D	8.0	0.3	7.0
44.00 to 45.00 D	8.1	0.35	7.0
42.00 to 43.75 D	8.2	0.4	7.0
Flatter than 42.00	8.3	0.4	7.1

Thicknesses: .07 to .11 mm.

Reprinted by permission from C. Moore, " A new concept for fitting ultrathin lenses." ***Int. Contact Lens Clinic*** **1:1974. Courtesy Con-Cise Contact Lens Co., San Leandro, Cal.**

5.29. Specialized Fitting Techniques (Dyer)

Table A. Base Curve

Primary Curve* in diopters	Base Curve in diopters corresponding to primary curve (40.00 D to 48.00 D) according to degree of astigmatism			
	0-.50 D	*.62-1.00 D*	*1.25-2.00 D*	*2.25-3.00 D*
40.00	40.25	40.50	40.75	41.00
40.25	40.50	40.75	41.00	41.25
40.50	40.75	41.00	41.25	41.50
40.75	41.00	41.25	41.50	41.75
41.00	41.25	41.50	41.75	42.00
41.25	41.50	41.75	42.00	42.25
41.50	41.75	42.00	42.25	42.50
41.75	42.00	42.25	42.50	42.75
42.00	42.25	42.50	42.75	43.00
42.25	42.50	42.75	43.00	43.25
42.50	42.75	43.00	43.25	43.50
42.75	43.00	43.25	43.50	43.75
43.00	43.25	43.50	43.75	44.00
43.25	43.50	43.75	44.00	44.25
43.50	43.75	44.00	44.25	44.50
43.75	44.00	44.25	44.50	44.75
44.00	44.25	44.50	44.75	45.00
44.25	44.50	44.75	45.00	45.25
44.50	44.75	45.00	45.25	45.50
44.75	45.00	45.25	45.50	45.75
45.00	45.25	45.50	45.75	46.00
45.25	45.50	45.75	46.00	46.25
45.50	45.75	46.00	46.25	46.50
45.75	46.00	46.25	46.50	46.75
46.00	46.25	46.50	46.75	47.00
46.25	46.50	46.75	47.00	47.25
46.50	46.75	47.00	47.25	47.50
46.75	47.00	47.25	47.50	47.75
47.00	47.25	47.50	47.75	48.00
47.25	47.50	47.75	48.00	48.25
47.50	47.75	48.00	48.25	48.50
47.75	48.00	48.25	48.50	48.75
48.00	48.25	48.50	48.75	49.00

Advise 1/3 of corneal astigmatism or toric contact lenses on 3.25 D of astigmatism and up

***If primary curve is a 0.12 D reading, use next steeper curvature.**

Table B. Corresponding Characteristics

Base Curve	*Diameter*	*O.Z.*	*I.P.C.*	*P.P.C.*
40.00 40.25	9.2	7.6	.2/36.50 .3/32.50	.3/27.50
40.50 40.75	9.1	7.5	.2/37.00 .3/33.00	.3/27.50
41.00 41.25	9.0	7.4	.2/37.50 .3/33.50	.3/27.50
41.50 41.75	8.9	7.3	.2/38.00 .3/34.00	.3/27.50
42.00 42.25	8.8	7.3	.2/38.50 .25/34.50	.3/27.50
42.50 42.75	8.7	7.3	.2/39.00 .2/35.00	.3/29.00
43.00 43.25	8.6	7.2	.2/39.00 .2/35.50	.3/29.00
43.50 43.75	8.5	7.1	.2/40.00 .2/36.00	.3/29.00
44.00 44.25	8.4	7.0	.2/40.50 .2/36.50	.3/30.00
44.50 44.75	8.3	6.9	.2/41.00 .2/37.00	.3/30.00
45.00 45.25	8.2	6.8	.2/41.50 .2/37.50	.3/31.00
45.50 45.75	8.1	6.7	.2/42.00 .2/38.00	.3/31.00
46.00 46.25	8.0	6.7	.15/42.50 .2/38.50	.3/33.00
46.50 46.75	7.9	6.7	.1/43.00 .2/39.00	.3/33.00
47.00 47.25	7.9	6.7	.1/43.50 .2/39.50	.3/33.00
47.50 47.75	7.9	6.7	.1/44.00 .2/40.00	.3/33.00
48.00 48.25	7.9	6.7	.1/44.50 .2/40.50	.3/33.00
48.50 48.75	7.9	6.7	.1/45.00 .2/41.00	.3/33.00
49.00 49.25	7.8	6.6	.1/45.50 .2/41.50	.3/35.00
49.50 49.75	7.8	6.6	.1/46.00 .2/42.00	.3/35.00
50.00 50.25	7.8	6.6	.1/46.50 .2/42.50	.3/35.00

5.30. Specialized Fitting Techniques (Aspheric Single Vision, Initial Lens Selection)

Table A. Diameter, Base Curve

Company: Name	*Average Diameter*	*Base Curve*
W/J: Dynacurve	8.2 mm	.37 D steeper than the flattest K
Compucon	B.C. + .6 mm	Apex is 1.25 D steeper than the flattest K
Neefe	Ave. 8.8 mm	Under 1.0 D cyl 1/4 D steeper Over 1.0 D cyl 1/2 the cyl.
Conforma: Ellip-see-con*	B.C. + 1.2 mm	Under 1.0 D .5 steeper than K Add .25 steeper each 1.25 D astigmatism
Milton Roy: Con-o-coid	B.C. + 1.0 mm	K + 1.75 D steeper
Wohlk:Parabolar	Corneal Diameter −2.25 mm Ave 9.0 mm	.1 mm flatter than K + steeper by 1/3 the astigmatism
Kelvin:Continuous curve*	9.4 to 9.7	standard: .05 mm steeper than K 4 edge lifts .05 to .2 av .1
	8.8 to 9.2	thin: .1 mm steeper than K 1 edge lift .15

*spherical at the apex

Table B. Spherical Equivalents for the Correction of Residual Astigmatism with Aspheric Anterior Surfaces

Cylinder	*Equivalent*
.50	.50
.75	.62
1.00	.75
1.25	.87
1.50	1.00
1.75	1.12
2.00	1.25

5.31. Specialized Fitting Techniques (Gas-Permeable Lenses)

Boston
Silicon Polymer
Base Curve: 0.5 steeper than K. Up to 1.50 D in astigmatism
Diameter: 8.5 to 9.0 single cut

Danker Labs
Meso (Cab)
Base Curve: 1.0 cyl, 1/2 steeper than K
1.0 cyl, 1/2 difference between meridians

Diameter: Add to radii:

42.75 or less	1.2
43.00 to 44.25	1.3
44.50 to 45.75	1.4
over 46.00	1.5

For aphakic power add an additional 0.5

Hydrocurve
Cabcurve (Porofocon B)
Base Curve:

41.00 to 42.75	steeper than PMMA design by .25 D
43.00 to 44.75	steeper than PMMA design by .50 D
45.00 to 45.75	steeper than PMMA design by .75 D

Diameter: 1.0 to 1.5 mm larger than the radius

Available Powers: Plano to −8.00
Radii: 7.18 to 8.23
Diameters: 8.8, 9.2, 9.6
Available Powers: +11.00 to +16.00
Radii 7.67 to 8.23 mm
Diameter 9.2 mm

Rynco
R_x56(Porofocon A)
Base Curve: 1/3 the difference between meridians

Diameter

40.25 to 43.00	9.4
43.25 to 45.50	9.2
45.75 to 48.00	9.0

Memlite: A thin R 56 (trial fit)
Available −1.00 to −6.00; Diameters 8.7 to 9.4

R_x56-TA: A thin aphakic fit as R_x56
Available: over +6.00; Diameter 9.5; Oz=7.50 mm

Syntex
Polycon (Silafocon) Silicon Methyl Methacrylate
Availabilities given are inventory

Diameter: 8.5 mm; Base Curve on K; Powers Available—plano to −8.00
Radii – 7.10 to 8.35; Optic Zone = 7.0 mm

Diameter: 9.5 Standard

> 1.50 cyl	.10 mm flatter
< 1.50 cyl	.05 flatter

Radii available: 7.20 to 8.6, Optic Zone 8.4
Powers available: Plano to −20.00

Diameter: 9.5 Aphakic

Radii available: 7.40 to 8.50 mm, Optic Zone 8.4 mm
Powers available: +20.00 to −20.00

Diameter: 10.0 Aphakic

Radii available: 7.60 to 8.65 mm, Optic Zone 8.6 mm
Powers available: +8.25 to +20.00

(continued)

Wohlk
Hartflex CAB
Diameter: 8.5 to 10.5 mm (.5 mm steps)
Base Curve: as Pmm Δ

Silflex (Silicone rubber)
Diameter: 11.7 to 13.2 mm (in .5 mm steps)
Base Curve: 0.2 to 0.4 mm flatter than K
Optic Zone: 8.00 mm

5.32. Specialized Fitting Techniques (Keratoconus: Hard, Corneal Lenses)

	Base Curve	*Diameter*	*O.Z.*	
Erwin H. Voss	Central touch with bearing	8.0 to 8.5		Fenestrations at edge of O.Z.
Maurice Poster	Apical clearance	Small as possible	From trial lens	Barely clears central area of cone (By trial lenses)
K.G. Hall	Central clearance	9.5 to 11.8 average 10.0	1 to 2 mm smaller than diameter	Maximum bearing
F.J.E. Sellers	Minimum apical clearance, about .1 mm steeper	About 9.0	6 to 7 mm	Fenestrates on occasion uses 4.0 to 6.0 mm diam. test lenses
Chiquiar-Arias	Apical touch with 2 supporting areas	For central cones 8.0 to 8.8. For eccentric cones to 10.0	4 to 5 mm	In some cases uses CA rings.
Donald A. Fonda	3 to 4 mm apical touch by trial lenses	<9.2	>7.0	In early cases may be .2 mm flat
R.A. Reynolds	2 mm apical feather touch by trial lenses	8.1 to 9.1	2.6 mm less than diam.	Nipple cones = 5.5 mm O.Z.

Reprinted from A.R. Reinke, Keratoconus: A review of research and current fitting techniques, *Int. Contact Lens Clinic,* Vol 2, #4 pp. 70-92 with the permission of the Professional Press, Inc., 101 East Ontario Street, Chicago, Illinois, 60611, U.S.A.

5.33. Specialized Fitting Techniques (Multifocals)

		Diagram Key
Nonconcentric		
Fused		
Base curve	*See* Table 5.38	1, 2, 3, 4
Diameter	9.3 to 9.8 mm truncated .4 to .6	
Optic zone	1.2 mm less than vertical diameter	
Seg. height	.2 to .3 mm into pupil	
Cut (front)		
Base curve	*See* Table 5.38	5, 6, 7, 8, 10*
Diameter	ca 9.65 Truncation .5	
Optic zone	ca. 7.8	
Seg. height	4 to 4.5 widths 8.0 to 8.5	
Prism	*See* Table 5.38	
Thickness	*See* Table 5.3	
Concentrics		
Front cut (Bicon)		
Base curve	.25 to .75 D flatter than K	11
Diameter	9.0 to 9.5 or .4 larger than SV	
Optic Zone	7.5 to 8.0	
DV Zone	*See* Table 5.2	
Peripheral curves	1.4 mm wide	
Add +.05 to standard thickness also −0.25 to DV and +0.50 to add		
Back Surface Concentric		
De Carle		15
Base curve	on K to .3 steeper (this the NV R_X)	
Diameter	9.0 to 10.5	
Optic Zone	8.0 mm	
DV Zone	.3 determined by add	
NV Zone	1.5 to 3.5 mm	
Can also be fit according to alternating vision principles. Base curve would then be on K and the DV zone enlarged to 5.0 mm.		
Moss-Arner (Optical Periphery)		11
Base curve	.15 steeper than K. Int. curve is the add	
Diameter	9.4 to 9.7	
Optic Zone		
DV Zone	1.0 to 1.5 over pupil size in ordinary room light Better for smaller pupils	
Front fused (reverse centrad)		9
Base curve	same as SV but centration required	
Optic zone	1.4 less than D always > 7.00 mm	
NV seg.	.1 to .2 smaller than pupil in bright illumination (2.2–3.0)	
Thickness	Plano = .18; see Table 5.1	
Segless		
Micropupil (Soehnges)	Graduated zones on front surface	13
Base curve	As SV	
Diameter	½ mm over SV, about 10.0	
DV zone	About 5 mm or pupil size in ordinary illumination	
Power	+100 over subjective NV	
Multirange	stenopaic slits in a 1.5 mm wedge	17
Aspherics	*See* Table 5.34	19

*No. 12 is a back seg design.

(continued)

	Diagram Key
Miscellaneous	
Sliding 4 to 5 mm by 9-11 horizontally. Fits below the pupil and steeper than K	14
Additive Back surface is .1 to 2 flatter than front surface of SV. 1/3 to 1/2 the overall size of the lens. Thickness .1 to .15 occasionally 1–2 Δ base down. Power is +0.50 over subjective.	20
Trifocal Trifocal segment .5 mm higher than bifocal seg. All other parameters as usual.	16
Pinhole 1 to 2.0 mm aperture	18

(continued)

5.33. Specialized Fitting Techniques (Multifocals) (continued)

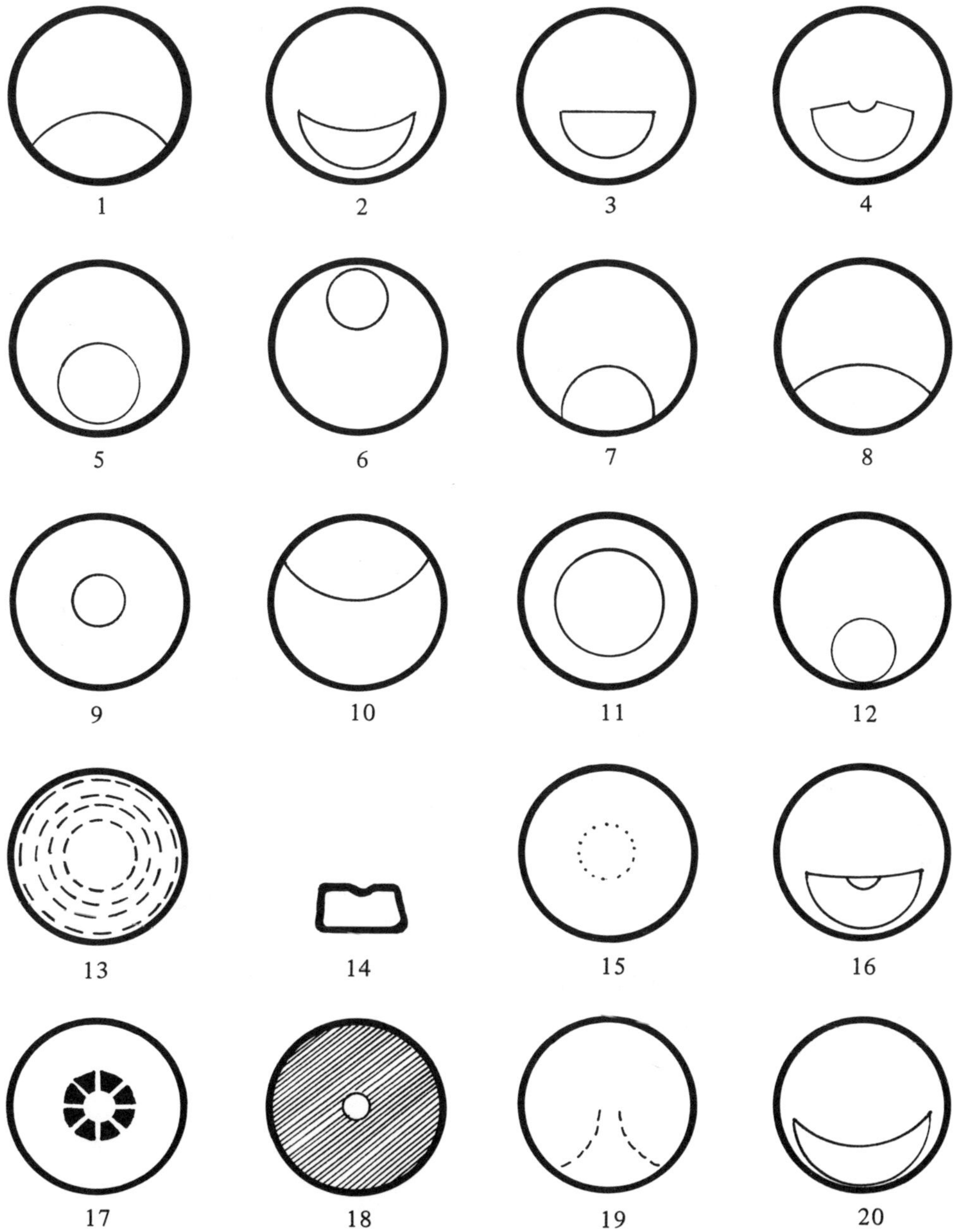

5.34. Specialized Fitting Techniques (Aspheric Multifocals)

Manufacturer/Lens	*Diam*	*Base Curve*
Conforma VFL	8.7	Steeper by 1/2 cyl + 1/2 D
Precision Cosmet[1] Varirange F	as SV	as SV
Neefe	8.8	Apex is 3 D steeper. Eccentricity varies from Apex to Edge.
Palco Palsite	9.0	Ave K + 2 D
Compucon Presbycon	B.C + .6	Base curve is peripheral area about 1.5 D flatter than K
W/J Autofocal		From P.E.K.
Contour Comfort Limitless	as SV	as SV
Breger Presbiflex	8.8 to 9.2	Apex is spherical. Peripheral area has eccentricity of .50 to .60.

[1] Add is on the front

5.35. Specialized Fitting Techniques (Orthokeratology)

	Base Curve diopters	*Base Curve* mm	*Power*	*Size*	*O.Z.*	*Peripheral curves*	*Thickness*
Ziff	44.50	7.58	−1.50	8.2	7.2	9.00/.2 11.50/.3	.009
May-Grant	44.50	7.58	−1.50	8.9	7.6	8.60/.3 9.10/.3	.007
Nolan	43.00	7.84	Plano	9.5 (approx.)	8.0	8.00/.4 12.25/.3	.008
Gates	43.50	7.75	− .50	8.7	7.3	14.00/.4	.008
Paige	44.0	7.67	−0.75	8.6	7.8		
Fontana (One-piece lathe-cut bifocal)	44.0		−1.00	9.6	6.0	7.50 1.0 10.00 .3 13.50 .5	

Theoretical Data: K = 45.00 × 46.00 R_x = −2.00

5.36 Specialized Fitting Techniques (Toric Base Curves, Hard)

Base Curve

Corneal Astigmatism		*Flatter Base Curve Meridian*
Between	2.00 D and 3.00	.025 D Steeper than k
	3.00 D and 5.00	.050 D Steeper than k
	5.00 D and 7.00	.075 D Steeper than k
	7.00 D and Up	1.00 D Steeper than k

STEEPER BASE CURVE MERIDIAN: Add 1/2 the difference between this and the corneal secondary meridian.

LENS SIZE AND OPTIC ZONE: See table 5.22: use the flatter base as a basis.

The front surface cylinder is a plus cylinder, one half the toroidal base curve cylinder with its axis along the flatter base curve.

5.37. Specialized Fitting Techniques (Aphakia)

Initial Lens Selection

Base curve	*Diameter*	*Secondary Curve*	*Peripheral Curve*	
Lenticular				
Flattest K +0.25 steeper for each diopter of astigmatism.	1.4 mm. larger than the base curve.	.9 mm. flatter than the base curve. .4 mm. wide.	3 mm. flatter than the base curve. .4 mm. wide.	Edge thickness approx. .12 mm. Flange radius 1.5 mm. flatter than the base curve. For central thicknesses see Table 89.
Single Cut				
Flattest K +0.25 steeper for each diopter of astigmatism.	.5 mm. larger than the base curve.		2.5 mm. flatter than the base curve. .4 wide blended to .5 mm.	For central thicknesses see Table 72.
Thin-Small Single Cut (After Welsh)				
Approximately .25 D steeper than k.	Approximately the same as the base curve.		12.25 mm. .3 wide blended to .4 mm.	For central thicknesses see Table 71.
Small Lenticular (After Polse)				
Approximately .25 D steeper than K.	Approximately 1.0 mm. larger than the base curve.	.8 mm. flatter than the base curve. .4 mm. wide.	3 mm. flatter than the base curve. .4 mm. wide.	Edge thickness .18 to .22 mm. Flange radius 1.8 mm. flatter than the base curve. Optic cap 6.5 to 7.5 mm depending on pupil size. For central thickness see Table 89. Deduct approximately .4 mm.

5.38. Specialized Fitting Techniques (Prism Ballast)

Table A. Base Curve

Amount of Corneal Toricity	*Base Curve Required*
Spherical to 0.50 D	Plano to 0.12 flatter than K
0.62 D to 1.50 D	On K
1.62 D to 3.37 D	One-third of the difference between K readings steeper
3.50 D and over	Consider toric base curve and delete prism

Table B. Optical Zone

Vertical Diameter of Lens	*Optical Zone Dimension*
8.0 mm	7.2 mm
8.2 mm	7.3 mm
8.4 mm	7.4 mm
8.6 mm	7.5 mm
8.8 mm	7.6 mm
9.0 mm	7.7 mm
9.2 mm	7.8 mm
9.4 mm+	7.9 mm

Table C. Prism

Power	*Prism Diopters Needed*
−8.00 D and over	2.50
−4.00 D to −7.87 D	2.25
−2.00 D to −3.87 D	2.00
Plano to −1.87 D	1.75
−2.00 D to −3.87 D	1.50
−4.00 D to −6.12 D	1.25
−6.25 D to −7.87 D	1.00
−8.00 D and over	0.75

Added Thickness: see Table 5.5 C

The usual amount of rotation, 15 degrees, yields a base-apex line along the 105-degree axis of the right eye and the 75-degree axis of the left.

Truncation: About .3 mm for plus lenses and .2 mm minus.

Overrefraction with a spherical diagnostic lens is recommended for determining the cylindrical component.

5.39. Specialized Fitting Techniques (Toric Peripheries)

Corneal Astigmatism	*Difference Between Meridians of the Peripheral Curve*
2.00 to 3.00 D	.4 mm
3.00 to 5.00 D	.7 mm
over 5.00 D	1.0 mm

The base curve should be .05 to .10 mm steeper than the best fitting spherical lens and the diameter about .5 mm larger.

5.40 Specialized Fitting Techniques (Hydrophilics)

Table A. Modifications to Standard Fitting Increments for Steep/Flat Radii

	Actual Radius				
Change in	7.0	7.3	7.7	8.1	8.4
Increment	+ 0.2	+ 0.1	0.0	– 0.1	– 0.2

Table B. Modifications to Standard Fitting Increment when Changing Diameter

	Change in Diameter			
Change in	∓ 0.5	∓ 1.0	∓ 1.5	∓ 2.0
Radius	∓ 0.2	∓ 0.5	∓ 0.8	∓ 1.2

Table C. Modifications to Overrefraction Findings: Aphakia

Overrefraction	*Minimum Amount Added to Overrefraction*
– 1.00 D	Add approximately – 0.25 D
– 1.25 to – 2.00 D	Add approximately – 0.50 D
– 2.25 to – 5.00 D	Add approximately – 0.75 D
+ 1.00 D	Add approximately + 0.25 D
+ 1.25 to + 2.00 D	Add approximately + 0.50 D
+ 2.25 to + 5.00 D	Add approximately + 0.75 D

For initial trial lens, see manufacturers' recommended fitting increments, Table # 5.49.

5.41. Specialized Fitting Techniques (Silicones)

Wohlk (Silflex)				
	Base Curve:	Flatter than K by:	*Radii*	*Increment*
			7.1 to 7.6	.40
			7.7 to 8.4	.30
			over 8.4	.20
	Diameter:	0.7 mm larger than horizontal iris diameter		
Danker				
	Base Curve:	Flatter than K for radii longer than 7.8 and on K for corneas steeper than this		
	Diameter:	11.0 mm		

5.42. Specialized Fitting Techniques (Cosmetics, Hard)

Base Curve: .10 to .20 mm flatter than the flattest corneal radii.
Diameter: 11.00 mm and up.
Optical Zone: About 8.00 mm.
Peripheral Curve: 0.3 mm at 12.25 mm.
Intermediate Curve: 0.4 mm at 10.00 mm.
Secondary: 1.2 mm flatter than the base curve.
There generally is a –10.00 D lenticular carrier included.
"Pupil" size should match that of the pupil in a well-illuminated room.

5.43. Axis Mislocation of the Toric Lenses

Table A. Mislocation and Overrefraction Location.*

ϕ *Overrefraction location (plus or minus) (overrefraction axis to required axix) (degrees)*	θ *Mislocation (sign as ϕ) (mislocation to required axis) (degrees)*
45	0
42.5	5
40	10
37.5	15
35	20
32.5	25
30	30
27.5	35
25	40
22.5	45
20	50
17.5	55
15	60
12.5	65
10	70
7.5	75
5	80
2.5	85
0	90

*On the basis that $F_R = F_1$ ϕ has a limiting value of 45 degrees; therefore, higher values are indicative that errors other than axis location are present. Application of linear interpolation is exact.

Reprinted from S.S. Dain, Overrefraction and Axis Mislocation of Toric Lenses, *International Contact Lens Clinic*, Vol. 6 #3, pp. 86-90, Professional Press with the permission of The Professional Press, Inc., 101 East Ontario Street, Chicago, Illinois 60611, U.S.A.

Table B. Mislocation and Cylinder Powers Ratio.*

Cylinder powers ratio	*Mislocation (to nearest degree)*
2.0	90
1.9	71
1.8	64
1.7	58
1.6	53
1.5	48
1.4	44
1.3	40
1.2	36
1.1	33
1.0	30
0.9	26
0.8	23
0.7	20
0.6	17
0.5	14
0.4	11
0.3	8
0.2	5
0.1	2
0.0	0

***Overrefraction cylinder power never exceeds twice correcting cylinder power. Application of linear interpolation is inexact.**

To interpolate take the values either side and add two-thirds of the difference to the lower value; i.e., 1.1 — 33; 1.2 — 36; therefore 1.15 — 33 + 2/3 of 3 = 35.

SAMPLE USE OF TABLE 5.43

Assumptions are made that the mislocated lens is in error only in its axis, that there is no lens flexure effect and that the lens is not toric on the back surface.

Required Lens R_x = +2.00 X 20°
Overrefraction = +0.37 +0.75 X 60°

Axis Method:

Overrefraction Location
+60° – 20° = +40°
Mislocation (Table 5.43A) = 10°
Mislocation Axis = 20° – 10° = 10°

Power Method:

$$\text{Ratio} = \frac{\text{overrefraction cylinder}}{\text{lens cylinder}}$$

$$= \frac{.75}{2.00} = .375$$

Mislocation (Table 5.43 B) = 10°
Mislocation Axis = 20° – 10° = 10° (Sign determined as above)
The mislocation axis will be in the opposite direction from the required axis than the overreaction axis.

If both axis and power methods are used and do not agree, this should be taken as an indication that the correcting lens also has incorrect power.

5.44. Set of Fenestrated Scleral Lenses for Optic Measurement

Back optic radius (mm)	*Back optic diameters (mm)*									
8.00	12.75	13	13.25	13.50	13.75	14				
8.25	12.75	13	13.25	13.50	13.75	14	14.25			
8.50	12.75	13	13.25	13.50	13.75	14	14.25	14.50		
8.75		13	13.25	13.50	13.75	14	14.25	14.50	14.75	
9.00			13.25	13.50	13.75	14	14.25	14.50	14.75	15
9.25				13.50	13.75	14	14.25	14.50	14.75	15
9.50							14.25	14.50	14.75	15

A set of 28 lenses (bold) constitutes the normal range of fitting lenses. 20 further lenses are specified where an extension is sought. The majority of back optic radii prescribed lie within the range of 8.75—9.25 mm.

Reprinted from N. Bier and G. Lowther, *Contact Lens Correction.* Woburn, Mass.: Butterworth Publishers, 1978.

5.45. Corneal Height as Related to Radius and Diameter

	Corneal Diameters (mm)										
Corneal Radius (mm)	*12.50*	*12.62*	*12.75*	*12.87*	*13.00*	*13.12*	*13.25*	*13.37*	*13.50*	*13.62*	*13.75*
8.00	3.01	3.09	3.17	3.25	3.34	3.43	3.52	3.61	3.71	3.80	3.91
8.12	2.93	3.01	3.09	3.17	3.25	3.34	3.43	3.51	3.60	3.70	3.81
8.25	2.86	2.93	3.01	3.09	3.17	3.25	3.33	3.42	3.51	3.60	3.70
8.37	2.80	2.87	2.95	3.02	3.10	3.18	3.26	3.34	3.42	3.51	3.60
8.50	2.74	2.80	2.87	2.94	3.02	3.09	3.17	3.25	3.33	3.42	3.51
8.62	2.68	2.75	2.82	2.89	2.96	3.03	3.11	3.19	3.27	3.35	3.43
8.75	2.63	2.69	2.75	2.82	2.89	2.96	3.03	3.10	3.18	3.26	3.34
8.87	2.58	2.64	2.71	2.77	2.84	2.91	2.98	3.05	3.12	3.19	3.27
9.00	2.52	2.58	2.65	2.71	2.78	2.84	2.91	2.98	3.05	3.12	3.20

5.46. Conical Concentric Polishing

With this method the lens is held in a series of female cone tools which have a soft pad material such as velveteen glued to the surface. The lens is first mounted by the concave surface so that the convex surface is placed down into the first three cones and then reversed and placed concave surface down into the next four cones. The lens is held in each cone for a specified time period as follows.

90 degrees tool (lens convex surface down)	10 seconds
60 degrees tool	5 seconds
180 degrees tool (lens concave surface down)	20 seconds
140 degrees cone	15 seconds
90 degrees cone	10 seconds
60 degrees cone	5 seconds
40 degrees cone	1 second

The cones rotate at 100 rev/min and the lens holder is held vertically in each case. The lens can be placed convex surface down into a 90-degree abrasive cone to thin the edge prior to going through the cone series if the lens originally has a thick edge.

Reprinted by permission from Norman Bier and Gerald Lowther, *Contact Lens Correction,* Woburn, Massachusetts: Butterworths Publishers, Inc., 1978.

5.47. Corneal Stains Associated with Contact Lens Wear

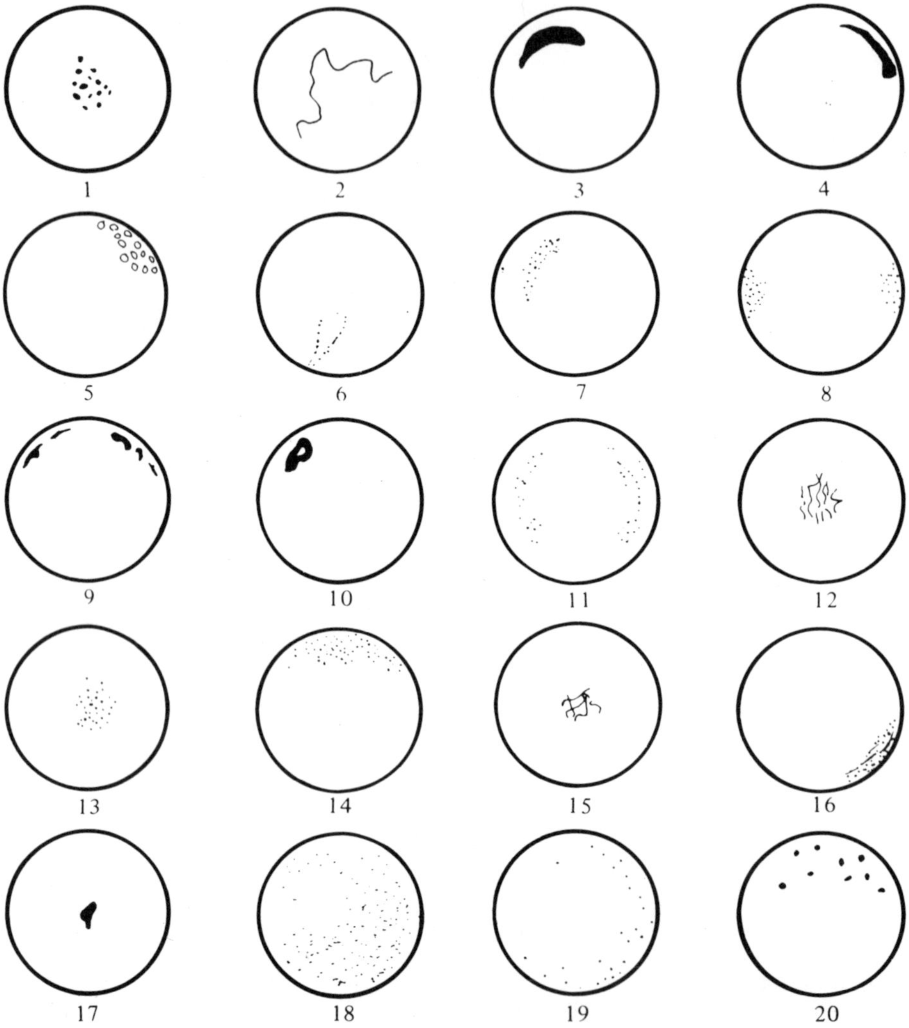

1. Central Punctate
2. Foreign Body
3. Archlike Coalesced
4. Insertion Stain
5. Dimple Vein
6. Removal Stain (S)
7. Defective Bevel
8. 3 O'clock – 9 O'clock Stain
9. Superior Pitting Stain (S)
10. Foreign Body
11. Tight Lens Stain
12. Flat Lens Abrasion
13. Central Stippling
14. Superior Stippling (S)
15. Foreign Body (S)
16. Arcuate (S)
17. Central Abrasion
18. Overall Stippling (S)
19. Mild Overall Stippling (S)
20. Superior Punctate (S)

(S) Usually found with flexible lens wear

See also Table 8.4E.

5.48. An Accurate Method of Measuring Soft Contact Lens Curvature

BCOR = R(Cell) × 1.334 + 0.057

R(Cell)	*BCOR*	*R(Cell)*	*BCOR*	*R(Cell)*	*BCOR*	*R(Cell)*	*BCOR*
5.00	6.727	5.50	7.370	6.00	8.040	6.50	8.710
5.01	6.740	5.51	7.383	6.01	8.053	6.51	8.723
5.02	6.754	5.52	7.397	6.02	8.067	6.52	8.737
5.03	6.767	5.53	7.410	6.03	8.080	6.53	8.750
5.04	6.780	5.54	7.424	6.04	8.094	6.54	8.764
5.05	6.794	5.55	7.437	6.05	8.107	6.55	8.777
5.06	6.807	5.56	7.450	6.06	8.120	6.56	8.790
5.07	6.820	5.57	7.464	6.07	8.134	6.57	8.804
5.08	6.834	5.58	7.477	6.08	8.147	6.58	8.817
5.09	6.847	5.59	7.491	6.09	8.161	6.59	8.831
5.10	6.860	5.60	7.504	6.10	8.174	6.60	8.844
5.11	6.874	5.61	7.517	6.11	8.187	6.61	8.857
5.12	6.887	5.62	7.531	6.12	8.201	6.62	8.871
5.13	6.900	5.63	7.544	6.13	8.214	6.63	8.884
5.14	6.914	5.64	7.558	6.14	8.228	6.64	8.898
5.15	6.927	5.65	7.571	6.15	8.241	6.65	8.911
5.16	6.940	5.66	7.584	6.16	8.254	6.66	8.924
5.17	6.954	5.67	7.598	6.17	8.268	6.67	8.938
5.18	6.967	5.68	7.611	6.18	8.281	6.68	8.951
5.19	6.980	5.69	7.625	6.19	8.295	6.69	8.965
5.20	6.994	5.70	7.638	6.20	8.308	6.70	8.978
5.21	7.007	5.71	7.651	6.21	8.321	6.71	8.991
5.22	7.020	5.72	7.665	6.22	8.335	6.72	9.005
5.23	7.034	5.73	7.678	6.23	8.348	6.73	9.018
5.24	7.047	5.74	7.692	6.24	8.362	6.74	9.032
5.25	7.061	5.75	7.705	6.25	8.375	6.75	9.045
5.26	7.074	5.76	7.718	6.26	8.388	6.76	9.058
5.27	7.087	5.77	7.732	6.27	8.402	6.77	9.072
5.28	7.101	5.78	7.745	6.28	8.415	6.78	9.085
5.29	7.114	5.79	7.759	6.29	8.429	6.79	9.099
5.30	7.127	5.80	7.772	6.30	8.442	6.80	9.112
5.31	7.141	5.81	7.785	6.31	8.455	6.81	9.125
5.32	7.154	5.82	7.799	6.32	8.469	6.82	9.139
5.33	7.167	5.83	7.812	6.33	8.482	6.83	9.152
5.34	7.181	5.84	7.826	6.34	8.496	6.84	9.166
5.35	7.194	5.85	7.839	6.35	8.509	6.85	9.179
5.36	7.207	5.86	7.852	6.36	8.522	6.86	9.192
5.37	7.221	5.87	7.866	6.37	8.536	6.87	9.206
5.38	7.234	5.88	7.879	6.38	8.549	6.88	9.219
5.39	7.247	5.89	7.893	6.39	8.563	6.89	9.233
5.40	7.261	5.90	7.906	6.40	8.576	6.90	9.246
5.41	7.274	5.91	7.919	6.41	8.589	6.91	9.259
5.42	7.287	5.92	7.933	6.42	8.603	6.92	9.273
5.43	7.301	5.93	7.946	6.43	8.616	6.93	9.286
5.44	7.314	5.94	7.960	6.44	8.630	6.94	9.300
5.45	7.327	5.95	7.973	6.45	8.643	6.95	9.313
5.46	7.341	5.96	7.986	6.46	8.656	6.96	9.326
5.47	7.354	5.97	8.000	6.47	8.670	6.97	9.340
5.48	7.367	5.98	8.013	6.48	8.683	6.98	9.353
5.49	7.381	5.99	8.027	6.49	8.697	6.99	9.367

There will be small individual differences from instrument to instrument. B+L keratometer will need a 25W source.

Reprinted from B. Holden, An Accurate Method of Measuring Soft Lens Curvature, *Australian J. of Optometry:* 58: pp 443-479.

5.49. Characteristics of Available Hydrophilic Lenses

Recommended fitting increment is given as ΔK.
See also Table 5.40.

Alcon Optics
- *Tresoft*
  - Lens Material: Ocufilon-A
  - Water content: 46%
  - Parameters:
    - Diameter: 13.5, 14, 14.5, 15 mm
    - Base curve: 8.2, 8.4, 8.6, 8.8
    - Power range: -20 to +20 DS
    - Center thickness: Minus .14 to .24; Plus .2 to .5
    - Optic zone: Varying 8 mm to 11 mm depending on power.
    - ΔK: 1.00 mm

American Hydron
- *Mini*
  - Lens Material: Polymacon
  - Water content: 38%
  - Parameters:
    - Diameter: 13.0 mm
    - Base curve: 8.1 to 8.9 mm in 0.2 mm steps
    - Power range: −20 to +20 DS
    - Center thickness: 0.12 mm minus
    - Optic zone: 11 mm at low minus
    - ΔK: 0.9 mm
- *Semi-scleral*
  - Parameters:
    - Diameter: 15.0 mm
    - Base curve: 9.0, 9.3, 9.6 mm
    - Power range: −30 to +30 DS
    - Center thickness: .12 mm minus, 0.26 mm low plus
    - Optic zone: 11 mm at low minus
    - ΔK: 1.4 mm
- *Toric*
  - Parameters:
    - Diameter: 13.5 to 14.5 mm, 1.0 to 1.5 mm truncation.
    - Base curve: 7.7 to 8.7 mm aspheric in 0.2 mm steps.
    - Power range: Sphere: −20 to +20 DS; Cylinder: −0.50 to −6.50 DS.
    - Center thickness: 0.16 mm (minus)
    - Optic zone: 9.0 mm
- *Zero 6*
  - Parameters:
    - Diameter: 14.0
    - Base curve: 8.4, 8.7, 9.0 mm
    - Power range: Plano to −6.00 DS
    - Center thickness: 0.06 mm
    - Optic zone: 11.00 mm

American Optical Corp.
- *Softcon Minus*
  - Lens material: Uifilcon A, HEMA povidone.
  - Water Content: 55%
  - Parameters:
    - Diameter and base curve: 13.5/7.8; 14.0/7.8; 14.0/8.1; 14.0/8.7; 14.0/8.4; 14.5/8.1; 14.5/8.4
    - Power range: plano to −8.00 DS (in .25 D steps)
    - Optic zone: 7.3 mm
    - Center thickness: .12 to .26 mm
    - ΔK: .3 mm
- *Softcon Plus*
    - Power range: 0 to +18.00 D (from +5JD in .50 D steps)

(continued)

Softcon Therapeutic Bandage Lens
Disinfection: Thermal – intermittent heating (bandage use only)
AOsoft
Lens material: Tetrafilcon A, three polymers (HEMA, NVP, MMA)
Water content: 42.5%
Parameters:
Diameter: 13 mm
Base curve: 7.8, 8.1, 8.4, 8.7, 9.0 mm
Power range: .25 to 9.75 D in .25 D steps
Center thickness: .12 mm to .22 mm
Optic zone: 8.9 to 12.25 mm
ΔK: .7 mm
AOsoft Low Plus
Parameters:
Diameter: 13 mm
Base curve: 7.8, 8.1, 8.4, 8.7, 9.0 mm
Power range: .25 to 6.50 D in .25 D steps
Center thickness: .14 to 28 mm
AOsoft Thin
Parameters:
Diameter: 13.8 mm
Base curve: 8.3, 8.6, 9.0 mm
Power range: –.25 to –7.75
Center thickness: .04 to .09 mm
Optic zone:

Bausch & Lomb
For standard lenses see table: 5.16
For basic fitting guide see table: 5.40
(Toric)
Lens material: Hefilcon B
Water content: 45%
Parameters:
Diameter: 14.0 mm
Base curve: 8.3, 8.6, 8.9 mm
Power range: Sphere +4.00 to –4.0 DS; Cylinder –1.25 and –1.75 DS
Axes: #20° from primary meridians in 10° increments
Prism: 1Δ, Chamfered

Comfortflex Hydrophilics
Lens material: Deltafilcon A
Water content: 43%
Parameters:
Diameter: 13.5 mm
Base curves: 38, 39, 40, 41, 42 D
Power range: –1.00 to –10.00
Center thickness: .10 mm
Optic zone: Variable

Cooper Labs
Permalens
Lens material: Perfilcon A
Water content: 71%
Parameters:
Diameter: 14.0, 14.5 mm
Base curve: 8.0, 8.3, 8.6, 8.9 mm
Power range: +11 to 17.00
Center thickness: .38 to .43
Optic zone: 6.6 to 7.4 mm

(continued)

Dow Corning Ophthalmics Inc.
Gelflex
Lens material: Dimefilcon A
Water content: 36%
Parameters:
Base curve: 7.6 to 8.6 mm in 0.2 mm steps
Power range: −20.00 to +20.0 DS in 0.25 DS steps.
Center thickness: 0.14 mm
Optic zone: Posterior 11.3 mm; Anterior 9.7 mm for minus, 8.8 mm for plus.
ΔK: .5 mm
Gelflex MT
Parameters:
Diameter: 13.6 mm
Base curve: 8.0, 8.3, 8.6 mm
Center thickness: 0.06 mm
Power range: to −10.00, −6.50 to −1.0 in 5 D steps
Optic zone: 11.3 mm anterior 10.4 mm
ΔK: .5 mm
Silsoft
Lens material: A silicon elastomer
Parameters:
Diameter: 11.3, 12.5 mm
Base curve: 8.0, 8.3, 8.6 mm
Center thickness: .10 (minus); .35 at +14.0
Power range: −1.00 to −4.50 D; +11.0 to +17.0 in .5 D steps
ΔK: 0 or .1
Silcon
Lens material: A silicon resin
Parameters:
Diameter: 8.9 mm (OZ = 7.8 mm)
Base curve: 7.26 to 8.13 mm (approx. .8 mm steps)
Center thickness: .14 (minus −2.50); .38 mm at +14
Power range: −0.50 to −4.50 D; +12.0 to +16.0 (.5 D steps)
ΔK: 0 or .1

Flexlens Inc.
Flexlens
Lens material: PHP (Hidilcon A)
Water content: 45.5%
Parameters:
Diameter: 12.5 to 16.5 mm in 0.5 mm steps
Base curve: 6.0 to 11.0 mm in 0.25 mm steps
Power range: unlimited
Center thickness: by prescription
Optic zone: by prescription
ΔK: 1.1 mm

Hoya
Hoya Soft Lens
Water content: 35%
Center thickness: .02 to .20 (minus); .22 to .56 (plus)

Hydrocurve Soft Lenses, Inc.
Lens material – all lenses: Bufilcon A; water content either 45 or 55%
Hydrocurve II – 45%
Parameters:
Diameter: 13.5, 15.5, 16.0 mm
Base curve: 13.5 mm diameter −8.6, 8.3 mm;
15.5 and 16.0 mm diameter −10.1, 9.8, 9.5 and 9.2 mm
Power range: 13.5 mm diam. 8.3 mm, −12.0 to +20 DS; 8.6 mm −12.0 to +9.75 D
15.5 and 16.0 mm diameters, −20.0 to +20.0

(continued)

Hydrocurve II–45% (continued)
Center thickness: minus lenses from .04 to .08 mm
Optic zone: at least 8 mm
ΔK for 15.5, 16.0 mm: 1.6 mm
for 13.5 mm: .8 mm
Hydrocurve II – 55% (extended wear)
Parameters:
Diameter: 14.0 mm, 14.5
Base curve:8.5 mm/14.0, 8.8/14.5
Power range: Plano to −12.00; +0.25 to +7.00 DS
Center thickness: .05 mm at −3.0
Optic zone: 8.25 mm
Hydrocurve II Toric
Parameters:
Radii: 8.6 mm and 13.5 mm; 8.9 mm and 14.0 mm radii are equivalents
Power range: spherical powers +3.00 to −6.00 D; cylinder power −1.25, −2.00 D
Optic zone: approx. 8 mm
Back surface cylinder ≠ 25° from major axes in 5° increments
Center thickness: .05 to .13 mm

Hydrocurve II – 55% for aphakic extended wear
Parameters:
Base curve/Diameter: 8.5 mm/13.5 mm; 8.9/14.0; 9.2/15.5 and 16.0 mm
9.2 mm/15.5 and 16.0; 9.5/15.5 and 16.0 mm
9.8/15.5 and 16.0 mm
Power range: +7.25 to +20.00 D
Center thickness: .29 to .47 mm
Hydrocurve II – 45% for aphakic extended wear
Parameters:
Diameter: 13.5 mm
Base curve: 8.6, 8.9 mm
Power range: +9.75 to +20.00 D
Center thickness: .25 to .42 mm

Hydro-Marc/Frontier Contact Lenses, Inc.
Hydro-Marc Spherical
Lens Material: Etafilcon A
Water content: 43%
Parameters:
Diameter: 13.5, 14.0, 14.5 and 15.0 mm
Base curve: 8.15, 8.30, 8.45, 8.60, 8.75, 8.90, 9.05, 9.50
Power range: −20.00 to +20.00 D
Center thickness: .09 to .52 mm
Optic zone: 8.0
ΔK: 1.00 mm
Hydro Marc Toric
Parameters:
Diameter: 14.0 to 14.5 mm
Base curves: I Flat, II Medium, III Steep
Power range: Cyl. .75 to 1.75D, 180°, 90°, +15°
−20.00 to +20.00 D
Center thickness: .09 to .52 mm
Optic zone: 9.0
Prism: 1.5 D
Hydro Marc SM Ultra Thin
Parameters:
Diameter: 14.0 mm
Base curve: 8.4 mm, also 8.8 mm
Power range: −0.75 to −5.75 D, +1.00 to +4.00
Center thickness: .06 to .07 mm

(continued)

Lombart Lenses Ltd.
AMSOF
Lens material: Deltafilcon A
Water content: 43%
Parameters:
Diameter: 13.5 mm
Base curve: 7.60 to 9.20 mm in 0.2 mm steps, Plus: 7.8 to 8.8 mm
Power range: +5.00 to −10.00 D
Center thickness: 0.09 to 0.25 mm
Optic zone: varies depending upon power (9.5 to 12.5 mm)
ΔK: .6 mm
AMSOF Thin
Parameters:
Diameter: 13.8 mm
Base curve: 8.3, 8.6 mm
Power range: −0.75 to −7.00 D
Center thickness: 0.6 mm
Optic zone: 7.55 mm (variable)
ΔK: .8mm (over 45.4 1mm under 41.50 .6 mm)

Medicornea, Inc.
Softflow
Lens material: Deltafilcon A
Water content: 43%
Parameters:
Diameter: 13.5, 14.0, 14.5 mm
Base curve: 8.00, 8.40, 8.80 mm
Power range: +20 to −20 D

Omega Optical Co.
Omega Soft
Lens material: Polymacon
Water content: 38.6%
Standard
Diameter: 13.0 mm
Base curve: 8.1 to 9.1 in .2 mm steps
Power range: +20.00 to −20.00
Cast molded
Thin
Diameter: 14.0 mm
Base curve: 8.4, 8.7, 9.0
Power range: Plano to −6.00
Thickness: .06
Lathe cut

Paris Contact Lens Lab
Softsite
Lens material: Hefilcon A PHP
Water content: 45%
Parameters:
Diameter: 13.5 mm
Base curve: 8.3 and 8.6 mm
Powers: low plus, high plus (aphakic); minus lenses
Power range: +10.0 to +20.0 D

Sauflon International
Sauflon 70
Lens material: Lidofilcon A
Water content: 70%
Parameters:
Diameter: 13.0, 13.7 mm
Base curve: 7.8 to 9.0 in .2 mm steps
ΔK: .5 mm

(continued)

Sauflon PW
Lens material: Lidofilicon B
Water content: 79%
Parameters:
Diameter: 13.0, 13.7 mm
Base curve: 7.5 to 8.2 mm in .2 mm steps
ΔK: K or flatter

Aphakia PW
Lens material: Lidofilcon B
Water content: 79%
Parameters:
Diameter: 14.4 mm
Base curve: 8.1, 8.4, 8.7 mm
Power range: +10.0 to +17.00
Center thickness: .46 to .67 mm
Optical zone: 8.0 mm
ΔK: .6 mm

Sof-Form Inc. (Div. Salvatori Ophthalmics)
Sof-Form
Lens material: Deltafilcon A
Water content: 43%
Parameters:
Diameter: 14.0 mm
Base curve: 8.30, 8.50, 8.70, 8.90 mm
Power range: ±0.50 to ±10.00 in 0.25 steps; +20.00 to −20.00 D available in 0.50 D steps
Center thickness: varies according to power and diameter; minus lens, 0.13 to 0.06 mm
Optic zone: varies from 8.6 to 7.4 mm
ΔK: .9 mm

Strieter Laboratories
Accugel
Lens material: Droxifilcon, HEMA, TGD and MA with residual amount PVP
Water content: 46.6%
Parameters:
Diameter: 13.5 mm, also 13.1 and 13.9
Base curve: 8.10 to 9.40 in 0.10 mm steps
Power range: ±20.00 D in spheres; toric available late 1979
Center thickness: 0.16 mm
Optic zone: 11.7 mm; Anterior: 8.0 mm
ΔK: .9 mm
Accugel[R] (Thin)
Diameter: 14.0 mm
Base curve: As standard thickness
Power range: As standard thickness
Center thickness: .07 for minus

Syntex Ophthalmics
CSI
Lens material: Crofilcon A Methyl and Glyceril Methacrylate
Water content: 38.5%
Parameters:
Diameter: 14.8 mm
Base curves: 8.6, 8.9, 9.35 mm
Power range: Plano to −6.00 +12.00 to +20.00 D
Center thickness: .05 to .2 mm .02 to .04

(continued)

UO Optics Inc.
Aquaflex Standard
Lens material:
Water content: 42.5%
Parameters:
Diameter: 13.0 mm
Base curve: vaults 0 thru IV; 9.0 to 7.8 mm in .3 mm steps
Power range: plano through −9.75 in .25 D steps
Center thickness: .10 to .18 mm (varies with power)
Optic zone: Posterior, 12.6 mm; minimum anterior, 9.00 mm (varies with power)
ΔK: .7 mm
Aquaflex Low Plus Super Thin Lenses
Parameters:
Diameter: 13.8 mm
Base curve: Vault II 8.80 mm; Vault III 8.50 mm
Power range: plano to +6.00 D in 0.25 D steps
Center thickness: .12 to .28 mm (varies with power)
Optic zone: Posterior 13.4 mm; anterior 9.0 mm
Aquaflex High Plus Lenses
Parameters:
Diameter: 13.8 mm
Base curve: Vaults 0 thru IV, 9.40 to 8.20 mm in .30 mm steps
Power range: +10.00 to +20.00 D in 0.25 D steps
Center thickness: .42 to .56 mm (varies with power)
Optic zone: Posterior, 13.4; minimum anterior 8.5 (varies with power)
Aquaflex Super Thin Minus
Parameters:
Diameter: 13.8 mm
Base curve: Vault II (8.80 mm)
Power range: −1.00 to −6.00 in .25 D steps
Center thickness: .05 to .07
Optic zone: 13.4 mm; Anterior 9.00 mm

Welcon
Lens material: HEMA
Water content: 40%
Parameters:
Diameter: 13.0, 14.0, 15.0 mm
Base curve: 8.4 to 9.4 mm in .2 mm steps
ΔK: 13.0 = .3 mm; 14.0 = .6 mm; 15.0 = .2 mm
Welcon Torics
Parameters:
Diameter: 15.0
Base curve: 8.4 to 9.4 mm in .2 mm steps
No prism or truncation; uses stabilization zones
ΔK: 1.2 mm

Wesley-Jessen
Lens material: Phemfilcon A
Water content: 30%
Durasoft (Blue Label)
Parameters:
Diameter: 12.8 mm
Base curve: 7.8, 8.0, 8.2, 8.45, 8.7, 9.0 mm
Power range: −20.0 to +20.0 D
Center thickness: 0.09 mm
Optic zone: 12.0 mm
ΔK: .6 mm

(continued)

Durasoft (Gold Label)
Parameters:
Diameter: 13.5 mm
Base curve: 8.3, 8.6, 9.0 mm
Power range: −20.0 to +20.0
Center thickness: 0.09 mm
Optic zone: 12.7 mm
ΔK: 1.0 mm
Durasoft TT (Toric lens for astigmatism)
Parameters:
Diameter: 12.8, 13.5 mm
Base curve: 7.8, 8.0, 8.2, 8.3, 8.45, 8.7, 9.0, 9.3 mm
Power range: Sphere, −20 to +20 D; Cylinder +0.75 to +4.0 D
Axes: 1° to 180°
Center thickness: 0.11 mm
Optic zone: 8.0 to 12.7 mm

Wohlk
Lens material: HEMA
Water content: 38.4%
Hydroflex M
Parameters:
Diameter: 12.5, 13.0 mm
Base curve: 7.5 to 8.6 mm in 0.1 mm steps
Power range: −20.0 to +20.0 D
Central thickness: 0.10 mm at −3.0
ΔK: 12.5 = 0.3 mm; 13.0 = 0.5 mm
Hydroflex
Parameters:
Diameter: 13.5 t0 16.0 mm in .5 mm steps
Base curve: 8.3 to 9.7 mm in .1 mm steps
Power range: −20.0 to +20.0 D
Central thickness: .2 to .3 in minus; up to .8 in plus
Hydroflex SD
Parameters:
Diameter: 13.0, 13.5, 14.5 mm
Base curve: 7.6, 8.0, 8.4 mm at 13.0 or 13.5; 8.4, 8.8, 9.2 mm at 14.5 mm
Power range: +10.0 to +20.0 D
Central thickness: .19 mm at +3.0; .08 mm in minus range
ΔK: .2 at 13.0/13.5; 1.0 at 14.5
Hydroflex TS (Toric optic zone with spherical surround)
Parameters:
Diameter: 14.0, 15.0 mm
Base curve: 8.1 to 10.0 in .1 mm steps
Truncated with 1 ΔBD
Power range: .5 to 6.0 cylinder in .5 mm steps; +20.0 to −20.0 D
ΔK: 1.1 mm
Hydroflex M-T (Toric optic zone with spherical surround)
Parameters:
1.5 ΔBD not truncated
Diameter: 12.0 to 13.5 mm in .5 mm steps
Base curve: 7.1 to 9.0 mm in .1 mm steps
ΔK: 12.5 mm = .3 mm

Low Vision 6

6.1. Low Vision Aids

Table A. Hand Magnifiers

True Dioptic Strength	*M Rating*	*Manufacturer or Supplier, and Magnification*
3 D	1.5–2.5	B&L
5 D	1.5–2.5	B&L, Selsi, Edroy, COIL Windsor Range
7 D	1.5–2.5	COIL Windsor Range
8 D	3	COIL Rectangular
10.00 D	4	COIL Square
11 D	4	Selsi B&L Packette
11.50 D	4	COIL 3X
12 D	4	COIL Windsor Range, Magnalite (LH)
14 D	5	Selsi
16 D	6	B&L 4X lens
20 D	7	COIL cataract reader, B&L Packette
21 D	8	Selsi 8X (two lenses)
27.60 D	10	B&L 7X (two lenses)
32 D	14	B&L 9X, Selsi 10X (two lenses)
36 D	14	B&L 12X
68 D	20	B&L 20X (three lenses)

Table B. Stand Magnifiers

3.8 v 3.0 h	1.5	COIL, Cross Cylinder
4.1	1.5	Selsi Bar Magnifier
4.7	1.5	COIL Junior Stand
4.7	1.5	Selsi Plano-Convex
5.3	2	COIL Large Stand Magnifier
5.3	2	Edmund 3X Plastic Base
6.2	2	COIL Optima*
8.3	3	COIL Small Stand Magnifier
8.7	3	Jupiter
8.7	3	COIL (Plasta Cataract Aspheric)*
11.5	4	COIL Raylite*
15	5	Sloan S-15*
18	7	COIL (Hi-Power Aspheric)
20		COIL (Cataract Stand)
29		COIL (Hi Power Stand)

***With illumination attachment eye at 40 cm from virtual image.**

Table C. Distance Telescopic Aids*

Manufacturer and Manufacturers' Designation	*Description*	
Designs for Vision	*Magnification*	*Approx. Total Object Field*
Full Field	1.3X	41°
	1.7X	37°
	2.2X	21°
	3.0X	11°
	4.0X	8°
	6.0X	4.5°
Wide Angle, Full Field	2.2X	23°
	3.0X	12°
Bioptic-Model I	2.2X	20.5° horizontal, 14.5° vertical
	3.0X	11° round
	4.0X	8° round
	6.0X	4.5° round
Wide Angle, Bioptic Model I	2.2X	22° horizontal, 11° vertical
	3X	9.9° horizontal, 7.4° vertical
Bioptic Model II	2.2X	18.5° round
Expanded Field	3X	13.4°
	4X	9.8°
	6X	6.5°
	8X	4°
Surgical Binoculars	*Work Distance*	*Monocular*
	2.5X 40 cm	6 cm horizontal, 5 cm vertical
	3.5X 35 cm	5 cm round
	4.5X 40 cm	4 cm round
Keeler		
LVA 31	Full field focusing telescope; 2X distance, 2.5X intermediate, 3X near.	
LVA 32	Focusing distance telescope miniature with 2X for distance and 3X for near (10″). For use on a ring finger.	
LVA 20	2X infinity telescope. +0.75, +4.00 caps.	
LVA 26	For distance, intermediate, and near use. 2.5X full field. +2.00, +3.00, +4.00 caps.	
Hamblin	*Magnification*	*Field of View*
Distance telescope	1.8X	18°
	2.0X	14°
Selsi	*Size*	*Specified Field*
	6 X 30 mm	7°28′
	8 X 30 mm	7°28′
	7 X 35 mm	6°29′
	7 X 50 mm	7°9′
	10 X 50 mm	5°24′
	12 X 50 mm	5°19′
	16 X 50 mm	4°10′
	20 X 50 mm	3°
	7 X –12 X 40 mm zoom	variable

(continued)

Table C. Distance Telescopic Aids* (continued)

Manufacturer and Manufacturers' Designation	*Description*			
	Size		*Specified Field*	
Walters, Sam	6 X 16	8 X 20	10 X 20	to 10″
	7 X 25	10 X 30		to 21″
	3 X 16			to 8″
	Variable focus telescopes, accessory lenses, and finger ring available.			

*The telescopics, made of glass and plastic combination, are available in full diameter or insert form. Bioptics feature a telescopic insert in a single vision lens, while trioptics feature an insert in a bifocal lens.

Table D. Reading Aids in Permanent Spectacles by Source

Manufacturer and Manufacturer's Designation	*Description*
American Optical	
Half lenses in frames	+6.00, +8.00, +10.00 with prism
Aspheric cataract lenses	+10.00, +12.00, +14.00, +16.00, +20.00 mag. 2.4 to 4.3; diameter 40 mm
Aspheric microscopic lenses	2X, 4X, 6X, 8X, 10X, 12X; spot diameters 40 to 25 mm
Glass microscopic lenses	2X, 4X, 6X, 8X; 81 mm blanks
Full diameter	2X, 4X, 6X, 10X, 12X, 14X, 16X, 20X
Designs for Vision	
Bifocal Type E 13 X 23	2X to 10X
Type R 19 X 25	2X to 10X
Half eye	2X to 10X
Wide angle	8X to 16X
Reading telescopes	2.5X, 3.5X, 4.5X
High Add	See Table 6.1 E
Aspheric Plastic Executive	See Table 6.1 E
T. Hamblin	
High definition telescopic spectacle for near	2X to 5X
DV telescope with cap added	1.8X, 2.0X, 2.7X, 3.0X, 3.6X, 4.0X, 4.5X, 5.0X
Half eye compound spectacle	
Trifocal A (compound near, conventional intermediate and distance correction)	
Trifocal B (compound near and intermediate and conventional distance correction)	
Compound Reading	2X, 3X, 4X, 6X, 8X, 12X, 15X, also 5X, 7X, 9X, 10X and 11X.
Fresnel	1.5X, 2.0X 2.5X, 5.0X; spot diameters 20 to 25 mm
Keeler	
LVA9; high powered compound	8X, 10X, 12X, 15X, 20X
LVA10; best for and aspheric magnifiers; full aperature or crescent	2X to 6X, 8X
LVA12; single lens aspheric button	2X to 9X, 15X
LVA21; monocular or binocular	2X to 5X; working distance 15.5
LVA22; full field	1.6X, 2X to 6X, 8X
LVA23; bifocal	1.6X, 2X to 5X
McLeod	
Igard hyperocular lenses	4X, 6X, 8X
Mentor	
Frenel press-on aspheric high plus adds.	1.25X, 2.5X, 3.5X, 5X
Shuron	
High power ultex bifocal adds	1.25X, 1.5X, 1.75X, 2.5X, 3X, 4X, 5X
Universal	6X, 8 X, 10X; spot diameters 25, 25, 20 mm.

Table E. Plastic High Add Bifocals

Aire-O-Lite	Adds available from +4.00 D to 10.00 D in 0.50 D steps, 22.0 mm round segment
American Optical	Adds available +6.00 D, +9.00 D, +12.00 D, and +18.00 D, 22.00 mm round segment; aspheric cataract high-add bifocal with adds +6.00 D, +12.00 D, and +18.00 D
Armorlite	Round seg lenticular, adds 4.50, 5.00, 6.50, 6.00; four base curves 10.00 to 16.00; Welsh four drop flattop, add 5.00 60 mm blank
BSA Industries	Adds available from +4.00 D to +6.00 D in 0.50 D steps, and +6.00 D to 10.00 D in 1.00 D steps, 22.0 mm round segment, or +4.00 to +6.00 D in 0.50 D steps, 22.0 mm flattop segment
Designs for Vision	High add executive bifocal, up to a total of +20.00 D; aspheric plastic executive bifocal microscope 2, 4, 6, 8X
Robinson-Houchin	CLX plus bifocal 38 X 33 seg CX plus bifocal 20 X 40 seg, adds 4.25 to 15.00; 5 base curves plano to 10.25
Shuron/Textron	Adds available from +4.00 D to +6.00 D in 0.25 D steps, 22.0 mm round segment, 25.0 or 28.0 mm flattop segments
Sola	Ultex A, adds 4.00, 6.00, 8.00, 12.00; 25 mm round, adds 4.00, 5.00, 6.00, 8.00, 12.00, 16.00

Table F. Miscellaneous Aids

Description	*Source*	*Transmittance*
Night Vision Enhancement Devices	Electro Optical Products National Institute for Rehabilitation Engineering	
Retinitis Pigmentosa Spectacles	Recreational Innov. (NO-IR #107) Carl Zeiss (Adrian Lens)	See Table 3.20T
Low Transmission Lenses	American Optical	
	Filterweld	1, 2, 5, 17%
	True Tone Aolite	5–50% (+8.0 to –8.0 cyl to –5.0) (at 550 NM)
	01o	1, 2, 4, 8, 10% 1, 2 and 10 are green 4 and 8% are amber (plano only)
	Recreational Innov.	
	No IR	1% (grey-green) 2% (green) 2% (amber) 10% (amber) 18% (grey-green)
	in R_X	#101 – 10%, 102 – 18% #107 – 2% amber (62 mm round blanks)

Table G. Nonoptical Aids

Description	*Source*
Reading Slit	Superior Optical
Reading Stand	Anco, N.Y. Lighthouse
Music Rack	American Printing House for the Blind
Tensorlite	Selsi
Jumbo Cards	American Foundation for the Blind
Large Number Telephone Dials	National Institute for Rehab. Eng.
Writing Guides	American Foundation for the Blind
Writing Paper	Nu Vu Products
Sure Guard Safety Goggles	American Optical
Watches	American Foundation for the Blind

Table H. Large Print Books

American Bible Society
1865 Broadway
New York, NY 10023

American Foundation for the Blind, Inc.
15 West 16 Street
New York, NY 10011

American Library Assoc.
50 East Huron Street
Chicago, IL 60611

American Printing House for the Blind
1839 Frankfort Avenue
Louisville, KY 40206

Better Vision Institute, Inc.
230 Park Avenue
New York, NY 10017

G. K. Hall & Co.
70 Lincoln Street
Boston, MA 02111

Keith Jennison Books
575 Lexington Avenue
New York, NY 10022

Large Print Ltd.
105 Pearl Street
Buffalo, NY 14202

Large Print Publications
11060 Fruitland Drive
North Hollywood, CA 91604

New York Times, Large Print Weekly
P.O. Box 2570
Boulder, CO 80302

Library of Congress
Division for the Blind &
Physically Handicapped
Washington, D.C.

The Lighthouse
New York Assoc. for the Blind
Low Vision Services
11 East 59 Street
New York, NY 10022

The Microfilm Co. of Calif.
1977 S. Los Angeles Street
Los Angeles, CA 90011

Miles Kimball
41 West Eighth Avenue
Oshkosh, WI 54901

National Aid to the Visually Handicapped
6201 Balboa Street
San Francisco, CA

Readers Digest
Pleasantville, NY 10570

Stanwix House Publishers
1306 Highland Building
Pittsburgh, PA

Xerox Corporation
Box 330 Dept. XB
Grand Central Station
New York, NY

Table I. Electronic Magnification Devices

Apollo Lasers, Incorporated 6357 Arizona Circle Los Angeles, CA 90045 (213)776-3343	Tele Com Enterprises, Incorporated 8610 Airport Boulevard Los Angeles, CA 90045 (213)641-4061, or (213)776-1553
Opaque Systems Limited 100 Taft Avenue Hempstead, NY 11550 (516)485-3322	Visualtek 1901 Olympic Boulevard Santa Monica, CA 90404 (213)829-3453
Pelco Sales Incorporated 351 East Alondra Boulevard Gardena, CA 90248 (213)321-5591	Warner Equipment Corp. 24001 Telegraph Rd. Southfield, MI 48075
Stimulation Learning Aids Ltd. 65 Grace Ave. Lynbrook, L.I., NY	X-Pert 6563 Mammoth Ave. Van Nuys, CA 91401

Table J. General Sources of Supply

Aids	*Source*	*Aids*	*Source*
5	The Albert Aloe Company 34 N. Brentwood St. Louis, MO 63105	2	Behr Manufacturing Co. 744 E. Wisconsin Ave. Oconomowoc, WI
4	Aire-O-Lite P.O. Box 2006 E 14 Street Alma, GA 31510	1,2,3,4,5	Bernell Corporation 316 South Eddy Street South Bend, IN 46617
4	American Bifocal Co., Inc. 1440 St. Clair Avenue Cleveland, OH	4	Bolsey Research and Development Windsor Park P.O. Box 248 Hartsdale, NY 10530
2,4	American Optical Co., Inc. 14 Mechanic Street Southbridge, MA 01550	4	B.S.A. Industries 2697 Cleveland Ave. Columbus, OH 43211
2	Amoriex-Ward Inst. Corp. 322 Belleville Pike North Arlington, NJ 07032	1,3	Burton Manufacturing Co. 7922 Haskell Avenue Van Nuys, CA 91406
2,3,4	Apex Specialties Co. 115 Douglas Avenue Providence, RI 02904	5	Bushnell 2828 E. Foothill Blvd. Pasadena, CA
4	Armorlite, Inc. 130 N. Brigham San Marcos, CA 92069	1,3,5	Colonial Optical Co., Inc. 1954 S. La Cienga Blvd. Los Angeles, CA
1,2,3,4,5	Bausch & Lomb, Inc. 635 St. Paul Street Rochester, NY 14602	2,3	Combined Optical Industries, Ltd. 200 Bath Road Slough SL1 4DW, England

1. Illumination Devices
2. Loupes
3. Magnifiers (various)
4. Microscopics (R_X)
5. Telescopes
6. Telescopes (R_X)
7. Pinhole Devices
8. Low Transmission Lenses

(continued)

Table J. General Source of Supply (continued)

Aids	*Source*	*Aids*	*Source*
1	Covington Plating Works, Inc. 331 Pike Street Covington, KY 41011	1,2,3,4,5	House of Vision 135-37 N. Wabash Ave. Chicago, IL 60602
1,3,4,5,6	Designs for Vision, Inc. 120 E. 23 Street New York, NY 10016	2	B. Jadow & Sons W 23 Street New York, NY 10010
2,3	Donegan Optical Co., Inc. 1405 Kansas Kansas City, MO 64127	1,2,3,4,5,6	Keeler Optical 456 Parkway Lawrence Park Industrial District Broomall, PA 19008
1	Eberson Enterprises P.O. Box 5516 Pasadena, CA	1,2,3,4,5	The Lighthouse New York Assn. for the Blind Low Vision Services 111 East 59th Street New York, NY 10022
1,2,3,4,5	Edmund Scientific Co. 602 Edscorp Building Barrington, NJ 08007	2	Magna-Add, Inc. 150 East Broad St. Suite 706 Columbus, OH 43215
1,2	Ednalite Corporation 200 North Water St. Peekskill, NY 10566	3,4	McLeod Optical Co., Inc. 100 Jefferson St. Warwick, RI 02888
1,2,3	Edroy Products Co., Inc. 130 W. 29th Street New York, NY 10001	8	National Institute for Rehabilitation Engineering 97 Decker Road Butler, NJ 17405
1,3	Fostoria-Fannon, Inc. 1200 North Main Street Fostoria, OH 44830		
4,6	Hamblin, Theodore, Ltd. 15 Wigmore Street London W1, England		

(continued)

Table J. General Source of Supply (continued)

Aids	*Source*	*Aids*	*Source*
7	Night Vision Aid Distributors P.O. Box 207 Randallstown, MD 21133	7	Pro-Optics 306 Busse Hwy. Park Ridge, IL 60068
1,2,3,4,5	New Era Optical Co. 17 N. Wabash Ave. Chicago, IL 60069	1,3	Ravadge Instruments 731 Biddle Road Glen Burnie, MD 21063
2	Nusinov, Charles & Sons, Inc. 1404 E. Baltimore Street Baltimore, MD 21231	8	Recreational Innovations P.O. Box 159 So. Lyon, MI 48178
1	Nu-Vue Visor Company P.O. Box 757 Fairhope, AL 36532	1,2,3,5	Selsi Company, Inc. 40 Veterans Blvd. Carlstadt, NJ 07072
5	Ocular Instruments Co. P.O. Box 1787 Los Gatos, CA 95030	4	Shuron-Continental P.O. Box 46367 9936 Princeton Pike Cincinnati, OH 45246
8	Olo Products, Ltd. Box 613 Manhasset, NY 11030	2	Sloan, Dr. Louise Wilmer Institute Johns Hopkins Hospital Baltimore, MD 21205
3,4	Optical Sciences Group, Inc. 2201 Webster Street San Francisco, CA 94115	1	Superior Optical Co. 1500 S. Hope Street Los Angeles, CA 90015
1,2,3,4,5	Prentiss Precision Div. of Transcontinental Sales Co. 1608 W. Pico Blvd. Los Angeles, CA 90015		

(continued)

Table J. General Source of Supply (continued)

Aids	*Source*	*Aids*	*Source*
3,5	Swift Instruments, Inc. 952 Dorchester Ave. Boston, MA 02125	1,7	Watchemoket Optical Co., Inc. 232 West Exchange Street Providence, RI 02903
1,2,3	Telesight, Inc. 1418 East 88 Street Brooklyn, NY 11236	1,2,3,5	Western Optical 1200 Mercer Street Seattle, WA 98109
4	Universal Ophthalmic Products P.O. Box 3144 Houston, TX 77001	1	Yorktowne Optical Co. 469 Market Street York, PA 17404
1	Visorette 3141 E. California Blvd. P.O. Box 5185 Pasadena, CA	1,3	Younger Manufacturing Co. 3788 S. Broadway Place Los Angeles, CA 90007
5	Walters, Sam 412 W 6th Street Los Angeles, CA 90014	1,2,3,4,5,6	Zeiss, Carl 444 Fifth Avenue New York, NY 10018

6.2. Effects of Reading Additions on Working Distance

Reading Addition (diopters)	*Working Distance (cm.)*	*Magnification*	*1.7× Telescopic Lens Field Diameter (cm.)*	*Magnification*	*2.2× Telescopic Lens field Diameter (cm.)*
+ 2	50	0.9	28.4	1.1	12.2
+ 3	33.33	1.3	19.0	1.7	8.1
+ 4	25	1.7	14.2	2.2	6.1
+ 5	20	2.1	10.9	2.8	5.1
+ 6	16.66	2.6	9.4	3.3	4.1
+ 8	12.5	3.4	6.9	4.4	3.0
+10	10	4.3	5.1	5.5	2.3
+12	8.33	5.1	3.6	6.6	1.8
+14	7.14	6.0	2.5	7.7	1.3

Reprinted by permission from N. Bier, *Correction of Subnormal Vision*, 2nd ed. London: Butterworths, 1970.

6.3. Design of Stigmagna Lenses (Lederer Principle)

Best Optical Form for Simple High Plus Lenses in a Spectacle Frame

Magnification	*Lens Power (diopters)*	*Lens Diameter*	*Center Thickness*	*Surface Powers (diopters)*
3×	+12 D.	42 mm.	6.80 mm.	+14.75 D. – 3.00 D.
4×	+16 D.	40 mm.	8.00 mm.	+16.00 D. plano
5×	+20 D.	38 mm.	9.00 mm.	+17.50 D. + 3.00 D.

Reprinted by permission form J. Lederer, "The Lederer lens: a new development in subnormal vision aids," *Aust. J. Opt.* 37: 1954. Reprinted in N. Bier, *Correction of Subnormal Vision*, 2nd ed. London: Buttersworths, 1970.

6.4. Total Magnification of Telescopic Distance Lenses Combined with Near Addition and Resultant Field of View with Object in Focal Plane

	With 1.80× Lens		*With 2× Lens*		*With 2.30× Lens*	
Near Addition	*Resultant Magnification*	*Field of View (cm.)*	*Resultant Magnification*	*Field of View (cm.)*	*Resultant Magnification*	*Field of View (cm.)*
+ 4 D.S.	1.8×	8	2×	7	2.3×	5.7
+ 6 D.S.	2.7×	6	3×	5	3.5×	4
+ 8 D.S.	3.6×	4.5	4×	4	4.6×	3
+10 D.S.	4.5×	3.5	5×	3	5.8×	2.5

The width of a normal newspaper column is 5 cm.

Reprinted by permission from N. Bier, *Correction of Subnormal Vision*, 2nd ed. London: Butterworths, 1970.

6.5. Determination of the Required Low Vision Add

Table A. Sloan Cards for Determining Required Reading Distance and Dioptric Power of Reading Aid

Size of Print in M Units Read at 40 cm.	*Equivalent Snellen Rating for Distance of 40 cm.*	*Reading Distance (cm.) Required for 1M Print*	*Dioptric Power of Required Reading Add**	*Equivalent Distance Acuity*
1.0	40/100	40	2.5	20/50
1.5	40/150	26.6	3.75	20/75
2.0	40/200	20	5.0	20/100
2.5	40/250	16	6.25	20/125
3.0	40/300	13.3	7.5	20/150
4.0	40/400	10	10.0	20/200
5.0	40/500	8	12.5	20/250
7.0	40/700	5.7	17.5	20/350
10.0	40/1000	4	25.0	20/500
14.0	40/1400	2.9	35.0	20/700
20.0	40/2000	2	50.0	20/1000

*These values assume that the reader supplies none of the required power by accommodation. The listed values can be reduced by the diopters that can be sustained by patients with active accomodation.

Adapted from *Recommended Aids for the Partially Sighted*, 2nd ed., rev., 1971, by permission from National Society for the Prevention of Blindness, Inc.

Table B. Print Size of Common Publications Correlated to Visual Acuity Needed

Diopters Addition for 1 M	*Distance Acuity*	*Print Correlated to Acuity*	*Metric*	*Point*
1.00	20/20	Mail order; medication labels	.4 M	3
1.25	20/25	Classified ads	.5 M	4
1.50	20/30	Telephone book	.6 M	5
2.00	20/40	Newspapers; paperback books	.8 M	6
2.50	20/50	Magazines; typing; books	1 M	8
3.00	20/60	Magazines; newspapers	1.2 M	9
3.50	20/70	Adult books	1.4 M	10
4.00	20/80	Books for ages 9–12	1.6 M	12
5.00	20/100	Books for ages 7–9	2 M	14
6.25	20/125	Books for ages 6–8; large print magazines	2.5 M	18
8.00	20/160	Large-print publications; pre-primer	3.2 M	
10.00	20/200	Children's books; subheadlines	4 M	24
12.00	20/250	Subheadlines	5 M	
15.00	20/300	Letters 9 mm high (lowercase)	6 M	
16.00	20/320		6.4 M	
20.00	20/400		8 M	
24.00	20/480	Letters 14 mm high (lowercase)	9.6 M (10 M)	
30.00	20/600	Letters 18 mm high (lowercase)	12 M	
40.00	20/800		16 M	
50.00	20/1000	Letters 30 mm high (lowercase)	20 M	
	(5/200)	Headlines over 1 inch; display ads		
74.00	3/200	Letters 45 mm high (lowercase)	30 M	

6.6. Field of View at Near

Table A. Approximate Linear Field for Full Diameter Microscopes (Morgan)

Magnification	*Linear Field*
2X	110 mm
4X	68 mm
6X	38 mm
8X	28 mm
10X	18 mm
12X	17 mm
14X	14 mm
16X	11 mm
20 X	8 mm

Table B. Size of Actual Reading Field

Working Distance (m)	*Working Distance* (cm)	*Compensating Addition* (D)	*Field Size of 10°* (in)	*Field Size of 10°* (cm)	*Field Size of 5°* (in)	*Field Size of 5°* (cm)	*Field Size of 3°* (in)	*Field Size of 3°* (cm)
40	100	1.00	7.0	17.5	3.5	8.75	2.1	5.25
16	40	2.50	3.0	7.5	1.5	3.75	.9	2.25
8	20	5.00	1.5	3.75	.75	1.9	.45	1.12
4	10	10.00	.75	1.9	.37	.92	.22	.55

Size of the central reading field at various distances from the eye for fields of 10°, 5°, and 3°. The 10° field at 1 meter measures 7 inches, or 17.5 cm. The size of a patient's reading field affects the amount of magnification he or she can appreciate.

Reprinted from E. Faye, *Clinical Low Vision.* Boston, Mass.: Little, Brown and Co., 1975.

6.7. Assessment of Visual Acuity and Magnification Required

	Magnification Required to Raise Acuity to:									
Acuity	*20/150*	*20/120*	*20/100*	*20/80*	*20/60*	*20/50*	*20/40*	*20/30*	*20/25*	*20/20*
20/20										
20/25										1.3
20/30									1.3	1.6
20/40								1.3	1.6	2.0
20/50							1.3	1.6	2.0	2.5
20/60						1.3	1.6	2.0	2.5	3.0
20/80					1.3	1.6	2.0	2.5	3.0	4.0
20/100				1.3	1.6	2.0	2.5	3.0	4.0	5.0
20/120			1.3	1.6	2.0	2.5	3.0	4.0	5.0	6.0
20/150		1.3	1.6	2.0	2.5	3.0	4.0	5.0	6.0	8.0
20/180	1.3	1.6	2.0	2.5	3.0	4.0	5.0	6.0	8.0	10.
20/240	1.6	2.0	2.5	3.0	4.0	5.0	6.0	8.0	10.	12.
20/300	2.0	2.5	3.0	4.0	5.0	6.0	8.0	10.	12.	15.
20/360	2.5	3.0	4.0	5.0	6.0	8.0	10.	12.	15.	18.
20/400	3.0	4.0	5.0	6.0	8.0	10.	12.	15.	18.	23.
20/600	4.0	5.0	6.0	8.0	10.	12.	15.	18.	23.	
20/800	5.0	6.0	8.0	10.	12.	15.	18.	23.		
20/1000	6.0	8.0	10.	12.	15.	18.	23.			
20/1400	8.0	10.	12.	15.	18.	23.				
20/2000	10.	12.	15.	18.	23.					
Reading Acuity at 25 cm.	J12	J10	J9	J6	J4	J2				

Acuities Refer to Near Vision

Adapted by permission from N. Bier, *Correction of Subnormal Vision,* 2nd ed. London: Butterworths, 1970.

6.8. Type Size Variability in Near Acuities

Measured heights of test digits, expressed in M notation (1 mm = 0.7 M), for near-point-acuity cards.

Table A. M Notation

Indicated M Size	*Measured Letter Height in M Notation*				
	Jaeger Card	*A.O. Card #1985-1A*	*Lighthouse Symbols*	*Lighthouse Card*	*M & F Card*
0.37	0.56	0.50			
0.40					
0.50	0.60	0.60	0.50	0.50	0.56
0.62	0.70	0.67			
0.75	0.88	0.84			
0.80			0.77	0.84	
1.00	0.98	1.05	0.91	1.05	1.05
1.25	1.33	1.47			
1.50			1.61		1.19
2.00			1.96	2.10	
3.00				3.15	
4.00			3.85	4.20	
6.00			6.30	6.30	

Table B. Points

Indicated Point Type	*Measured Digit Height in M Notation*		
	Feinbloom Digits	*M & G Card*	*Lebensohn Chart*
3		0.56	0.42
4	0.77	0.77	0.56
5	1.05	0.91	0.77
6		1.12	0.84
7	1.33		
8		1.47	1.05
9	1.61		1.12
10		1.75	1.33
12	2.10		1.68
14	2.80	2.52	1.96
18	3.64		2.73
24			3.43

Table C. "Point-Type"

Indicated Point Type	A.O. Wells #9012	Lighthouse Symbols	Good-Lite Card
	Measured Letter Height in M Notation		
4	0.70	0.49	0.42
5			0.56
6			0.63
7	1.05	0.77	
8			0.84
10	1.26		1.05
11	1.40		
12	1.47		1.12
18	2.03	1.96	1.96
24			2.52

Table D. Snellen Notation

Indicated Snellen Notation 20/	Reduced Snellen	Tumbling E	M & G Card	Lighthouse Symbols	Lighthouse Card	Lebensohn Chart
	Measured Letter Height in M Notation					
20	0.42	0.42	0.60			0.42
25		0.56	0.77	0.50	0.50	0.56
30	0.67	0.67	0.91	0.77		0.77
40	0.91	0.84	1.12		0.84	0.84
50		1.00	1.47	0.91	1.05	1.05
60	1.33	1.26			1.33	
80	1.75	1.61		1.61	1.54	1.68
100			2.59	1.96	2.20	1.82
120	2.66	2.38				
160		3.15		3.15		
200	4.34	3.85	3.71	3.92	4.20	

Adapted with permission from R.T. Jose and R.M. Acheson, "Type Size Visibility in Near Accuracy Tests," tables 1, 4, 5. *American Journal of Optometry and Physiologic Optics*, September 1977.

6.9. Determination of the Correct Angle for Bioptic Telescopes

Normal Distance Viewing Point	Backward Head Tilt for Carrier Lens Viewing	Forward Head Tilt for Telescopic Viewing	Telescope Angle if Pantoscopic Tilt = 5°
6 mm	28°	−8°	3° down
8 mm	24°	−4°	1° up
10 mm	20°	0°	5° up
12 mm	16°	4°	9° up
14 mm	12°	8°	13° up
16 mm	8°	12°	17° up
18 mm	4°	16°	21° up
20 mm	0°	20°	25° up

This table assumes that the telescopic and carrier viewing points will be 10 mm and 20 mm, respectively, from the eyewire.

Reprinted from Optometric Monthly (June, 1979, pp. 131–138) published by the Professional Press, Inc., 101 East Ontario Street, Chicago, Illinois 60611.

6.10. Decentrations for Telescopic Devices Used at Near

Distance P.D. (mm.)	Near P.D. (mm.) For Magnifications 1.6×	2×	3×	4×	5×
56	50	49		47	
58	52	51		49	
60	53	52		50	
62	55	54		52	
64	57	56		54	
66	59	58		55	
68	61	59		57	
70	62	61		59	
72	64	63		60	

Courtesy Hamblin Instruments, Ltd., Hamblin House, London, England.

6.11. Magnification of Telescopic Loupes

Table A. Reading Caps Needed for Particular Magnifications

MAG:	*2×*	*2.5×*	*3×*	*4×*	*5×*	*6×*
T.S.						
1.3×	+3.84	+4.80	+5.76	+7.70	+9.60	+11.50
1.7×	+2.92	+3.68	+4.40	+5.87	+7.35	+ 8.80
2.2×	+2.27	+2.84	+3.30	+4.55	+5.70	+ 6.81
3.0×	+1.67	+2.08	+2.50	+3.33	+4.14	+ 5.00
4.0×	+1.25	+1.56	+1.87	+2.50	+3.12	+ 3.75

Table B. Magnification Produced by Telescope and Reading Cap Combinations

CAP:	*+2.00*	*+4.00*	*+6.00*	*+8.00*	*+10.00*
T.S.					
1.3×	1.04×	2.08×	3.12×	4.16×	5.20×
1.7×	1.36×	2.72×	4.08×	5.44×	6.80×
2.2×	1.76×	3.52×	5.28×	7.04×	8.80×
3.0×	2,40×	4.80×	7.20×	9.60×	12.00×
4.0×	3.20×	6.40×	9.60×	12.80×	16.00×

Reprinted by permission from D. R. Williams, "Magnification of telescopic loupes," *J. Am. Opt. Assoc.* 45: 1974.

Table C. Determining the Magnifying Power of Galilean Telescopes

Determining the magnifying power of Galilean telescopes by measuring telescope length and the amount of change in back vertex power that results from adding a +1.00 D lens to the objective.

Change in BVP when +1.00 D added to objective (D)	*Telescope magnification (X)*					
	Length of telescope (mm)					
	10	*20*	*30*	*40*	*50*	*60*
1	1.00	0.99	0.99	0.98	0.98	0.97
2	1.39	1.39	1.38	1.37	1.36	1.36
3	1.72	1.70	1.69	1.67	1.66	1.64
4	1.98	1.96	1.94	1.92	1.90	1.88
5	2.21	2.19	2.16	2.14	2.11	2.09
6	2.42	2.39	2.36	2.33	2.30	2.28
7	2.61	2.58	2.54	2.51	2.48	2.44
8	2.79	2.75	2.71	2.67	2.64	2.60
9	2.96	2.91	2.87	2.83	2.78	2.74
10	3.11	3.06	3.02	2.97	2.92	2.88
11	3.26	3.21	3.16	3.10	3.05	3.00
12	3.40	3.35	3.29	3.23	3.17	3.12
13	3.54	3.47	3.42	3.35	3.30	3.24
14	3.67	3.60	3.54	3.47	3.41	3.35
15	3.80	3.72	3.65	3.58	3.52	3.45
16	3.92	3.84	3.77	3.69	3.62	3.55
17	4.04	3.96	3.88	3.80	3.72	3.64
18	4.15	4.07	3.98	3.90	3.82	3.74
19	4.26	4.17	4.08	4.00	3.91	3.83
20	4.37	4.28	4.18	4.09	4.00	3.91
21	4.48	4.38	4.28	4.18	4.09	4.00
22	4.58	4.48	4.37	4.27	4.17	4.08
23	4.68	4.57	4.46	4.36	4.26	4.16
24	4.78	4.66	4.55	4.44	4.34	4.23
25	4.88	4.76	4.64	4.52	4.41	4.31

Reprinted from Bailey, I.L.: *A Lensometer Method for Checking Telescopes*, Optometric Monthly (March, 1979, pp. 99–102) published by Professional Press, Inc., 101 East Ontarior Street, Chicago, IL 60611.

6.12. Classification of Handicapped Persons by Visual Acuity*

Common definition	*Snellen index*	*Practical test*	*Legal significance*
No light perception (total blindness)	—	Cannot see light	Totally blind
Light perception only	Less than 1/60 (3/200)	Unable to see hand movement at 1 meter	Satisfies all criteria for legal blindness**
Form and motion	Less than 2/60 (6/200)	Hand movement visible, but unable to count fingers at 1 meter	Total disability for Social Security Administration
Travel vision	Less than 3/60 (10/200)	Unable to read newspaper headlines	Legal blindness
Minimal reading	Less than 6/60 (20/200)	Reads headlines, but not 14-point (4.7 mm) type	Maximum acuity for legal blindness for Internal Revenue Service and most state industiral commissions
Partially seeing (borderline)	More than 6/60 (20/200), but less than 6/24 (20/70)	Cannot read 10-point (3.4 mm) type without marked difficulty	Not legally blind, but eligible for some services

***Better eye with best possible correction**
****Legal blindness also present if visual field is contracted to 20° or less**
Reprinted from P.C. Wheeler, *Missouri Med.*, Vol. 64, p. 315, 1967.

6.13. Determination of Visual Efficiency

Table A. Central Vision Loss

Distance		
Snellen		*Loss of Central Vision, %*
English	*Metric*	
20/16	6/5	0
20/20	6/6	0
20/25	6/7.5	5
20/32	6/10	10
20/40	6/12	15
20/50	6/15	25
20/64	6/20	35
20/80	6/24	40
20/100	6/30	50
20/125	6/38	60
20/160	6/48	70
20/200	6/60	80
20/300	6/90	85
20/400	6/120	90
20/800	6/240	95

Near			
Snellen	*Jaeger*	*Point*	*Loss of Central Vision, %*
14/14	1–	3	0
14/18	2–	4	0
14/22	. . .	5	5
14/28	3	6	10
14/35	6	8	50
14/45	7–	9+	60
14/56	8	12	80
14/70	11	14	85
14/87	. . .	. . .	90
14/112	14	22	95
14/140	. . .	. . .	98

Central vision loss = $\frac{\text{Distance loss + Near loss}}{2}$

Example: 20/160, 14/35 = $\frac{70\% + 50\%}{2}$ = 60%

Central vision efficiency = 100% — loss = 40%

AMA council on Industrial Health, 1955

Table B. Visual Field Loss

Minimal Normal Extent of Visual Field From Point of Fixation	*Degrees*
Temporally	85
Down temporally	85
Down	65
Down nasally	50
Nasally	60
Up nasally	55
Up	45
Up temporally	55
Total	500

3 mm white disk at a distance of 330 mm

Example: A concentric contraction to 25° is a cumulative loss of:
60°, + 60° + 40° + 25° + 35° + 30° + 20° + 30° = 300° (60% of 500°)
efficiency VF_E = 40%

Table C. Ocular Motility Loss

	20°	*30°*	*40°*
Right	100%	20%	10%
Left	100%	20%	10%
Down	100%	50%	30%
Up	100%	10%	10%
Oblique up	100%	10%	10%
Oblique down	100%	20%	20%

Use the point from center of fixation at which diplopia occurs (target small test light)

Sample use: The only loss is up and oblique at 40° from center of fixation = 10% OME = 90%

Visual efficiency of one eye = $CVE \times VFE \times OME = .40 \times .40 \times .90 = 14\%$

Visual efficiency of two eyes = $\frac{3 \times VE \text{ better eye} + VE \text{ poorer eye}}{4}$

If the corrected vision of bilateral aphakia has been used, impairment of the visual system is increased by 25%.

Pharmacology 7

7.1. Generic Name/Brand Name Table of Ocular Side Effects of Systemic Drugs

Generic Name	*Brand Name*	*Ocular Side Effects*
Acetazolamide	Diamox	Myopia, loss of accommodation, anterior lens displacement, ocular hypotony, retinal edema, changes in refractive power
ACTH	Acthar	Transient myopia, subcapsular cataract, glaucoma, potentiation of viral, bacterial and fungal ocular infection
Allopurinol	Zyloprim	Cataracts
Amitriptyline	Elavil	Blurred vision, mydriasis
Amphetamines	(Many Mfrs.)	Mydriasis, cycloplegia, widening of palpebral aperture, glaucoma
Amprotropine	Syntropan	Angle closure glaucoma, mydriasis, cycloplegia, difficulty with near vision, diminished lacrimal secretion, diplopia, hallucinations
Antimony compounds		Toxic amblyopia, yellowing of skin and sclera
Antipyrine	(Many Mfrs.)	Urticaria of lids, keratoconjunctivitis, toxic amblyopia
Arsenicals		Toxic amblyopia, transient myopia, retinal and vitreous hemorrhages, keratoconjunctivitis secondary, to arsenical dermatitis
Aspidium		Toxic amblyopia, mydriasis, optic atrophy and occasional permanent blindness
Atropine	(Many Mfrs.)	Mydriasis, risk of angle closure glaucoma, cycloplegia, hallucinations, difficulty with diminished lacrimal secretion near vision, diplopia
Bemethan	Vasculat	Increased blood flow through eye, increased IOP
Barbiturates	(Many Mfrs.)	Transient loss of vision, nystagmus, extraocular palsies, ptosis, diplopia, allergic conjunctivitis
Betamethasone	Celestone	See cortisone
Bethanechol	Urecholine	Miosis, low IOP, ocular pain, myopia, ciliary spasm, impaired day vision
Biperidin	Akineton	Blurred vision
Caffeine	NoDoz, also found in cola drinks, tea, coffee (Many Mfrs.)	Transient rise in IOP
Carbachol	Carcholin	See bethanecol
Carbromal	Adalin	Cataracts
Chloral hydrate	Noctec, Somnos (Many Mfrs.)	Diplopia, miosis, mydriasis with overdose, allergic conjunctivitis, transient amaurosis
Chloramphenicol	Chloromycetin	Optic neuritis, loss of vision, blurred vision, scotoma, internal ophthalmoplegia of iris, various neuropathies, toxic amblyopia, paralysis of extraocular muscles, nystagmus
Chlordiazepoxide	Librium	Blurred vision, decreased saccadic eye movements
Chlorthalidone	Hygroton	Xanthopsia, transient myopia

(continued)

7.1. Generic Name/Brand Table of Ocular Side Effects of Systemic Drugs (continued)

Generic Name	*Brand Name*	*Ocular Side Effects*
Chlorisondamine	Ecolid	Low IOP, loss of vision, amblyopia, difficulty with near vision, glaucoma, cycloplegia, diminished lacrimal secretion, mydriasis, difficulty in accommodation, conjunctival suffusion
Chloroquin	Aralen	Blurred vision, loss of vision, halos around lights, scotoma, constriction of peripheral fields, 6th cranial nerve paralysis, optic pallor, retinal edema, photophobia, premature graying of eye lashes, corneal pigmentation, pigmentary degeneration, ocular palsies, ptosis, decreased corneal sensitivity, corneal edema, keratopathy, pigmentary retinopathy and macular degeneration
Chlorothiazide	Diuril	Yellow vision, transient myopia, retinal edema, flattening of cornea with contact lens
Chlorpromazine	Thorazine	See phenothiazines
Chlorpropamide	Diabinese	Central scotoma, loss of vision, hyperopia with overdose, mydriasis, diplopia, hallucinations, toxic amblyopia, exudative pemphigoid conjunctivitis, changes in refractive power
Cholestyramine	Questran	Arcus juvenilis, uveitis
Clorazepate dipotassium	Tranxene	Blurred vision, diplopia
Clortermine	Voranil	Euphoria, dysphoria, glaucoma
Chrysarobin		Conjunctivitis, keratitis
Clomiphene	Clomid	Cataracts, loss of central vision, scintillating scotoma
Cocaine		Allergic conjunctivitis, mydriasis, cycloplegia, ptosis, transitory amblyopia
Cortisone (Corticosteroid Drugs)	Cortogen, Cortone (Many Mfrs.)	*Systemic Administration*—Optic nerve changes, increased IOP (less than with Topical), posterior subcapsular cataracts, lens changes, papilledema with pseudotumor cerebri, transient myopia *Topical Administration*—increased IOP, may induce and aggravate wide angle glaucoma, potentiation of viral, bacterial and fungal ocular infections
Cyclandelate	Cyclospasmol	Increased IOP
Dantrolene sodium	Dantrium	Visual disturbances, diplopia, hyperlacrimation
Dexamthasone	Decadron, Maxidex	See cortisone
Dextroamphetamine	Dexedrine (Many Mfrs.)	Mydriasis
Dextrothyroxine	Choloxin	Ptosis
Diazepam	Valium	Diplopia, blurred vision, decreased saccadic eye movements
Diazoxide	Hyperstat	Cataracts, euphoria
Dichlorphenamide	Daranide	Transient myopia, retinal edema, ocular hypotony, loss of accommodation, anterior lens displacement
Dicyclomine	Bentyl	See atropine

(continued)

7.1. Generic Name/Brand Table of Ocular Side Effects of Systemic Drugs (continued)

Generic Name	*Brand Name*	*Ocular Side Effects*
Digitalis	Digitalis	Green-yellow vision (sometimes red, brown, white), snowy vision, photophobia, halos around lights, blurred vision, sparks, scintillating scotoma, amblyopia, low IOP, paralysis of extraocular muscles, retrobulbular neuritis, cortical blindness, conjunctivitis, toxic amblyopia
Digitoxin	Purodigin, Crystodigin	See digitalis
Digoxin	Lanoxin	See digitalis
Diisopropylfluorophosphate; DFP	Floropryl	See isoflurophate
Dinoprost tromethamine	Prostin F2 Alpha	Burning sensation of the eye, diplopia, glaucoma
DMSO		Blurred vision, changes in transparency and refractive power of lens
Doxepin	Sinequan, Adapin	Blurred vision, photophobia, glaucoma
Echothiophate	Phospholine	See bethanechol
Ephedrine	Ephedrine	Mydriasis
Ergonovine	Ergotrate	Blurred vision, optic edema, concentric constriction of vision fields
Ergotamine	Cafergot*	Bilateral papillitis
Ethambutol	Myambutol	Toxic amblyopia
Ethoxzolamide	Cardrase	See dichlorphenamide
Fenfluramine	Pondimin	Blurred vision, nystagmus, ocular burning, dilated, non-reactive pupils with overdosage
Flavoxate	Urispas	Blurred vision
Flucytosine	Ancobon	Hallucinations
5-Fluorouracil	Fluoracil	Hyperlacrimation
Flurazepam	Dalmane	Focusing difficulty, blurred vision, ocular burning
Furosemide	Lasix	Altered color vision
Gold compounds	(Many Mfrs.)	Chrysiasis of conjunctiva, cornea and lens, keratoconjunctivitis, involvement of lids by exfoliative dermatitis, ocular palsies, nystagmus secondary to encephalitis
Guanethidine	Ismelin	Blurred vision, ptosis
Haloperido	Haldol	Blurred vision
Heroin	*Heroin*	Anisocoria upon withdrawal
Hexamethonium	Methium	See chlorisondamine
Hometropine	(Many Mfrs.)	See atropine
Hydrochlorothiazide	HydroDiuril	See chlorothiazide
Hydrocortisone	Cortef, Cortril (Many Mfrs.)	See cortisone
Hydromorphone	Dilaudid	Pinpoint pupils
Hydroxychloroquin	Plaquenil	See chloroquin

(continued)

7.1. Generic Name/Brand Table of Ocular Side Effects of Systemic Drugs (continued)

Generic Name	*Brand Name*	*Ocular Side Effects*
Hyoscine (Scopolamine)	(Many Mfrs.)	See atropine
Hyoscyamine	(Many Mfrs.)	See atropine
Imipramine	Tofranil	Blurred vision, toxic amblyopia, mydriasis, cycloplegia, diplopia, glaucoma
Indomethacin	Indocin	Deterioration of visual acuity, visual field, dark adaptation, and scotopic ERG and EOG ratio decreased after initial blurred vision, mydriasis, toxic amblyopia, diplopia
Insulin	(Many Mfrs.)	Hyperopia with overdose
Iodides (iodide salts [such as potassium iodide] and radioactive iodine)		Amblyopia, green vision, conjunctivitis, keratitis, hypopyon, iridocyclitis, topical dermatitis of lens, retinal hemorrhage which may lead to retinal degeneration and optic neuritis, risk of precipitating malignant exophthalmos and ophthalmoplegia, iritis, intraocular hemorrhage, lacrimation chemosis
Iodochlorhydroxyquin	Vioform	Sub-acute myeloptic neuropathy leading to blindness
Isocarboxazid	Marplan	See MAO inhibitors
Isoflurophate	Floropryl	Iris cysts, retinal detachment, ciliary spasm myopia, ocular pain, impaired day vision, miosis, low IOP
Isoniazid	INH	Toxic amblyopia
Isorbide dinitrate	Isordil	See nitrates
Isoxsuprine	Vasodilan	Increased IOP
Lead compounds		Toxic amblyopia, ocular palsies, papilledema, mydriasis, cycloplegia
Levodopa	Dopar; Larodopa	Blurred vision, diplopia, mydriasis, activation of latent Horner's syndrome
Lithium carbonate	Eskalith; Lithane	Blurred vision, scotomata
LSD_{25}		Mydriasis, pupillary dilation of unequal size, unpredictable pupillary response to light
Marijuana	*Cannabis*	Visual disturbances, conjunctivitis, anisocoria
Meclizine	Antivert, Bonine	Blurred vision
Mellaril	Thioridazine	See phenothiazines
Mephenesin	Tolserol	Diplopia, nystagmus
Meprobamate	Equanil, Miltown	Loss in accommodative power for near objects
Mercury salts	(Many Mfrs.)	Visual hallucinations, lid and conjunctival discolorations, metallic deposits in cornea and conjunctiva, discoloration of anterior chamber, photophobia
Mesoridazine	Serentil	See phenothiazines
Methacholine	Mecholyl	See bethanechol
Methantheline	Banthine	See atropine
Methixene	Trest	Blurred vision
Methylphenidate	Ritalin	Mydriasis
Methylprednisone	Medrol	See cortisone

(continued)

7.1. Generic Name/Brand Table of Ocular Side Effects of Systemic Drugs (continued)

Generic Name	*Brand Name*	*Ocular Side Effects*
Metolazone	Zaroxolyn	Xanthopsia
MAO inhibitors (monoamine oxydase inhibitors)	Eutonyl, Nardil, Niamid, Marplan, Parnate	Toxic amblyopia, blurred vision, cycloplegia, disturbed color vision, extraocular muscle palsies, mydriasis, nystagmus
Morphine		Pinpoint constriction of pupils
Nalidixic acid	NegGram	Papilledema, altered color vision, blurred vision, diplopia, photophobia, accommodation difficulties
Neostigmine	Prostigmin	See bethanechol
Nialamid	Niamid	See MAO inhibitors
Nicotinyl alcohol	Roniacol	See nicotinic acid
Nicotinic acid	(Many Mfrs.)	Amblyopia, hyperlacrimation, mydriasis, toxic maculopthy
Nitrates	Isordil, Nitroglycerin, Peritrate	Increased IOP
Nitrites		Increased IOP
Nitroglycerin	(Many Mfrs.)	See nitrates
Nylidrin	Arlidin	Increased blood flow through eye, increased IOP
OC's (oral contraceptives)	C-Quens, Enovid, Norinyl, Norlestrin, Norquen, Oracon, Ortho-Novum, Ovral, Ovulen, Provest, Micronor, Loestrin, Zorne	Lowering of IOP with wide angle glaucoma, neuro-ocular lesions, retinal thrombosis, optic neuritis, photophobia, diplopia, retinal edema, proptosis, drop in visual acuity, homonymous hemianopia
Oxygen		Conjunctival edema, dilated and fixed pupils, retinal detachment, taporetinal degeneration, retrolental fibroplasia in premature infants, blurred vision, constriction of visual fields, ocular irritation
Oxyphenbutazone	Tandearil	Conjunctivitis, toxic amblyopia, Stevens-Johnson syndrome, adhesion of lids to eyeballs, gross scarring of lids, corneal ulceration and scarring, vascularization of cornea, loss of vision, possible retinal hemorrhage
Para-aminosalicylic acid (PAS)		Ocular itching and burning
Pargyline	Eutonyl	See MAO inhibitors
Pentaerythritol tetranitrate	Peritrate	See nitrates
Pentazocine	Talwin	Visual hallucinations, visual blurring, focusing difficulty
Perphenazine	Trilafon	See phenothiazines
Phenelzine	Nardil	See MAO inhibitors
Phenmetrazine	Preludin	Central and paracentral corneal curvature

(continued)

7.1. Generic Name/Brand Table of Ocular Side Effects of Systemic Drugs (continued)

Generic Name	*Brand Name*	*Ocular Side Effects*
Phenothiazines	Thorazine, Phenergan, Sparine, Trilafon, Stelazine, Mellaril, Serentil and others (Many Mfrs.)	Transient blurred vision, amblyopia, night blindness, central scotoma, loss of peripheral vision, possible corneal flattening, blue-grey pigmentation of eyelids, photosensitization, corneal and lenticular opacities, oculogyric crisis in a parkinsonian-type extra-pyramidal syndrome, ocular melanosis, miosis, temporary cycloplegia, possible glaucoma, drop in visual acuity
Phenoxybenzamine	Dibenzyline	Miosis
Phenylbutazone	Butazolidin	See oxyphenbutazone
Phenylephrine	Neosynephrine	"Whitens" inflamed or reddened conjunctiva
Phenylpropanolamine	Propadrine	Mydriasis
Physostigmine (Eserine)	(Many Mfrs.)	See bethanechol
Pilocarpine	(Many Mfrs.)	See bethanechol
Piperactazine	Quide	See phenothiazines
Polymyxin B sulfate	Aerosporin	Blurred vision
Prednisolone	Meticortelone	See cortisone
Primidone	Mysoline	Edema of lids and orbit, visual hallucinations, diplopia
Promazine	Sparine	See phenothiazines
Promethazine	Phenergan	See phenothiazines
Propoxyphene napsylate with acetaminophen	Darvocet N*	Pupillary constriction, visual disturbances
Propranolol	Inderal	Visual disturbances, hallucinations
Protriptyline	Vivactil	Blurred vision, mydriasis
Quinidine		Amblyopia, optic and retinal ischemia
Quinine		Diplopia, toxic amblyopia which may lead to blindness, scotoma, disturbed color perception, night blindness, photophobia, paralysis of extraocular muscles, mydriasis, retinal edema, optic pallor, narrowing of arterioles, peripheral contraction of visual fields, ocular anesthesia, iris atrophy
Radioactive iodides		See iodides
Reserpine	Serpasil (Many Mfrs.)	Glaucoma, uveitis, optic atrophy, blurred vision, conjunctivitis, ptosis
Resorcinol	(Many Mfrs.)	Conjunctivitis, keratitis
Salicylates	(Many Mfrs.)	Toxic amblyopia, possible cortical blindness, mydriasis, allergic conjunctivitis, nystagmus, ocular hypotony, hallucinations
Scopolamine (Hyoscine)	(Many Mfrs.)	See atropine
Sex hormones, female, including OC's	(Many Mfrs.)	Cyclitis, cycloplegia, diplopia, lowering of IOP with angle glaucoma, hallucinations, homonymous hemianopia, ocular palsies, optic neuritis, mydriasis, neuro-ocular lesions, nystagmus, papilledema, phosphenes, photophobia, proptosis, retinal edema, retinal perivasculitis, retinal thrombosis, scotoma, drop in visual acuity

(continued)

7.1. Generic Name/Brand Table of Ocular Side Effects of Systemic Drugs (continued)

Generic Name	*Brand Name*	*Ocular Side Effects*
Silver compounds	Argyrol	Discoloration of vision, corneal discoloration, metallic deposits in and discoloration of conjunctiva
Steroids		See cortisone (corticosteroids)
Streptomycin	(Many Mfrs.)	Optic neuritis, optic atrophy, toxic amblyopia, loss of vision, scotoma
Succinylcholine	Anectine	Diplopia, increased IOP, contraction of extraocular muscles
Sulfadimethoxine	Madribon	Stevens-Johnson syndrome, exudative pemphigoid conjunctivitis, transient myopia, ocular palsies, iritis, retinal edema and hemorrhage, toxic amblyopia, injection of conjunctiva and sclera
Sulfamethoxazole	Gantanol	See sulfadimethoxine
Sulfamethoxypyridazine	Kynex, Midicel	See sulfadimethoxine
Sulfisoxazole	Gantrisin	See sulfadimethoxine
Thallium		Cataracts, ptosis, extraocular muscle palsies, mydriasis, central scotoma
Thiazides	(Many Mfrs.)	See chlorothiazide
Thoridazine	Mellaril	Pigmentary degeneration of retina, occasional blindness, see also under phenothiazines
Tolazoline	Priscoline	Increased IOP
Tranylcypromine	Parnate	See MAO inhibitors
Triamcinolone	Aristocort, Kenacort	See cortisone
Trifluoperazine	Stelazine	See phenothiazines
Trihexyphenidyl	Artane	Blurred vision, mydriasis, increased IOP
Trimethadione	Tridione	Unusual sense of brightness, hallucinatory snow-storm effects, photophobia, diplopia, impaired color vision
Triparano	MER-29	Cataracts
Tryparsamide		Shimmering effect, narrowing field of vision, optic neuritis and atrophy, if not withdrawn may lead to blindness
Vitamin A	Alphalin (Many Mfrs.)	Excessive dose can cause papilledema, retinal detachment, epithelial lesions, loss of brows and eyelashes, ocular palsies, nystagmus, exophthalmos, retinal hemorrhage, yellow vision
Vitamin C (Ascorbic acid)		Decreased IOP
Vitamin D	(Many Mfrs.)	Excessive dose can cause calcium deposits in cornea and conjunctiva, band shaped corneal degeneration

*Multi-component drug

Reprinted with permission from H. I. Silverman, "The adverse effects of commonly used systemic drugs on the human eye. Part II," *Am. J. Optom.* **49**: 1972; and H. I. Silverman and R. J. Harvie, "The adverse effects of commonly used systemic drugs. Part III," *Am. J. Optom.* **52**: 1975.

7.2. Pharmacological Table of Ocular Side Effects of Systemic Drugs

Pharmacological Classification	*Generic Name*	*Brand Name*	*Ocular Effect*
Sympathomimetics (Adrenergics)	Amphetamine	Benzedrine	Mydriasis, possible glaucoma, cycloplegia, widening of palpebral aperture
	Clortermine	Voranil	Euphoria, dysphoria, glaucoma
	Dextroamphetamine	Dexedrine	Mydriasis
	Ephedrine	Tedral*, Primatene*, Quadrinal*, Bronakaid*	
	Fenfluramine	Pondimin	Blurred vision, nystagmus, burning sensation of the eye, dilated, non-reative pupils with overdosage
	Methylphenidate	Ritalin	
	Phenylpropanolamine	Propadrine	
	Levodopa	Dopar, Larodopa	Blurred vision, diplopia, mydriasis, activation of Horner's syndrome
	Phenmetrazine	Preludin	Central and paracentral corneal curvature
	Phenylephrine	Neosynephrine	Mydriasis, "whitens" inflamed or reddened conjunctiva
Sympatholytics Alpha blocker	Ergotamine	Bellergal*, Gynergen Cafergot*	Blurred vision, optic edema, concentric constriction of visual fields, bilateral papillitis
	Phenoxybenzamine	Dibenzylene	Miosis
Beta blocker	Propranolol	Inderal	Visual disturbances, hallucinations
Parasympathomimetics (Cholinergics)	Bethanechol	Urecholine	Ciliary spasm, myopia, ocular pain, impaired day vision, miosis, low IOP. Iris cysts and retinal detachment have also been reported with Floropryl.
	Carbachol	Carcholin	
	Echothiophate	Phospholine	
	Isoflurophate (DFP)	Floropryl	
	Methacholine		
	Neostigmine	Prostigmine	
	Physostigmine	Eserine	
	Pilocarpine		
Parasympatholytics–1 (strong)	Atropine		Risk of precipitating angle closure glaucoma, mydriasis, cycloplegia, difficulty with near vision, diminished lacrimal secretion, diplopia, visual hallucinations
	Homatropine		
	Hyoscyamine		
	Scopolamine (hyoscine)		
Parasympatholytics–2 (weak)	Mephenesin	Tolserol	Diplopia, nystagmus

(continued)

7.2. Pharmacological Table of Ocular Side Effects of Systemic Drugs (continued)

Pharmacological Classification	*Generic Name*	*Brand Name*	*Ocular Effect*
Antispasmodics	Amprotropine	Syntropan	See atropine
	Dicyclomine	Bentyl	
	Flavoxate	Urispas	Blurred vision
	Methantheline	Banthine	Blurred vision, mydriasis
	Methixene	Trest	Blurred vision
Antihistaminic	Meclizine	Antivert, Bonine	Blurred vision
	Promethazine	Phenergan	
Antipsychotics (See also under tranquilizers)			
Anti-depressants	Amitriptyline	Elavil	Blurred vision, mydriasis
	Protriptyline	Vivactil	
	Imipramine	Tofranil	Blurred vision, toxic amblyopia, mydriasis, cycloplegia, diplopia, glaucoma, difficulty in accommodation
	Doxepin	Sinequan, Adapin	Blurred vision, photophobia, glaucoma
	Phenothiazines	(Many Mfrs.)	Mydriasis, miosis
	MAO inhibitors		Mydriasis, cycloplegia, disturbed color vision, nystagmus, extraocular muscle palsies, toxic amblyopia, blurred vision
	Isocarboxazid	Marplan	
	Nialamid	Niamid	
	Pargyline	Eutonyl	
	Phenelzine	Nardil	
	Tranylcypromine	Parnate	
Anti-parkinsonism	Biperiden	Akineton	Blurred vision
	Trihexyphenidyl	Artane	Blurred vision, mydriasis, increased IOP
Ganglionic blockers	Chlorisondamine	Ecolid	Low IOP, loss of vision, toxic amblyopia, difficulty with near vision, glaucoma, cycloplegia, diminished lacrimal secretion, mydriasis, difficulty in accommodation, conjunctival suffusion
	Hexamethonium	Methium	
CNS stimulants (See also under sympathomimetics)	Caffeine	Cola beverages, tea, coffee, NoDoz	Transient rise in IOP
CNS depressants	Barbiturates	Nembutal Phenobarbital (Many Mfrs.)	Transient loss of vision, nystagmus, extraocular palsies, ptosis, diplopia, allergic conjunctivitis
	Carbromal	Adalin	Cataracts

(continued)

7.2. Pharmacological Table of Ocular Side Effects of Systemic Drugs (continued)

Pharmacological Classification	*Generic Name*	*Brand Name*	*Ocular Effect*
	Chloral hydrate	Noctec, Somnos	Diplopia, ptosis, miosis; mydriasis with overdose, allergic conjunctivitis, transient amaurosi
	Flurazepam	Dalmane	Focusing difficulty, blurred vision, ocular burning
Neuromuscular blockers (Skeletal muscle relaxants)	Dantrolene	Dantrium	Visual disturbances, diplopia, excessive tearing
	d-Tubocurarine		Ptosis, relaxation of extraocular muscles
	Mephenesin	Tolserol	Diplopia, nystagmus
	Succinylcholine	Anectine	Diplopia, increased IOP, contraction of extra-ocular muscles
Analgesics	Antipyrine		Urticaria of lids, keratoconjunctivitis, toxic amblyopia
	Hydromorphone	Dilaudid	Pinpoint constriction of pupils
	Morphine and its semi-synthetic cogeners	(Many Mfrs.)	Pinpoint constriction of pupils
	Oxyphenbutazone	Tandearil	Conjunctivitis, toxic amblyopia, Stevens-Johnson syndrome, adhesion of lid to eyeball, gross scarring of lids, corneal ulceration and scarring, vascularization of cornea, loss of vision, possible retinal hemorrhage
	Phenylbutazone	Butazolidin	
	Propoxyphene napsylate with acetaminophen	Darvocet N*	Pupillary constriction, visual disturbances
	Pentazocine	Talwin	Visual hallucinations, visual blurring, focusing difficulty
	Salicylates		Toxic amblyopia, possible cortical blindness, mydriasis, allergic conjunctivitis, nystagmus, ocular hypotony, visual hallucinations
Anti-inflammatory agents	*Corticosteroid drugs*		*Systemic*: Optic nerve changes, increased IOP, cataracts, lens changes, papilledema with pseudotumor cerebri, transient myopia *Topical*: Increased IOP, induces and aggravates wide angle glaucoma, potentiation of ocular infections
	Betamethasone	Celestone	
	Cortisone	(Many Mfrs.)	
	Dexamethasone	Decadron, Mexidex	
	Hydrocortisone	(Many Mfrs.)	
	Methylprednisone	Medrol	
	Prednisolone	Meticortelone	
	Prednisone	Meticorten	
	Triamcinolone	Aristocort, Kenacort	
	Indomethacin	Indocin	Mydriasis, diplopia, toxic amblyopia
Antimalarials	Chloroquin	Aralen	Blurred vision, halos around lights, scotoma, constriction

(continued)

7.2. Pharmacological Table of Ocular Side Effects of Systemic Drugs (continued)

Pharmacological Classification	*Generic Name*	*Brand Name*	*Ocular Effect*
	Hydroxychloroquin	Plaquenil	of peripheral fields, optic pallor, retinal edema, photophobia, premature greying of eyelashes, corneal pigmentation, pigmentary degeneration, ocular palsies, ptosis, decreased corneal sensitivity, corneal edema, keratopathy, pigmentary retinopathy, macular degeneration
	Quinine		Diplopia, toxic amblyopia, scotoma, disturbed color perception, night blindness, photophobia, paralysis of extraocular muscles, mydriasis, retinal edema, optic pallor, narrowing of arterioles, peripheral contraction of visual fields, ocular anesthesia, iris atrophy
Antidiabetics	Chlorpropamide	Diabinese	Central scotoma, changes in refractive power, mydriasis, diplopia, visual hallucinations, toxic amblyopia, exudative pemphigoid conjunctivitis, hyperopia with overdose
	Insulin	(Many Mfrs.)	Hyperopia with overdose
Cardiovascular drugs	Digitalis		Disturbed color vision where objects appear green or yellow, snowy vision photophobia, halos around lights, blurred vision, scotoma, toxic amblyopia, low IOP, paralysis of extraocular muscles, retrobulbular neuritis, cortical blindness, conjunctivitis
	Digitoxin	Purodigin, Crystodigin	
	Digoxin	Lanoxin	
Antiarrythmic	Quinidine		Amblyopia, optic and retinal ischemia
Hallucinogen	Heroin	*Heroin*	Anisocoria in withdrawals
	Marijuana	*Cannabis*	Anisocoria
	LSD_{25}		Mydriasis, pupillary dilation of unequal size, unpredictable pupillary response to light
Anti-infectives Antibiotics	Chloramphenicol	Chloromycetin	Optic neuritis, loss of vision, blurred vision, scotoma, internal ophthalmoplegia of iris, various neuropathies, toxic amblyopia, paralyses of extraocular muscles, nystagmus
	Streptomycin	(Many Mfrs.)	Optic neuritis, optic atrophy, toxic amblyopia, loss of vision, scotoma
Sulfonamides	Sulfadimethoxine	Madribon	Stevens-Johnson syndrome, myopia, conjunctivitis, ocular

(continued)

Pharmacological Classification	*Generic Name*	*Brand Name*	*Ocular Effect*
(Especially long acting types)	Sulfamethoxazole	Gantanol, Septra, Bactrim	palsies, iritis, retinal edema and hemorrhage, toxic amblyopia, exudative pemphigoid conjunctivitis, injection of conjunctiva and sclera
	Sulfamethoxypyridazine	Kynex, Midicel	
	Sulfisoxazole	Gantrisin	
Anti-amoebics	Iodochlorhydroxyquin	Vioform	Sub-acute myeloptic neuropathy leading to blindness
	Tryparsamide	(Many Mfrs.)	Shimmering effect, narrowing field of vision, optic neuritis
Miscellaneous	Ethambutol	Myambutol	Toxic amblyopia
	Isoniazid (INH)	(Many Mfrs.)	
	Para-aminosalicylic acid	(Many Mfrs.)	Ocular itching and burning
Anti-convulsants	Primidone	Mysoline	Edema of lids and orbit, visual hallucinations
	Trimethadione	Tridione	Unusual sense of brightness, snow-storm effects, photophobia, diplopia, impaired color vision
Diuretics			
Thiazides	Chlorothiazide	Diuril	Yellow vision, transient myopia, retinal edema, flattening or cornea with contact lens
	Hydrochlorothiazide	HydroDiuril	
	Metolazone	Zaroxolyn	Xanthopsia
Urinary Antiseptic	Nalidixic acid		Papilledema, altered color vision, blurred vision, diplopia, photophobia, accommodation difficulties
Anthranilic Ac. Deriv.	Furosemide	Lasix	Altered color vision
Carbonic Anhydrase inhibitors	Acetazolamide	Diamox	Retinal edema, loss of accommodation, anterior lens displacement, transient myopia, ocular hypotony, changes in refractive power
	Dichlorphenamide	Daranide	
	Ethoxzolamide	Cardrase	
Sulfonamide Deriv.	Chlorthalidone	Hygroton	Xanthopsia, transient myopia
Oral contraceptives (see also under Hormones)		C-Quens, Enovid, Loestrin, Norinyl, Norlestrin, Norquen, Oracon, Ortho-Novum, Ovral, Ovulen, Provest	Low IOP with wide angle glaucoma, neuro-ocular lesions, retinal thrombosis, optic neuritis, photophobia, diplopia, retinal edema, protosis, drop in visual acuity, homonymous hemianopia
Heavy Metals	Antimony compounds		Toxic amblyopia, yellowing of skin and sclera
	Arsenicals		Toxic amblyopia, myopia, retinal hemorrhage, keratoconjunctivitis
	Gold compounds		Chryiasis of conjunctiva, cornea and lens, keratoconjunctivitis, ocular palsies, nystagmus
	Lead compounds		Toxic amblyopia, ocular palsies, papilledema, mydriasis, cycloplegia

(continued)

7.2. Pharmacological Table of Ocular Side Effects of Systemic Drugs (continued)

Pharmacological Classification	*Generic Name*	*Brand Name*	*Ocular Effect*
	Mercury salts		Visual hallucinations, lid and conjunctival discolorations, metal deposits in cornea and conjunctiva, photophobia, discoloration of anterior chamber
	Silver compounds	Argyrol	Discoloration of vision, corneal discoloration, metal deposits in conjuctiva, discoloration of conjunctiva
	Thallium		Cataracts, ptosis, extraocular muscle palsies, mydriasis, toxic amblyopia
Gas	Oxygen–100%		Conjunctival edema, mydriasis, retinal detachment, tapeoretinal degeneration, retrolental fibroplasia in premature infants, blurred vision, constriction of visual fields, ocular irritation
Inorganic halide	Iodides (Iodide salts such as potassium iodide and radioactive iodine)	(Many Mfrs.)	Amblyopia, green vision, conjunctivitis, keratitis, hypopyon, iridocyclitis, topical dermatitis of lens, retinal hemorrhage which may lead to retinal degeneration and optic neuritis, risk of precipitating malignant exophthalmos and ophthalmoplegia, iritis, intraocular hemorrhage
Tranquilizers			
Propanediol	Meprobamate	Equanil Miltown	Loss of accommodation for near objects
Dibenzazepines	Amytriptyline	Elavil	Mydriasis, blurred vision
	Protriptyline	Vivactil	
	Imipramine	Tofranil	Difficulty in accommodation, toxic amblyopia, mydriasis, cycloplegia, diplopia, glaucoma, blurred vision
Benzodiazepine	Chlorazepate	Tranxene	Diplopia, blurred vision, decreased saccadic eye movements
	Chlordiazepoxide	Librium	
	Diazepam	Valium	
Phenothiazines	Chlorpromazine	Thorazine	Blurred vision, amblyopia, night blindness, scotoma, loss of peripheral vision, corneal flattening, blue-grey pigmentation of eyelids, photosensitization, corneal and lenticular opacities, oculogyric crisis resulting in a parkinsonian-type extrapyramidal syndrome, ocular melanosis, miosis, cycloplegia, possible glaucoma, drop in visual acuity
	Mesoridazine	Serentil	
	Perphenazine	Trilafon	
	Piperactazine	Quide	
	Promazine	Sparine	
	Promethazine	Phenergan	
	Trifluoperazine	Stealzine	

(continued)

7.2. Pharmacological Table of Ocular Side Effects of Systemic Drugs (continued)

Pharmacological Classification	*Generic Name*	*Brand Name*	*Ocular Effect*
	Prochlorperazine	Compazine	
	Fluphenazine	Prolixin	
	Thioridazine	Mellaril	Pigmentary degeneration of retina and occasional blindness in addition to above
Butyrophenone	Haloperidol	Haldol	Blurred vision
Vasodilators	Nitrates and nitrites	Peritrate, Nitrogylcerin, Isordil	Increased IOP
	Nicotinic acid	(Many Mfrs.)	Amblyopia, hyperlacrimation, mydriasis
	Nicotinyl alcohol	Roniacol	
	Bamethan	Vasculate	Increased IOP
	Cyclandelate	Cyclospasmol	
	Isoxuprine	Vasodilan	
	Nylidrin	Arlidin	
	Tolazoline	Priscoline	
Antihypertensive	Reserpine	Serpasil	Glaucoma, uveitis, optic atrophy, blurred vision, conjunctivitis, ptosis
	Diazoxide	Hyperstat	Cataracts, blurred vision, euphoria
Anti-neoplastic	5-Fluorouracil	Fluoracil	Excessive lacrimation
Vitamins	Nicotinic acid	(Many Mfrs.)	See vasodilators
	Vitamin A	Alphalin (Many Mfrs.)	Excessive dose can cause papilledema, retinal detachment, epithelial lesions, loss of brows and eyelashes, ocular palsies, nystagmus, exophthalmos, retinal hemorrhage, yellow vision
	Vitamin C	Ascorbic acid	Decreased IOP
	Vitamin D		Calcium deposits in cornea and conjunctiva, band shaped corneal degeneration
Oxytocic	Denoprost tromethamine	Prostin F2 Alpha	Burning sensation of the eye, diplopia, glaucoma
	Ergonovine	Ergotrate	Blurred vision, optic edema, concentric constriction of visual fields
Local anesthetic	Cocaine		Allergic conjunctivitis, mydrisis, cycloplegia, ptosis, transitory amblyopia

(continued)

7.2. Pharmacological Table of Ocular Side Effects of Systemic Drugs (continued)

Pharmacological Classification	*Generic Name*	*Brand Name*	*Ocular Effect*
Hormones	ACTH Steroids	(Many Mfrs.)	Transient myopia, posterior subcapsular cataract, glaucoma, potentiation of viral, bacterial and fungal ocular infections
	Female sex hormones (See also under oral contraceptives)		Cyclitis, cycloplegia, diplopia, lowering of IOP with wide angle glaucoma, hallucinations, homonymous hemianopia, ocular palsies, optic neuritis, mydriasis, neuro-ocular lesions, nystagmus, papilledema, phosphenes, photophobia, proptosis, retinal edema, retinal perivasculitis, retinal thrombosis, scotoma, drop in visual acuity
Unclassified drugs	Clomiphene	Clomid	Cataracts, loss of central vision, scintillating scotoma
	DMSO		Blurred vision, changes in transparency and refractive power of lens with high doses
	MER-29†	Triparanol	Cataracts
Miscellaneous	Cholestyramine	Questran	Arcus juvenilis, uveitis
	Chrysarobin		
	Resorcinol		
	Dextrothyroxine	Choloxin	Ptosis
	Guanethidine	Ismelin	Blurred vision, ptosis
	Lithium carbonate	Eskalith, Lithane	Blurred vision, scotomata
	Reserpine	Serpasil	Glaucoma, uveitis, optic atrophy, blurred vision, conjunctivitis
	Zyloprim	Allopurinol	Cataracts

*Multi-component drug
†No longer manufactured

Reprinted with permission from H. Silverman, "The adverse effects of commonly used systemic drugs on the human eye. Part II," *Am. J. Optom.* **49:** 1972; and H. I. Silverman and R. J. Harvie, "The adverse effects of commonly used systemic drugs on the human eye. Part III," *Am. J. Optom.* **52:** 1975.

7.3. Ocular Side Effects and Drugs Eliciting Same

Accommodation, difficulty in
  Chlorisondamine (Ecolid)
  Hexamethonium (Methium)
  Imipramine (Tofranil)
  Nalidixic acid (NegGram)
  Phenothiazines
Accommodation, loss of
  Acetazolamide (Diamox)
  Dichlorphenamide (Daranide)
  Ethoxzolamide (Cardrase)
  Meprobamate (Equanil)
Adhesion of lids to eyeballs
  Oxyphenbutazone (Tandearil)
  Phenylbutazone (Butazolidin)
Amaurosis, transient
  Chloral hydrate (Noctec, Somnos)
Amblyopia, toxic
  Antimony compounds
  Antipyrine
  Arsenicals
  Aspidium
  Chloramphenicol (Chloromycetin)
  Chlorisondamine (Ecolid)
  Chlorpromazine (Thorazine)
  Chlorpropamide (Diabinese)
  Digitalis
  Digitoxin (Purodigin, Crystodigin)
  Digoxin (Lanoxin)
  Ethambutol (Myambutol)
  Hexamethonium (Methium)
  Imipramine (Tofranil)
  Indomethacin (Indocin)
  Iodides
  Isoniazid (INH)
  Lead compounds
  MAO inhibitors
  Mesoridazine (Serentil)
  Nicotinic acid
  Nicotinyl alcohol (Roniacol)
  Oxyphenbutazone (Tandearil)
  Perphenazine (Trilafon)
  Phenothiazines
  Phenylbutazone (Butazolidin)
  Piperactazine (Quide)
  Promazine (Sparine)
  Promethazine (Phenergan)
  Quinidine
  Quinine
  Salicylates
  Streptomycin
  Sulfadimethoxine (Madribon)
  Sulfamethoxazole (Gantanol)
  Sulfamethoxypyridazine (Kynex, Midicel)
  Thallium
  Thioridazine (Mellaril)
  Trifluoperazine (Stelazine)
Amblyopia, transitory
  Cocaine
Anisocoria
  Heroin (upon withdrawal)
  Marijuana (*Cannabis*)
Anterior chamber, discolored
  Mercury salts
Anterior lens displacement
  Acetazolamide (Diamox)
Arcus Juvenilis
  Cholestyramine (Questran)
  Dichlorphenamide (Daranide)
  Ethoxzolamide (Cardrase)
Arterioles, narrowing of
  Quinine
Band shaped corneal degeneration
  (See under corneal degeneration)
Bilateral papillitis
  Ergotamine (Cafergot)
Blindness
  (See under vision)
Blood flow, increase
  Bamethan (Vasculat)
  Nylidrin (Arlidin)
Blurred vision
  Amitriptyline (Elavil)
  Biperidin (Akineton)
  Chlorazepate (Tranxene)
  Chloremphenicol (Chloromycetin)
  Chlordiazepoxide (Librium)
  Chloroquin (Aralen)
  Chlorpromazine (Thorazine)
  Diazepam (Valium)
  Diazoxide (Hyperstat)
  Digitalis
  Digitoxin (Purodigin, Crystodigin)
  Digoxin (Lanoxin)
  DMSO
  Doxepin (Sinequan, Adapin)
  Fenfluramine (Pondimin)
  Flavoxate (Urispas)
  Ergonovine (Ergotrate)
  Ergotamine (Bellergal, Gynergen)
  Flurazepam (Dalmane)
  Haloperidol (Haldol)
  Hydroxychloroquin (Plaquenil)
  Imipramine (Tofranil)
  Indomethacin (Indocin)
  Levodopa (Dopar, Larodopa)
  Lithium carbonate (Eskalith, Lithane)
  MAO inhibitors
  Meclizine (Antivert, Bonine)
  Mesoridazine (Serentil)
  Methantheline (Banthine)
  Methixene (Trest)
  Nalidixic acid (NegGram)
  Oxygen
  Oxyphenbutazone (Tandearil)
  Pentazocine (Talwin)
  Perphenazine (Trilafon)
  Phenylbutazone (Butazolidin)
  Phenothiazines
  Piperactazine (Quide)
  Polymyxin B sulfate (Aerosporin)

(continued)

Promazine (Sparine)
Promethazine (Phenergan)
Protriptyline (Vivactyl)
Reserpine (Serpasil)
Thioridazine (Mellaril)
Trifluoperazine (Stelazine)
Trihexyphenidyl (Artane)
Brightness, unusual sense of
Trimethadione (Tridione)
Burning, ocular
Dinoprost tromethamine (Prostin F2 Alpha)
Flurazepam (Dalmane)
Para-aminosalicylic acid
Calcium deposits in cornea and conjunctiva
Vitamin D
Cataracts
ACTH (Acthar)
Allopurinol (Zyloprim)
Bethamethasone (Celestone)
Carbromal (Adalin)
Clomiphene (Clomid)
Corticosteroid drugs
Cortisone
Dexamethasone (Decadron, Maxidex)
Hydrocortisone
MER-29 (Triparanol)
Methylprednisone (Medrol)
Predisolone (Meticortelone)
Prednisone (Meticorten)
Thallium
Triamcinolone (Aristocort, Kenacort)
Central vision, loss of
Clomiphene (Clomid)
Chemosis
Iodides
Chrysiasis of conjunctiva, cornea and lens
Gold compounds
Ciliary spasm
Bethanechol (Urecholine)
Carbachol (Carcholine)
Echothiophate (Phospholine)
Isoflurophate (Floropryl)
Methacholine (Mecholyl)
Neostigmine (Prostigmine)
Physostigmine (Eserine)
Pilocarpine
Color perception, disturbed or altered
Quinine
Color vision, disturbed or altered
Chlorothiazide (Diuril)
Digitalis
Digitoxin (Purodigin, Crystodigin)
Digoxin (Lanoxin)
Furosemide (Lasix)
Hydrochlorothiazide (HydroDiuril)
Iodides
MAO inhibitors
Marijuana (*Cannabis*)
Metolazone (Zaroxolyn)
Nalidixic acid (NegGram)
Thiazides
Trimethadione (Tridione)
Vitamin A
Concentric constriction of visual fields
(See under peripheral fields)
Conjunctiva, discolored
Mercury salts
Conjunctiva, metallic deposits in
Mercury salts
Silver compound
Conjunctiva, "whitening" of reddened or inflamed
Phenylephrine (Neosynephrine)
Conjunctival edema
Oxygen
Conjunctival suffusion
Chlorisondamine (Ecolid)
Conjunctivitis
(See also under exudative pemphigoid conjunctivitis)
Chlorprompamide (Diabinese)
Chrysarobin
Digitalis
Digitoxin (Purodigin, Crystodigin)
Digoxin (Lanoxin)
Iodides
Marijuana (*Cannabis*)
Oxyphenbutazone (Tandearil)
Phenylbutazone (Butazolidin)
Radioactive iodine
Reserpine (Serpasil)
Resorcinol
Sulfadimethoxine (Madribon)
Sulfamethoxazole (Gantanol)
Sulfamethoxypyridazine (Kynex, Midicel)
Conjunctivitis, allergic
Barbiturates
Chloral hydrates (Noctec, Somnos)
Cocaine
Salicylates
Cornea, central and paracentral curvature
Phenmentrazine (Preludin)
Corneal degeneration, band shaped
Vitamin D
Corneal discoloration
Silver compounds
Corneal edema
Chlorquin (Aralen)
Hydroxychloroquin (Plaquenil)
Corneal flattening
Chlorothiazide (Diuril)
Chlorpromazine (Thorazine)
Hydrochlorothiazide (HydroDiuril)
Mesoridazine (Serentil)
Perphenazine (Trilafon)
Phenothiazines
Piperactazine (Quide)
Promazine (Sparine)
Promethazine (Phenergan)

(continued)

Thioridazine (Mellaril)
Trifluoperazine (Stelazine)
Corneal pigmentation
Chloroquin (Aralen)
Hydroxychloroquin (Plaquentil)
Corneal sensitivity, decreased
Chloroquin (Aralen)
Hydroxychloroquin (Plaquenil)
Corneal ulceration and scarring
Oxyphenbutazone (Tandearil)
Phenylbutazone (Butazolidin)
Corneal vascularization
Oxyphenbutazone (Tandearil)
Phenylbutazone (Butazolidin)
Cortical blindness
Digitalis
Digitoxin (Purodigin, Crystodigin)
Digoxin (Lanoxin)
Salicylates
Cyclitis
Oral contraceptives
Sex hormones, female
Cycloplegia
Amphetamines
Amprotropine (Syntropan)
Atropine
Chlorisondamine (Ecolid)
Chlorpromazine (Thorazine)
Cocaine
Dicyclomine (Bentyl)
Hexamethonium (Methium)
Homatropine
Hyoscyamine
Imipramine (Tofranil)
Lead compounds
MAO inhibitors
Mesoridazine (Serentil)
Oral contraceptives
Perphenazine (Trilafon)
Phenothiazines
Piperactazine (Quide)
Promazine (Phenergan)
Scopolamine (Hyoscine)
Sex hormones, female
Thioridazine (Mellaril)
Tirfluoperazine (Stelazine)
Dark adaptation difficulty
Indomethacin (Indocin)
Day vision, impaired
Bethanechol (Urecholine)
Carbachol (Carcholin)
Echothiophate (Phospholine)
Isoflurophate (Floropryl)
Neostigmine (Prostigmine)
Physostigmine (Eserine)
Pilocarpine
Dermatitis of lens, topical
Iodides
Dilated non-reactive pupils (in overdosage)
Fenfluramine (Pondimin)
Diplopia
Amprotropine (Syntropan)
Atropine
Barbiturates
Chloral hydrate (Noctec, Somnos)
Chlorazepate (Tranxene)
Chlordiazepoxide (Librium)
Chlorpropamide (Diabinese)
Dantrolene (Dantrium)
Diazepam (Valium)
Dicyclomine (Bentyl)
Dinoprost tromethamine (Prostin F2 Alpha)
Homatropine
Hyoscyamine
Imipramine (Tofranil)
Indomethacin (Indocin)
Levodopa (Dopar, Larodopa)
Mephenesin (Tolserol)
Mysoline (Primidone)
Nalidixic acid (NegGram)
Oral contraceptives
Quinine
Scopolamine (Hyoscine)
Sex hormones, female
Succinylchloride (Anectine)
Trimethadione (Tridione)
Dysphoria
Clortermine (Voranil)
Edema of lids and orbit
Primidone (Mysoline)
Epithelial lesions
Vitamin A
Euphoria
Clortermine (Voranil)
Diazoxide (Hyperstat)
Eyebrows and lashes, loss of
Vitamin A
Eyelashes, greying of
Chloroquin (Aralen)
Hydroxychloroquin (Plaquenil)
Eyelids, blue-grey pigmentation
Chlorpromazine (Thorazine)
Mesoridazine (Serentil)
Perphenazine (Trilafon)
Phenothiazines
Piperactazine (Quide)
Promazine (Sparine)
Promethazine (Phenergan)
Thioridazine (Mellaril)
Trifluoperazine (Stelazine)
Exophthalmos
Iodides
Vitamin A
Extraocular muscles, contraction of
Succinylchloride (Anectine)
Extraocular palsies
Barbiturates
Thallium
Exudative pemphigoid conjunctivitis

(continued)

Chlorpropamide (Diabinese)
Sulfadimethoxine (Madribon)
Sulfamethoxazole (Gantanol)
Sulfamethoxypyridazine (Kynex, Midicel)
Flashing lights phenomenon
Clomiphene (Clomid)
Focusing, difficulty in
Flurazepam (Dalmane)
Pentazocine (Talwin)
Glaucoma
ACTH (Acther)
Amphetamines
Amprotropine (Syntropan)
Atropine
Bethamethasone (Celestone)
Chlorisondamine (Ecolid)
Chlorpromazine (Thorazine)
Clortermine (Voranil)
Corticosteroid drugs (Mainly Topical Applications)
Cortisone
Dexamethasone (Decadron, Maxidex)
Diclomine (Bentyl)
Dinoprost tromethamine (Prostin F2 Alpha)
Doxepin (Sinequan, Adapin)
Hexamethonium (Methium)
Homatropine
Hydrocortisone
Hyoscyamine
Imipramine
Mesoridazine (Serentil)
Methylprednisone (Medrol)
Perphenazine (Trilafon)
Phenothiazines
Piperactazine (Quide)
Prednisolone (Meticortelone)
Prednisone (Meticorten)
Promazine (Sparine)
Promethazine (Phenergan)
Reserpine (Serpasil)
Scopolamine (Hyoscine)
Thioridazine (Mellaril)
Trimcinolone (Aristocort, Kenacort)
Trifluoperazine (Stelazine)
Green vision
(See also under color vision)
Iodides
Green-yellow vision
(See also under color vision)
Digitalis
Digitoxin (Purodigin, Crystodigin)
Digoxin (Lanoxin)
Hallucinations
Amprotropine (Syntropan)
Atropine
Chlorpropamide (Diabinese)
Dicyclomine (Bentyl)
Flucytosine (Ancobon)
Heroin
Homatropine
Hyoscyamine
Marijuana (*Cannabis*)
Mercury salts
Oral contraceptives
Pentazocine (Talwin)
Primidone (Mysoline)
Salicylates
Scopolamine (Hyoscine)
Sex hormones, female
Sulfadimethoxine (Madribon)
Halos around lights
Chloroquin (Aralen)
Digitalis
Digitoxin (Purodigin, Crystodigin)
Digoxin (Lanoxin)
Hydorxychloroquin (Plaquenil)
Homonymous hemianopia
Oral contraceptives
Sex hormones, female
Horner's Syndrome, latent, activation of
Levodopa (Dopar, Larodopa)
Hyperlacrimation
Nicotinic acid
Nicotinyl alcohol (Roniacol)
Hyperopia (Hypermetropia)
Chlorpropamide (with overdose) (Diabinese)
Insulin (with overdose)
Hypopyon
Iodides
Injection of conjunctiva and sclera
Sulfadimethoxine (Madribon)
Sulfamethoxazole (Gantanol)
Sulfamethoxypyridazine (Kynex, Midicel)
Intraocular hemorrhage
Iodides
Intraocular pressure, decrease
Bethanechol (Urecholine)
Carbachol (Carcholin)
Chlorisondamine (Ecolid)
Digitalis
Digitoxin (Purodigin, Crystodigin)
Digoxin (Lanoxin)
Echothiophate (Phospholine)
Hexamethonium (Methium)
Isoflurophate (Floropryl)
Methacholine (Mecholyl)
Neostigmine (Prostigmine)
Oral contraceptives
Physostigmine (Eserine)
Pilocarpine
Sex hormones, female
Vitamin C
Intraocular pressure, increase
Bamethan (Vasculat)
Betamethasone (Celestone)
Caffeine
Corticosteroid drugs (MAINLY TOPICAL APPLICATION)

(continued)

Cortisone
Cyclandelate (Cyclospasmol)
Dexamethasone (Decadron, Maxidex)
Hydrocortisone
Isoxsuprine (Vasodilan)
Methylprednisone (Medrol)
Nitrates
Nitrites
Nylidrin (Arlidin)
Prednisolone (Meticortelone)
Prednisone (Meticorten)
Succinycholine (Anectine)
Tolazoline (Priscoline)
Triamcinolone (Aristocort, Kenacort)
Trihexyphenidyl (Artane)

Iridocyclitis
Iodides

Iris, atrophy of
Quinine

Iris cysts
Echothiophate (Phospholine)
Isoflurophate (Floropryl)
Neostigmine (Prostigmine)
Physostigmine (Eserine)

Iritis
Iodides
Sulfadimethoxine (Madribon)
Sulfamethoxypyridazine (Kynex, Midicel)

Itching, ocular
Para-aminosalicylic acid

Keratitis
Chrysarobin
Iodides
Resorcinol

Keratoconjunctivitis
Antipyrine
Arsenicals
Gold compounds

Keratopathy
Chloroquin (Aralen)
Hydroxychloroquin (Plaquenil)

Lacrimal secretion, diminished
Amprotropine (Syntropan)
Atropine
Chlorisondamine (Ecolid)
Dicyclomine (Bentyl)
Hexamethonium (Methium)
Homatropine
Hyoscyamine
Scopolamine (Hyoscine)

Lacrimation (hyper)
Iodides
Dantrolene (Dantrium)
5-Fluorouracil (Fluoracil)
Nicotinic acid

Lens changes
Betamethasone (Celestone)
Corticosteroid drugs
Cortisone
Dexemethasone (Decadron, Maxidex)
Hydrocortisone
Methylprednisone (Medrol)
Prednisolone (Meticortelone)
Prednisone (Meticorten)
Triamcinolone (Aristocort, Kenacort)

Lids, discoloration of
Mercury salts

Lids, scarring of
Oxyphenbutazone (Tandearil)
Phenylbutazone (Butazoldin)

Loss of vision
Oral contraceptives

Macular degeneration
Chloroquin (Aralen)
Hydoxychloroquin (Plaquenil)

Maculopathy, toxic
Nicotinic acid

Malignant exophthalmus
Iodides

Metal deposits in cornea
Mercury salts

Miosis
Bethenechol (Urecholine)
Carbachol (Carcholin)
Chloral hydrate (Noctec, Somnos)
Chlorpromazine (Thorazine)
Echothiophate (Phospholine)
Isoflurophate (Floropryl)
Mesoridazine (Serentil)
Methacholine (Mecholyl)
Neostigmine (Prostigmine)
Perphenazine (Trilefon)
Phenothiazines
Phenoxybenzamine (Dibenzyline)
Phenylbutazone (Butazolidin)
Physotigmine (Eserine)
Piperactazine (Quide)
Promazine (Sparine)
Promethazine (Phenergan)
Thioridazine (Mellaril)
Trifluoperazine (Stelazine)

Mydriasis
Amitriptyline (Elavil)
Amphetamines
Amprotropine (Syntropan)
Aspidium
Atropine
Chloral hydrate (with overdoses) (Noctec, Somnos)
Chlorisondamine (Ecolid)
Chlorpromazine (Thorazine)
Chlorpropamide (Diabinese)
Cocaine
Dextroamphetamine
Dicyclomine (Bentyl)
Ephedrine
Hexamethonium (Methium)
Homatropine
Hyoscyamine
Imipramine (Tofranil)

(continued)

Indomethacin (Indocin)
Lead compounds
Levodopa (Dopar, Larodopa)
LSD_{25}
MAO inhibitors
Mesoridazine (Serentil)
Methantheline (Benthine)
Methylphenidate (Ritalin)
Nicotinic acid
Nicotinyl alcohol (Roniacol)
Oral contraceptives
Perphenazine (Trilafon)
Phenothiazines
Phenylephrine (Neosynephrine)
Phenylpropanolmine (Propadrine)
Piperactazine (Quide)
Promazine (Sparine)
Promethazine (Phenergan)
Protriptyline (Vivactil)
Quinine
Selicylates
Scopolamine (Hyoscine)
Sex hormones, female
Thallium
Trifluoperazine (Stelazine)
Trihexyphenidyl

Myeloptic neuropathy, sub-acute
Iodochlorhydroxyquin (Vioform)

Myopia
Acetazolamide (Diamox)
ACTH
Arsenicals
Bethanechol (Urecholine)
Carbachol (Carcholin)
Chlorothiazide (Diuril)
Chlorthalidone (Hygroton)
Dichlorphenamide (Daranide)
Echothiophate (Phospholine)
Ethoxzolamide (Cardrase)
Hydrochlorothiazide (HydroDiuril)
Isoflurophate (Floropryl)
Methocholine (Mecholyl)
Neostigmine (Prostigmine)
Physostigmine (Eserine)
Pilocarpine
Sulfadimethoxine (Madribon)
Sulfamethoxazole (Gantanol)
Sulfamethoxypyridazine (Kynex, Midicel)
Thiazides

Narrowing of field of vision
(See under peripheral fields; peripheral vision)

Near vision, difficulty with
Amprotropine (Syntropan)
Atropine
Chlorisondamine (Ecolid)
Dicyclomine (Bentyl)
Hexamethonium (Methium)
Homatropine
Hyoscyamine
Scopolamine (Hyoscine)

Neuro-ocular lesions
Oral contraceptives
Sex hormones, female

Neuropathies
Chloramphenicol (Chloromycetin)

Night blindness
Chlorpromazine (Thorazine)
Mesoridazine (Serentil)
Perphenazine (Trilafon)
Phenothiazines
Piperactazine (Quide)
Promazine (Sparine)
Promethazine (Phenergan)
Quinine
Thioridazine (Mellaril)
Trifluoperazine (Stelazine)

Nystagmus
Barbiturates
Chloramphenicol (Chloromycetin)
Gold compounds
MAO inhibitors
Mephenesin (Tolserol)
Oral contraceptives
Salicylates
Sex hormones, female
Vitamin A

Ocular anesthesia
Quinine

Ocular hypotony
Acetazolamide (Diamox)
Dichlorphenamide (Daranide)
Ethoxzolamide (Cardrase)
Salicylates

Ocular infection, potentiation of
ACTH
Steroids

Ocular irritation
Oxygen

Ocular itching and burning
Para-aminosalicylic acid

Ocular melanosis
Chlorpromazine (Thorazine)
Mesoridazine (Serentil)
Perphenazine (Trilafon)
Phenothiazines
Piperactazine (Quide)
Promazine (Sparine)
Promethazine (Phenergan)
Thioridazine (Mellaril)
Trifluoperazine (Stelazine)

Ocular pain
Bethanechol (Urecholine)
Carbachol (Carcholin)
Echothiophate (Phospholine)
Insoflurophate (Floropryl)
Methacholine (Mecholyl)
Neostigmine (Prostigmine)
Physostigmine (Eserine)
Pilocarpine

(continued)

7.3. Ocular Side Effects and Drugs Eliciting Same (continued)

Ocular palsies
- Chloroquin (Aralen)
- Gold compounds
- Hydroxychloroquin (Plaquenil)
- Lead compounds
- MAO inhibitors
- Oral contraceptives
- Sex hormones, female
- Sulfadimethoxine (Madribon)
- Sulfamethoxazole (Gantanol)
- Sulfamethoxypyridazine (Kynex, Midicel)
- Vitamin A

Oculogyric crisis in a parkinsonian-type extrapyramidal syndrome
- Chlorpromazine (Thorazine)
- Mesoridazine (Serentil)
- Perphenazine (Trilafon)
- Piperactazine (Quide)
- Phenothiazines
- Promazine (Sparine)
- Promethazine (Phenergan)
- Thioridazine (Mellaril)
- Trifluoperazine (Stelazine)

Opacities, corneal and lenticular
- Phenothiazines

Ophthalmoplegia
- Carbimazole
- Chloramphenicol (Chloromycetin)
- Iodides

Optic atrophy
- Aspidium
- Reserpine (Serpasil)
- Streptomycin
- Tryparsamide

Optic edema
- Ergonovine (Ergotrate)
- Ergotamine (Bellergal, Gynergen)

Optic nerve changes
- Betamethasone (Celestone)
- Corticosteroid drugs
- Cortisone
- Dexamethasone (Decadron, Maxidex)
- Hydrocortisone
- Methylprednisone (Medrol)
- Prednisolone (Meticortolone)
- Prednisone (Meticorten)
- Triamcinolone (Kenacort, Aristocort)

Optic and retinal ischemia
- Quinidine

Optic neuritis
- Chloramphenicol (Chloromycetin)
- Iodides
- Oral contraceptives
- Oxyphenbutazone (Tandearil)
- Phenylbutazone (Butazolidin)
- Sex hormones, female
- Streptomycin
- Tryparsamide

Optic pallor
- Chloroquin (Aralen)
- Hydroxychloroquin (Plaquenil)
- Quinine

Palpebral aperture, widening of
- Amphetamines

Papilledema
- Betamethasone (Celestone)
- Corticosteroid drugs
- Cortisone
- Dexamethasone (Decadron, Maxidex)
- Hydrocortisone
- Lead compounds
- Methylprednisone (Medrol)
- Nalidixic acid (NegGram)
- Oral contraceptives
- Prednisolone (Meticortelone)
- Prednisone (Meticorten)
- Sex hormones, female
- Triamcinolone (Aristocort, Kenacort)
- Vitamin A

Paralysis of extraocular muscles
- Chloramphenicol (Chloromycetin)
- Digitalis
- Digitoxin (Purodigin, Crystodigin)
- Digoxin (Lanoxin)
- Quinine

Periorbital edema
- Sulfadimethoxine (Madribon)

Peripheral fields, constriction of
- Chloroquin (Aralen)
- Ergonovine (Ergotrate)
- Ergotamine (Bellergal, Gynergen)
- Hydroxychloroquin (Plaquenil)
- Oxygen
- Quinine
- Tryparsamide

Peripheral vision, loss of
- Chlorpromazine (Thorazine)
- Mesoridazine (Serentil)
- Perphenazine (Trilafon)
- Phenothiazines
- Piperactazine (Quide)
- Promazine (Sparine)
- Promethazine (Phenergan)
- Thioridazine (Mellaril)
- Trifluoperazine (Stelazine)

Phosphenes
- Oral contraceptives
- Sex hormones, female

Photophobia
- Chloroquin (Aralen)
- Digitalis
- Digitoxin (Purodigin, Crystodigin)
- Digoxin (Lanoxin)
- Doxepin (Sinequin, Adapin)
- Hydroxychloroquin (Plaquenil)
- Mercury salts
- Nalidixic acid (NegGram)
- Oral contraceptives

(continued)

Phenothiazines
Quinine
Sex hormones, female
Trimethadione (Tridione)
Photosensitization
Chlorpromazine (Thorazine)
Mesoridazine (Serentil)
Perphenazine (Trilafon)
Phenothiazines
Piperactazine (Quide)
Promazine (Sparine)
Promethazine (Phenergan)
Thioridazine (Mellaril)
Trifluoperazine (Stelazine)
Pigmentary degeneration
Chloroquin (Aralen)
Hydroxychloroquin (Plaquenil)
Thoridazine (Mellaril)
Pigmentary retinopathy
Chloroquin (Aralen)
Hydroxychloroquin (Plaquenil)
Phenothiazines
Pigmentation (blue-grey) of eyelids
Phenothiazines
Posterior subcapsular cataract
ACTH
Steroids
Proptosis
Oral contraceptives
Sex hormones, female
Ptosis
Barbiturates
Chloral hydrate (Noctec, Somnos)
Chloroquin (Aralen)
Cocaine
Guanethidine (Ismelin)
Hydroxychloroquin (Plaquenil)
Lithium carbonate (Eskalith, Lithane)
Reserpine (Serpasil)
Thallium
Pupil, constriction pin-point
Hydromorphone (Dilaudid)
Morphine (and semi-synthetic cogeners)
Propoxyphene napsylate with acetaminophen (Darvocet N)
Pupil, dilated and fixed
Oxygen
Pupillary response to light, unpredictable
LSD_{25}
Pus, in anterior chamber
(See under hypopyon)
Refractive power of lens, changes in
Acetazolamide (Diamox)
Chlorpropamide (Diabinese)
DMSO
Retinal degeneration
Iodides
Retinal detachment
Echothiophate (Phospholine)
Isoflurophate (Floropryl)
Neostigmine (Prostigmine)
Oxygen
Physostigmine (Eserine)
Retinal edema
Acetazolamide (Diamox)
Chloroquin (Aralen)
Chlorothiazide (Diuril)
Dichlorphenamide (Daranide)
Ethoxzolamide (Cardrase)
Hydrochlorothiazide (HydroDiuril)
Hydroxychloroquin (Plaquenil)
Oral contraceptives
Phenothiazines
Quinine
Sex hormones, female
Sulfadimethoxine (Madribon)
Sulfamethoxazole (Gantanol)
Sulfamethoxypyridazine(Kynex, Midicel)
Thiazides
Retinal hemorrhage
Arsenicals
Iodides
Oxyphenbutazone (Tandearil)
Phenylbutazone (Butazolidin)
Sulfadimethoxine (Madribon)
Sulfamethoxazole (Gantanol)
Sulfamethoxypyridazine (Kynex, Midicel)
Vitamin A
Retinal perivasculitis
Oral contraceptives
Sex hormones, female
Retinal thrombosis
Oral contraceptives
Sex hormones, female
Retrobulbular neuritis
Digitalis
Digitoxin (Purodigin, Crystodigin)
Digoxin (Lanoxin)
Retrolental fibroplasia (premature infants)
Oxygen
Saccadic eye movements, decreased
Clorazepate (Tranxene)
Chlordiazepoxide (Librium)
Diazepam (Valium)
Scarring of lids
Oxyphenbutazone (Tandearil)
Phenylbutazone (Butazolidin)
Scintillating scotoma
Clomiphene (Clomid)
Sclera, yellowing of
Antimony compounds
Scotoma
Chloramphenicol (Chloromycetin)
Chloroquin (Aralen)
Chlorpromazine (Thorazine)
Chlorpropamide (Diabinese)
Clomiphene (Clomid)
Digitalis

(continued)

Digitoxin (Purodigin, Crystodigin)
Digoxin (Lanoxin)
Hydroxychloroquin (Plaquenil)
Lithium carbonate (Eskalith, Lithane)
Mesoridazine (Serentil)
Oral contraceptives
Perphenazine (Trilafon)
Phenothiazines
Piperactazine (Quide)
Promazine (Sparine)
Promethazine (Phenergan)
Quinine
Sex hormones, female
Streptomycin
Thallium
Thioridazine (Mellaril)
Trifluoperazine (Stelazine)

Scotopic ERG and EOG ratio, decreased
Indomethacin (Indocin)

Shimmering effect
Tryparsamide

Snow-storm effects
(See under snowy vision)

Snowy vision
Digitalis
Digitoxin (Purodigin, Crystodigin)
Digoxin (Lanoxin)
Trimethadione (Tridione)

Sparks
(See under snowy vision)

Stevens-Johnson syndrome
Oxyphenbutazone (Tandearil)
Phenylbutazone (Butazolidin)
Sulfadimethoxine (Madribon)
Sulfamethoxazole (Gantanol)
Sulfamethoxypyridazine (Kynex, Midicel)

Tapetoretinal degeneration
Oxygen

Topical dermatitis of lens
Iodides

Transparency of lens, changes in
DMSO

Urticaria of lids
Antipyrine

Uveitis
Cholestyramine (Questran)
Reserpine (Serpasil)

Vision, blurred
(See under blurred vision)

Vision, discoloration of
Silver compounds

Vision, loss of (transient or permanent)
(See also under peripheral fields: peripheral vision)
Aspidium
Barbiturates
Chloramphenicol (Chloromycetin)
Chlorisondamine (Ecolid)
Chloroquin (Aralen)
Chlorpropamide (Diabinese)
Chlorpromazine (Thorazine)
Clomiphene (Clomid)
Hexamethonium (Methium)
Hydroxychloroquin (Plaquenil)
Mesoridazine (Serentil)
Oxyphenbutazone (Tandearil)
Perphenazine (Trilafon)
Phenothiazines
Piperactazine (Quide)
Promazine (Sparine)
Promethazine (Phenergan)
Quinine
Streptomycin
Thioridazine (Mellaril)
Trifluoperazine (Stelazine)
Tryparsamide

Visual acuity, drop in
(See also under peripheral fields; peripheral vision)
Chlorpromazine (Thorazine)
Indomethacin (Indocin)
Mesoridazine (Serentil)
Oral contraceptives
Perphenazine (Trilafon)
Phenothiazines
Piperactazine (Phenergan)
Promazine
Promethazine (Phenergan)
Sex hormones, female
Thioridazine (Mellaril)
Trifluoperazine (Stelazine)

Visual disturbances
Dantrolene (Dantrium)
Marijuana (*Cannibis*)
Propranolol (Inderal)
Propoxyphene napsylate with acetaminophen (Darvocet N)

Visual field, decreased
Indomethacin (Indocin)

Yellow sclera
Antimony compounds

Yellow vision (Xanthopsia)
(See also under color vision)
Chlorothiazide (Diuril)
Chlorthalidone (Hygroton)
Hydrochlorothiazide (HydroDiuril)
Thiazides
Vitamin A

Reprinted by permission from H.I. Silverman, "The adverse effects of commonly used systemic drugs on the human eye. Part II," *Am. J. Optom.* **49**: 1972; and H.I. Silverman and R.J. Harvie, "The adverse effects of commonly used systemic drugs on the human eye. Part III," *Am. J. Optom.* **52**: 1975.

7.4. Commonly Used Ophthalmological Drugs by Brand Name

Brand Name	*Main Use*	*Generic Name, Class*
Achromycin	Bacterial endophthalmitis	Tetracycline, AB
Actest	Anti-inflammatory	ACTH, C
Acthar	See Actest	
Actrope	See Actest	
Adrenatrate	Open angle glaucoma	Epinephrine, mydriatic
Adsorbonac	Reduction of corneal edema	Saline (25%)
Adsorbotear	Mucomimetic, corneal wetting	Artificial tears
Aerosporin	Conjunctivitis, corneal ulcers	Polymyxin B, AB
Albalon	Vasoconstrictor, decongestant	Naphazoline
Alidase	Enzyme with local anesthesia	Hyaluronidase
Allerest 20/20	See Albalon	
Alpha Chymar	Dissolution of zonlar fibers	Alpha-chymol-pepsin
Amphicol	Superficial ocular infections	Chloramphenicol, AB
Aucobon	Candida endopthalmitis	Flucytosine
Anicel	Surface anesthetic	Tetracaine
Antazoline	Antihistamine	
Antibiopto	See Amphicol	
Antistine	Allergic reactions	Antazoline, AN
Aristocort	Anti-inflammatory	Cortisone, Triamcinolone G, C
Atropine	Cycloplegic, mydriatic	
Atromide-S	Reducing cholesterol levels	Clofibrate
Aureomycin	Infections, antibacterial	Chlorotetracycline, AB
Bacitracin	Antibacterial, conjunctiva, lids	AB
Bleph 10, 30	Antibacterial	Sodium sulfacetamide
Blephamide	Antibacterial, antiseborrheic	S. sulfacetamide, predniso-lone, phenylepherine
BSS	Irrigant	Balanced salt solution
Bro-lac	See Adsorbotear	
Bufopto Atropine	Cycloplegic	Atropine sulfate
Butazolidin	Uveitis	Phenylbutazone
Carbacel	Open angle glaucoma	Carbachol
Carbocaine	Local anesthetic	Mepiuacaine HCl
Carbamiotin	See Carbacel	
Carcholin	See Carbacel	
Cardrase	Diuretic, primary and secondary glaucoma	Ethoxzolamide
Celestone	Anti-inflammatory	Betamethazone, C
Cetamide	Wide range antibacterial	Sodium-sulfa cetamide, AB
Cetapred	Antibacterial, anti-inflammatory	Sodium-sulfa and predniso-lone
Chloromycetin	See Amphicol	
Chloroptic	See Amphicol	
Citanest	Local anesthetic	Phylocaine HCl
Coly-mycin	Gram neg. Antibacterial (incl. pseu-domonas)	Colistin, AB
Corphos	Anti-inflammatory	Hydracortisone, C
Cortigel	See Actest	
Cortisporin	Anti-inflammatory, antibacterial	Hydrocortisone, aerosporin, Neomycin, AB, C
Cortone	See Corphos	
Cortril	See Corphos	
Cortrophin	See Actest	

AB: Antibiotic
C: Corticosteroid
AN: Antihistamine

(continued)

7.4. Commonly Used Ophthalmological Drugs by Brand Name (continued)

Brand Name	*Main Use*	*Generic Name, Class*
Coumadin	Retinal venous occlusions	Warfarin
Cyclogel	Cycloplegic	Cyclopentolate
Cytoxan	Immune reactions of the uvea	Cyclophosphomide
Daranide	Narrow angle and secondary glaucoma	Dichlorphenamide
Daraprim	Uveitis and retinitis	Priminethamine
Decadron	Inflammations of conjunctiva and cornea	Dexamethasone, C
Dendrin	Herpes simplex, vaccina keratitis	Idoxuridine
Depo-ACTH	See Actest	
Diamox	Antiglaucomatous	Acetazolamide
Dicumarol	Retinal occlusions	Bishydroxycoumarin
DFP	Antiglaucomatous, useful in aphakia	Iso flurophate
Dorsacaine	Local anesthetic	Benoxinate
Doryl	Open angle glaucoma	Carbachol
E_1, E_2	Antiglaucomatous	Epinepherine
E-carpine	See Adrenate	
Echodide	Antiglaucomatous, miotic	Echothlopate iodide
Econochlor	Antibiotic	Chloramphenicol
Econopred	Anti-inflammatory	Prednisolone
E-pilo	See Adrenate	
EDTA	Anti-calcium	
Efricel	Vasoconstrictor	Phenylephrine
EL	See Adrenate	
Endrate	See EDTA	
Enuclene	Isotonic for artificial eyes	
Epifrin	See Adrenate	
Epinal	See Adrenate	
Epitrate	Antiglaucomatous	Epinephrine bitartrate
EPPY	See Adrenate	Erythromycin, AB
Erythrocin	Antibacterial	Erythromycin, AB
Eserine	Antiglaucomatous	Physostigmine
Ethamide	See Cardrase	
Ether	Herpes simplex, keratitis	
Euphthalmine	Mydriasis without cycloplegia	Eucatropine HCl
Florinef	Anti-inflammatory	Fludrocortisone, C
Floropryl	See DFP	
Fluorescein	Diagnostic stain	
Fluor-I	See Fluorescein	
Ful-Glo	See Fluorescein	
Fluress	Rapid topical anesthetic and stain	Fluorescein and Benoxi-
FML	Inflammations of conjunctiva	Fluorometholone, C
Fungizone	Mycotic infections	Amphotericin B, AB
Gantrisin	Anti-infectious (Gram pos.)	Sulfisoxazole, AB
Garamycin	Broad spectrum antibacterial	Gentamycin, AB
Glaucon	See Adrenate	
Glyrol	Narrow angle and malignant glaucoma	Glycerine
Haldrane	Anti-inflammatory	Paramethasone, C
Heparin	Retinal venous occlusions	
Herplex	See Dendrin	
Hexadrol	See Decadron	
Hexplex	See Dendrin	
HMS	Allergic conjunctivitis	Medrysone, C
Homatrocel	Cycloplegic and mydriatic	Homatropine hydro br.

AB: Antibiotic
C: Corticosteroid
AN: Antihistamine

(continued)

7.4. Commonly Used Ophthalmological Drugs by Brand Name (continued)

Brand Name	*Main Use*	*Generic Name, Class*
Homatropine	See Homatrocel	
Humersol	Open angle glaucoma	Demacarium br.
Hydreltasol	Inflammations of anterior segment	Prednisolone, C
Hydrocortone	See Corphos	
Hydronol	Secondary glaucoma	Isosorbide
Hyoscine	Iritis	Scoplamine, mydriatic
IDU	See Dendrin	
Ilosone	See Erythrocin	
Ilotycin	See Erythrocin	
Imuran	Suppress immune reactions	
Indocin	Uveitis	Indomethacin
Inflamase	See Hydreltasol	
Iodine	Herpes simplex keratitis	
Iodo-niacin	Hemorrhages, floaters, etc.	Iodine and niacin
Iso-hist	Decongestant, antiallergic	Chlorpheniramine, AN
IUDR	See Dendrin	
Kantrex	Anti-infectious	Kanamycin, AB
Kenalog	Anti-inflammatory	Triamcinoloneacetonide, C
Lacril	See Adsorbotear	
Lacri-lube	Lubricant	
Lavoptic	Eyewash	
Lanoxin	Open angle glaucoma	Digoxin
Leritine	Analgesic, nausea and vomiting	Anileridine
Leukeran	Inflamatory disorders	Chlormabucil
Lyophorin	See Adrenate	
Maxidex	See Decadron	
Maxitrol	Infections, inflammation	Maxidex and neomyci
Medrocort	See HMS	
Methulose	See Adsorbotear	
Metimyd	Inflammatory, allergic conditions of lid	Prednisolone, sulfased mide
Metreton	Anti-inflammatory	Prednisolone
Metrocortelone	See Hydreltasol	
Metycaine	Local anesthetic	Piperocaine
Miocel	Antiglaucomatic	Pilocarpine +
Miochol	Rapid miosis for surgery	Acetylcholine
Mi-pilo	Open angle glaucoma	Pilocarpine
Miotat	Miotic	Carbachol
Mistura E	Open angle glaucoma	Epinephrine
Mistura C	See corbachol	
Mustargen	Retinoblastoma	Mechlorethanine HCl
Murine	Eye wash	
Mychel	See Amphicol	
Mycostatin	Mycotic infections of cornea	Nystatin
Mydriacyl	Rapid mydriatic and cycloplegic	Tropicamide
Mytrate	See Adrenate	
Mydfrin	Vasoconstrictor, mydriatic	Phenylepherine
Naphcor	Vasoconstrictor	Naphazoline
Neo-cortef	Anti-inflammatory, antibacterial	Neomycin, hydrocortisone
Neo-flow	Irrigant	
Neomycin	Antibacterial	AB
Neo-propisol	See Albalon	

AB: Antibiotic
C: Corticosteroid
AN: Antihistamine

(continued)

7.4. Commonly Used Ophthalmological Drugs by Brand Name (continued)

Brand Name	*Main Use*	*Generic Name, Class*
Neosporin	Superficial external infections	Polymyxin, neomycin, gramicidin, AB
Neo-synerphrine	Mydriatic	Phenylephrine
Neozin	Antiseptic, decongestant, astringent	Phenylephrine, zinc sulfate
Neptazane	Antiglaucomatous	Methazolamide
Nilstat	See Mycostatin	
Nitroglycerin	Retinal arterial spasm	
Nitrogen mustard	See Mustargen	
Novocain	Local anesthetic	Procaine
Ocusert Pilozo	Antiglaucomatous	Pilocarpine
Ophthaine	Surface local short term anesthetic	Proparacaine
Ophthetic	See Ophthaine	
Ophthochlor	See Amphicol	
Op-isophrin	Congestion of the conjunctiva	Phenylephrine +
Opsulfa 10, 30	Superficial ocular infections	Sulfacetamide, AB
Optef	See Corphos	
Optihist	See Iso-hist	
Optimyd	See Metimyd	
Optival	See Hydeltrasol	
Oratrol	See Daranide	
Osmitrol	Acute glaucoma, diuretic	Mannitol
Osmoglyn	See Glyrol	
Oxylone	See FML	
P1E1 to P6E1	See Adrenatrate	
Panmycin	See Achromycin	
Paredrine	Mydriatic	Hydroxyamphetamir hydro br.
Physostigmine	Miotic	
Phospholine I.	Resistant open angle glaucoma	Echothiophate I.
Pilo B	Open angle glaucoma	Pilocarpine
Pilocar	See Pilo B	
Pilocel	See Pilo B	
Pilofrin	Open angle glaucoma	Pilocarpine and phenylephrine
Pontocaine	Long lasting corneal anesthetic	Tetracaine
Polycycline	See Achromycin	
Polyspectrin	Superficial infections	Polymyxin, neomycin, bacitracin, AB
Polysporin	Infections conjunctiva, cornea	Polymyxin, bacitracin, AB
Pred Forte	Anti-inflammatory	Prednisilone
Prednefrin	See Hydreltasol	
Predulose	Anti-inflammatory	Prednisalone, pilocarpine,C
Prefrin	See Efricel	
Priscoline	Central retinal artery occlusions	Tolazoline HCl
Prostigmin	Antiglaucomatous	Neostigmine
Purinethol	Unresponsive uveitis	Mercaptopurine
PVCarbachol	See Carbacel	
PVCarpine	See Pilo B	
Quimotrase	See Alpha Chymar	
Scopolamine	Iritis, mydriasis	
Sodium edetate	See EDTA	

AB: Antibiotic
C: Corticosteroid
AN: Antihistamine

(continued)

Sodium sulamyd	Superficial infections caused by micro-organisms	Sulphasedamide, AB
Solacthyl	See Actest	
Staphage lysate	Blepharitis, hordeola, etc.	Vaccine, staphylococcal phage
Statrol	Antibiotic	Neomycin
Steclin	See Achromycin	
Stoxil	See IDU	
Streptomycin	Anti-infectious	AB
Succus Cineravia Maritima	Lymphaoque	
Sulapred	Anti-inflammatory, decongestant, anti-bacterial	Sulfasedamyde, prednisolone, phenylephrine, AB
Sulfacel-15	See Sodium Sulamyd	
TEM	Retinal blastoma	Tri ethylenemelamine
Terramycin	See Achromycin	
Tetracyn	See Achromycin	
Thiotepa	Recurring pterygia	Triethylenethiophose
Thrombolysin	Retinal venous occlusions	Fibrinolysin, human
Travenol	See Osmitrol	
Timoptic	Antiglaucomatous	Timolol maleate
Ureaphil	Unresponsive glaucoma	Urea
Urevert	See Ureaphil	
Vancocin	Antibacterial	Vancomycin, AB
Vasocidin	Decongestant, antiallergic	Phenylephrine, predniso-lone, C, AN
Vasocon	See Albalon	
Vasocon A	Vasoconstrictor, anti-inflammatory	Naphazoline, antazoline, AN
Vasospred	See Hydreltasol	
Vasosulf	See Bleph	
Vernacel	Decongestant, antiallergic	Pheniramine, AN
Versenate	See EDTA	
VIG	Vaccina lesions	Vaccine immune globulin
Visculose	See Adsorbotear	
Visine	Decongestant	Tetrahydrozoline, AN
Xylocaine	Rapid local anesthetic	Lydocaine HCl
Zephiran	Antiseptic, nonspecific conjunctivitis	Benzoconium
Zingfrin	Astringent, decongestant	Phenylephrine, zinc sulfate
Zinc sulfate	Nonspecific conjunctivitis	
Zolyse	See Alpha Chymar	

7.5. Pharmaceutical Adjuncts Found in Commercial Ophthalmic Solutions

Tonicity Agents

Sodium chloride
Potassium chloride
Glycerin
Mannitol
Magnesium chloride

Surface Active Agents

Benzalkonium chloride
Polysorbate 80
Polyoxyl-40 stearate
Polyoxypropylene-polyoxyethendiol
Myristyl-gamma-picolinium Cl

Suspending Systems

Cetyl alcohol
Glyceryl monostearate
Liquid petrolatum
Polyoxyl-40 stearate
Propylene glycol
PEG 4000
Aluminum tristearate

Antioxidants

Sodium bisulfite
Ascorbic acid

Viscosity Agents

Carboxymethylcellulose
Gelatin
Hydroxypropylmethylcellulose
Methylcellulose
Polyethylene glycol
Polyvinyl alcohol
Polyvinyl glycol
Povidone

Vasoconstrictors

Neosynephrine (phenylephrine)
Privine (naphazoline)
Tyzine (tetrahydrozoline)

Preservatives

Benzakonium Cl .09%
Benzethonium Cl .025%
Butylparaben .0005%
Cetypyridinium Cl .02%
Chlorobutanol .25 to .5%
Methyl paraben .1%
Phenyl mercuric nitrate .013%
Phenol .25%
Phenylethyl alcohol
Sodium EDTA
Thimerosal .01%
Zinc sulfanilate

Buffers

Acetic acid
Barbital
Boric acid
Hydrochloric acid
Potassium acid phosphate
Sodium acetate
Sodium barbital
Sodium biphosphate
Sodium borate
Sodium carbonate
Sodium citrate
Sodium hydroxide
Sodium phosphate

7.6. Ophthalmological Drugs by Function

Table A. Miscellaneous

Analgesics	Acetaminophen (Tylenol) Anileridine (Uritine) Aspirin Codeine Dextropropoxyphene (Darvon) Meperidine (Demerol) Morphine Pentazocine (Talwin)
Anticoagulant	Heparin Sodium Bishydroxycoumarin (Dicumarol) Warfarin Sodium (Coumadin)
Antifungal	Amphotericin B (Fungizone) Flucytosine (Anacoban) Griseofulvin (Fulvicin-U/F, Grifulvin V, Grisactin) Miconazole Nystatin (Mycostatin, Nilstat) Pimarcin
Antihelmintics	Diethylcarbamazine citrate (Hetrazan) Gentian violet Piperazine (Antepar, Multifuge oxocide, Parazine, Vermizine) Pyrvinium pamoate (Povan) Thiabendazole (Mintezoc)
Antihistamines	Antazoline Chlorpheniramine (Chlor-trimeton, Teldrin) Cyclizine (Marazine) Cyproheptadine (Periactin) Dimenhydrinate (Dramamine) Diphenildramine (Bendryl) Hydroxyzine (Atarax, Vistaril) Promethazine (Phenergan) Pyribenzamine
Anti-inflammatory	Acetylsalicylic Acid (Aspirin) Betamethasone (Celestone) Corticotropin (ACTH, Actest, Acthar, Actrope, Cortigel, Cortotrophin, Depto ACTH, Solacthyl) Cortisone Acetate (Cortone Acetate) Dexamethasone (Decadron, Deronil, Dexameth, Gamacorten, Hexadrol) Fluprednisolone (Alphadrol) Fludracortisone (Florine F) Hydrocortisone (Cortef, Cortril, Hydrocortone) Indomethacin (Indocin) Methyprednisolone (Medrol, Stamex) Paramethasone Acetate (Haldrone) Prednisone (Delta-dome, Deltasone, Lisacort, Meticorten, Orasovel, Paracort, Servisone) Phenylbutazone (Butazolidin) Triamcinolone (Aristocort, Kenacort)

(continued)

Table A. Miscellaneous (continued)

Antineoplastic	Azathioprine (Imuran) Chlorambucil (Leukeran) Cyclophosilomide (Lytoxan) Mechlorthamine (Mustargen, Nitrogen Mustard) Mercaptopurine (Purinethol) Triethyenemelamine (Tem) Triethylenethio (Thio-tem)
Antiprotozoan	Clindamycin Diiodydroxyquin (Diodoquin) Pryrimethamine Quinacrine (Atabrine) Trisulfapyrimidines
Antiviral	Adenine Arabinoside (Ara A) Amantadine (Symmetrel) Idoxuridine (IDU, IUDR, Herplex, Stoxil)
Chelating and Epitheliolytic	Ethylenediamine Tetra-Acetate (EDTA, Sodium Edetate, Endrate, Versenate Sodium) Iodine Ether
Enzymes	Alpha-Chromotrypsin (Alpha-Chymar, Quimatrase, Zolyse) Fibrinolysin (Thrombolysin) Hyaluronidase (Alidase, Hyazyme, Wydase)
Sedatives	Chloral Hydrase Pentobartibal (Nembutal) Phenobarbital Secobarbital (Seconal)
Tranquilizers	Chlordiazepoxide (Librium) Chlorapromazine (Thorazine) Diazepam (Valium) Hydroxyzine (Atarax, Vistaril) Prochorperazine (Compazine) Promethazine (Phenergan) Triflupromazine (Vesprin)

Table B. Antibiotics and Chemotherapeutic Agents

Amphotericin B (Fungizone)
p-Aminosalicylic acid (PAS)
Bacitracin
Cefazolin (Ancef, Kefazol)
Cephalexin (Keflex)
Cephaloridine (Loridine)
Cephalothin (Keflin sodium)
Cephapirin (Cefadyl)
Cephradine (Anspor, Velosef)
Chloramphenicol (Amphicol, Chloro mycetin, Mychel)
Clindamycin (Cleocin)
Colistin (Coly-Mycin)
Erythromycin (Erythocin, Ilotycin, Ilosone)
Flucytosine (Ancobon)
Gentamicin (Garamycin)
Griseofulvin (Fulvicin, Grifilvin, Grisactin)
Isoniazid
Kanamycin (Kantrex)
Lincomycin (Lincocin)
Neomycin
Nitrofurantoin (Furadantin)
Nystatin (Mycostatin, Nilstat)
Penicillin G
Penicillin V
Semisynthetic penicillins
1. Methicillin sodium (Staphcillin)
2. Oxacillin sodium (Bactocil, Prostaphlin)
3. Ampicillin (Amcil, Omnipen, Pen A, Polycillin, Penbritin, Pensyn, Principen, Procillin, QIDamP, Supen)

Semisynthetic penicillins (continued)
4. Amoxicillin (Amoxil, Larotid, Polymox)
5. Nafcillin sodium (Unipen)
6. Dicloxacillin (Dynapen, Pathocil, Veracillin)
7. Cloxacillin (Tegopen)
8. Carbenicillin (Geopen, Pyopen)

Polymyxin B (Aerosporin)
Rifampin (Rifadin, Rimactane)
Steptomycin
Sulfacetamide (Sulamyd Sodium)
Sulfadiazine or sulfamerazine; mixed sulfonamides
Sulfadimethoxine (Madribon)
Sulfamethoxypyridazine (Midicel, Acetyl)
Sulfa-trimethoprim and sulfamethoxazole combination (Bactrim, Septra)
Sulfisoxazole (Gantrisin)
Tetracycline group (Aureomycin, Terramycin, Achromycin, Terracyn, Mysteclin, Sumycin, Panmycin)
Tetracycline group
Doxycycline (Doxy-H, Vibramycin)
Minocycline (Minocin, Vectrin)
Tobramycin (Nebcin)
Troleandomycin (TAO, Cyclamycin)
Vancomycin (Vancoein)

Table C. Antiglaucomatous Agents

Local treatment	**General Treatment**	**Various agents**
Parasympathomimetic agents	**Carbonic anhydrase inhibitors**	**Central nervous system**
Direct-acting (cholinergic agents)	Acetazolamide (Diamox)	**depressants**
Acetylcholine	Dichlorphenamide (Daranide;	*Analgetics*
Methacholine (Mecholyl)	Oratrol)	Morphine
Pilocarpine	Methazolamide (Neptazane)	Morphine derivatives
Aceclidine	Ethoxzolamide (Cardrase;	*Sedatives*
Carbachol	Ethamide)	*Tranquilizers*
Indirect-acting (cholinesterase	**Aldosterone antagonists**	Meprobamate
inhibitors; anticholinesterase	Spironolactone (Aldactone)	Benzodiazepine derivatives
agents)	Triamterene	*Neuroleptics*
Reversible Inhibitors	**Hyperosmotic agents**	Chlorpromazine
Physostigmine (Eserine)	*Intravenous*	Reserpine
Neostigmine (Prostigmin)	Mannitol	*Antidepressant agents*
Pyridostigmine (Mestinon)	Urea	**Local anesthetics**
Distigmine bromide	Sodium ascorbate	**Cardiac glycosides**
Demecarium bromide	*Oral*	**Ganglionic blocking agents**
(Tosmilen; Humorsol)	Glycerol	**Ferments**
Irreversible Inhibitors	Isosorbide	
Isoflurophate (DFP; Floropryl)	Ethyl alcohol	
Paraoxon	Beta Adrenergic	
Echothiophate (Phospholine iodide)	Timoptic	
Sympathomimetic agents		
Epinephrine		
Analog agents		
Phenylephrine (Neo-Synephrine)		
Isoproterenol		
Salbutamol		
Sympatholytic agents		
N,N-dibenzyl-beta-chloraethyl-amine		
Propranolol		
Guanethidine (Ismelin)		
6-Hydroxydopamine		
Clonidine		

Reprinted from Hans Heilman, *Glaucoma: Concepts of a Disease*, Toronto: W.B. Saunders, 1970.

Table D. Miotics

Generic Name	*Brand Names**	*Concentration*	*Duration of Miotic Action*
		%	
Cholinergic Drugs			
Carbachol	Carbacel, Carcholin, Carbamiotin, Moryl, Doryl, Coletyl, Isopto Carbachol, Jestryl, P.V. Carbachol, Lentin	0.75–3	2 hours to 2 days
Pilocarpine	Almocarpine, E-Carpine, Epicar, E-Pilo, Isopto Carpine, Mi-Pilo, Miocel, Pilocar, Pilomiotin, Pilofrin, Pilovise, P.V. Carpine, Pilo-B, Pilocel	0.25–10	4 to 8 hours
Anticholinesteratic Drugs			
Demecarium bromide	Humorsol, Tosmilen	0.125–0.25	days to weeks
Diisopropyl fluorophosphate (DFP)	Dyflos, Floropryl, Isoflurophate	0.01–0.1	days to weeks
Echothiophate iodide	Phospholine iodide	0.03–0.25	days to weeks
Neostigmine bromide	Prostigmin, Proserine bromide, Eustigmine bromide, Philostigmine bromide	3.0–5.0	hours to days
Physotigmine (eserine)	Miocel, Physostol	0.25–1.0	hours to days

*Many preparations have more than one active ingredient. An exhaustive search of drug indexes might reveal brand names of less commonly used miotics.

Table E. Mydriatics and Cycloplegics – Sympathomimetic Drugs

	Maximum Mydriasis	*Duration of Mydriasis*	*Percent*
Phenylephrine	20 minutes	3 hours	10
Adrenaline			1/1000
Hydroxyamphetamine	40 minutes		1
Cocaine	20 minutes	2 hours	2–4
Ephedrine	30 minutes	3 hours	5

Table F. Mydriatics and Cycloplegics – Parasympatholytic Drugs

	Max. Mydriasis *Max. Cycloplegia*	*Duration Mydriasis* *Duration Cycloplegia*	*Percent*
Atropine	30–40 minutes several hours	12 days 2 weeks	0.25–4
Homatropine	10–30 minutes 30–90 minutes	6 hours–4 days 10–48 hours	1–5
Scopolamine	15–30 minutes 30–45 minutes	several days 5–7 days	0.25–0.5
Cyclopentolate	15–30 minutes 15–45 minutes	24 hours 24 hours	0.5–2
Tropicamide	20–30 minutes 20–25 minutes	4 hours 6 hours	1–2
Oxyphenonium	Comparable to atropine	4 days 12 days	1&5
Eucatropine	30 minutes poor cycloplegia	4 hours	5&10

Table G. Local Anesthetics for Topical Use

Generic Name	*Trade Name*	*Usual Concentration*
tetracaine hydrochloride	Pontocaine	0.5%
proparacaine hydrochloride	Ophthaine	0.5%
benoxinate	Dorsacaine	0.4%
cocaine		0.5%
dibucaine hydrochloride	Nupercaine	0.1%
piperocaine	Metycaine	2.0%
phenacaine hydrochloride	Holocaine	1.0%
naepaine	Amylsine	4.0%
dyclonine hydrochloride	Dyclone	0.5%

Table H. Local Anesthetics for Injection

Generic Name	*Trade Name*	*Usual Concentration*	*Duration of Action (min.)*
procaine	Novocaine	1.0%	30 60*
lidocaine	Xylocaine	1.0%	60 120*
mepivacaine	Carbocaine	2.0%	120
hexylcaine	Cyclaine	1.0%	60
bupivacaine	Marcaine	0.25%	400*
tetracaine	Pontocaine	0.25%	120*
prilocaine	Citanest	1.0–2.0%	120*

*Indicates the duration of action when epinephrine is present in the solution.

7.7. Index of Side Effects

Abnormal Conjugate Deviations
Abnormal Visual Sensations
Absence of Foveal Reflex
Absence of Pupillary Reaction to Light
Accommodative Spasm
Achromatopsia, Blue-Yellow Defect
Achromatopsia, Red-Green Defect
Anisocoria
Blepharitis
Blepharoclonus
Blepharoconjunctivitis
Blepharospasm
Blindness
Cataracts
Cenral Serous Retinopathy
Colored Haloes around Lights
Congenital Cataracts
Conjunctival Deposits
Conjunctival Hyperemia
Conjunctivitis–Follicular
Conjunctivitis–Nonspecific
Constriction of Visual Fields
Corneal Deposits
Corneal Edema
Corneal Opacities
Cortical Blindness
Decreased Accommodation
Decreased Anterior Chamber Depth
Decreased Convergence
Decreased Corneal Reflex
Decreased Dark Adaptation
Decreased Depth Perception
Decreased Intraocular Pressure
Decreased Lacrimation
Decreased Pupillary Reaction to Light
Decreased Resistance to Infection
Decreased Spontaneous Eye Movements
Decreased Tolerance to Contact Lenses
Decreased Vision
Delayed Corneal Wound Healing
Diplopia
Dyschromatopsia
Enlarged Blind Spot
Exophthalmos
Eyelid Deposits
Eyelids – Depigmentation
Eyelids – Erythema
Eyelids – Exfoliative Dermatitis
Eyelids – Urticaria
Eyelids or Conjunctiva – Allergic Reactions
Eyelids or Conjunctiva – Angioneurotic Edema
Eyelids or Conjunctiva – Discoloration
Eyelids or Conjunctiva – Edema
Eyelids or Conjunctiva – Erythema Multiforme
Eyelids or Conjunctiva – Hyperpigmentation
Eyelids or Conjunctiva – Lupoid Syndrome
Eyelids or Conjunctiva – Lyell's Syndrome
Eyelids or Conjunctiva – Purpura
Eyelids or Conjunctiva – Stevens-Johnson Syndrome
Heightened Color Perception
Hemianopsia
Hippus
Horner's Syndrome
Hypermetropia
Hypopyon
Increased Intraocular Pressure
Iris or Ciliary Body Cysts
Iritis
Jerky Pursuit Movements
Keratitis
Keratoconjunctivitis
Lacrimation
Lens Deposits
Loss of Eyelashes or Eyebrows
Macular Edema
Macular or Paramacular Degeneration
Miosis
Myasthenic Neuromuscular Blocking Effect
Mydriasis
Myopia
Narrowing or Occlusion of Lacrimal Canaliculi or Punctum

(continued)

7.7. Index of Side Effects (continued)

Night Blindness
Nonrhegmatous Retinal Detachment
Nystagmus
Objects Have Blue Tinge
Objects Have Brown Tinge
Objects Have Green Tinge
Objects Have Red Tinge
Objects Have Violet or Purple Tinge
Objects Have White Tinge
Objects Have Yellow Tinge
Ocular Exposure – Irritation
Ocular Teratogenic Effects
Oculogyric Crises
Optic Atrophy
Oscillopsia
Papilledema
Papilledema Secondary to Pseudotumor Cerebri
Paralysis of Accommodation
Paralysis of Extraocular Muscles
Paresis of Extraocular Muscles
Periorbital Edema
Photophobia
Photosensitivity
Ptosis
Random Ocular Movements
Retinal Degeneration
Retinal Edema
Retinal or Macular Pigmentary Changes or Deposits
Retinal Vascular Disorders
Retrobulbar or Optic Neuritis
Scleral Deposits
Scotomas
Strabismus
Subconjunctival or Retinal Hemorrhages
Subconjunctival or Retinal Hemorrhages Secondary to Drug-induced Anemia
Symblepharon
Systemic Administration – Nonspecific Ocular Irritation
Uveitis
Visual Agnosia
Visual Hallucinations

Reprinted from F.T. Fraunfelder, *Ocular side effects and drug interactions.* Philadelphia: Lea and Febiger, 1976.

7.8. Chromatopsias and Drugs That May Cause Them

1. Chromatopsia, type not described
   (a) drugs–bromides, eosine, paramethadione, piperazine citrate, phenylbutazone, sulthiame, trimethadione, barbiturates, mescaline, nicotine
   (b) disease conditions–with hysteria, neurosis, epilepsy, migraine
   –pathologic central processes caused by vascular diseases or tumors
   –electrical stimulation of areas 17 or 18 in the occipital lobe

2. Ianthinopsia–violet vision
   (a) drugs–cannabis, santonin, quinacrine, fungus poisoning, mescaline, nicotine
   (b) disease conditions–with hysteria
   –with retinal detachment
   –with diseases of retina and choroid
   –tabetic optic atrophy

3. Cyanopsia–blue vision
   (a) drugs–ethyl alcohol, amyl alcohol, methylene blue, digitalis, amphetamines, mescaline, quinacrine, tetramethylbutanediamine, carbon disulfide, nalidixic acid, nicotine. Drugs or conditions which produce corneal cloudiness will cause objects to appear bluish.
   (b) disease conditions–syphilitic optic atrophy
   –with diseases of retina and choroid
   –following cataract surgery
   –with retinal detachment
   –with hysteria

4. Glaucopsia–blue-gray vision
   (a) drugs–ethanolamine, tobacco smoking, nicotine; possibly mescaline.

5. Chloropsia–green vision
   (a) drugs–epinephrine, acridines, quinine, quinacrine, barbiturates, lead, strychnine, carbon sulfite, carbon disulfide, digitalis, griseofulvin, iodides, mescaline, nicotine.
   (b) disease conditions–with hysteria
   –with diseases of retina and choroid
   –with retinal detachment
   –following retinal hemorrhage
   –tabetic optic atrophy
   –phototraumatism
   –following cataract surgery, some see a greenish haze

6. Xanthopsia–yellow vision
   (a) drugs–fluorescin, arsenic, barbiturates, trinitrophenol (picric acid), carbon monoxide, picrotoxin, lead, salicylates, santonin, mushroom toxins, carbon dioxide, carbon disulfide, chlorthalidone, acetophenetidin, amyl nitrate, aspidium, streptomycin and dihydrostreptomycin, sulfonamides, digitalis, quinacrine, quinethazone, compounds of chrome, thiabendazole, thiazide diuretics, pentylenetetrazol, Vitamin A, chloroquine, DDT, aconite, ethyl alcohol, chlorothiazide, chromic acid, methazolamide, thioridazine, silver preparations, rauwolfia derivatives, mescaline, nicotine, phenacetin, marihuana, snake venoms.
   (b) disease conditions–congenital jaundice
   –hyperbilirubinemia
   –dyspepsia
   –blood in the aqueous
   –when recovering from ether anesthesia
   –diabetic retinopathy
   –with hysteria, mental disturbances
   –siderosis
   –with sarcoma of the choroid
   –with chorioretinitis

7. A brownish discoloration of vision has been reported with:
   (a) drugs–digitalis, thioridazine, chlorpromazine, phenothiazines, myristicine, mescaline, nicotine; and following topical application of fluorescein, argyrol or mild silver proteinate to the eye.
   (b) disease conditions–a vitreous hemorrhage
   –hysteria

8. Erythropsia
   (a) drugs–amyl alcohol, atropine, duboisine, hyoscyamine, ergotamine, creosote, quinine, chloroquine, DDT, chromic acid, digitalis, quinacrine, veratrine, eosine, carbon disulfide, mescaline, nicotine, and rarely sulfonamides.
   (b) disease conditions
   –phototraumatism, (due to excess ultraviolet), snow blindness.

   With snow blindness the color vision defect can be permanent. Luminous surfaces appear purpurine-red and shadows show the complementary color, emerald green. Some report chloropsia or a R-G type defect. Exposure to excess light causes erythropsia or green-red disturbances. In these cases red vision is attributed to visual pigment exhaustion or to a prolongation of the red phase of the afterimage. Francois and Verriest describe a pseudo-erythropsia produced by light entering the eye through the sclera.

   –exposure to intense blue light caused long lasting damage to the color vision of monkeys
   –electric shock
   –during development of cataract
   –following cataract surgery
   –following iridectomy
   –development of pigmentary retinopathy
   –following cerebral thrombosis
   –syphilitic optic atrophy
   –attacks of hysteria
   –Vitamin A deficiency
   –blood in the anterior chamber
   –hemorrhage into retina, or vitreous or preretinal

(continued)

Drugs which may cause retinal hemorrhage include arsenicals, ethyl alcohol, aniline dyes, methyl bromide, procarbazine, mercury poisoning, phosphorus poisoning, snake bite toxins. Other drugs which can cause retinal or vitreous hemorrhages include sulfonamides, iodides, phenylbutazone, oxyphenbutazone.

Vitamin A excess, can cause retinal hemorrhages.

Anticoagulants can result in retinal or vitreous hemorrhages.

Indomethacin (Indocid) can cause a vitreous hemorrhage. Retinal hemorrhages are a feature of many disease conditions including diabetes mellitus, papilledema, hyptertension, hypotension, venous occlusions, thrombosis of the cavernous sinus, disseminated lupus erythematosus, polyarteritis nodosa, erythroblastosis fetalis, serum sickness, retinal vessel atheroma or embolism, phlebitis, cachexia, hypoxia, traumatic asphyxia, blast injuries, coughing, vomiting, scurvy, cystic fibrosis, subacute bacterial endocarditis, blood dyscrasias, anemia, leukemia, thrombocytopenic purpura, polycythemia, macroglobulinemia, cryoglobulinemia, hemophilia, sickle cell disease; Coats' disease, Eales' disease; and various infectious diseases, e.g. malaria, pneumonia, septicemia, influenza, rickettsial infections, infectious mononucleosis, meningitis, typhoid, whooping cough, filariasis, yellow fever. Retinal hemorrhages may follow cataract surgery or an iridectomy or trauma, or occur with subarachnoid hemorrhages or with papilledema.

–Retinal hemorrhages also occur with these syndromes according to Geeraets:
–Addison
–Bourneville
–carotid artery–cavernous sinus fistula
–Ehlers-Danlos
–Hand-Schuller-Christian
–Herrick
–von Hippel-Lindau
–Leber
–Waldenstrom

The following subgroups are not truly chromatopsias but are listed here for comparison.

1. White snowstorm-like effect may occur with:
   (a) drugs–trimethadione, tobacco smoking, nicotine, digitalis, paramethadione, diphenylhydantoin, mescaline.
   (b) disease conditions–lesions affecting the chiasma can cause a vague whiteness or a visual glow, or a film of water appearance to objects
   –phototraumatism
   –hysteria
2. Seeing colored haloes, iridescent vision, (outer ring blue-violet, inner ring reddish and sometimes green between the two).
   (a) disease conditions–glaucoma, cataract, corneal opacities, edema of corneal epithelium, changes in corneal endothelium, excess mucous on the cornea.
   (b) drugs and chemicals–ointment on the cornea, amyl nitrate, amodiaquin, birth control pills, quinacrine, chloroquine, chlorine, digitalis, alkaloids, dimethylamino propylamine, hydrogen sulfide, indomethacin, nitroglycerine, osmium tetroxide, oxygen, oxalyl chloride, phenothiazines, squill, tetramethylbutanediamine, volatile heterocyclic amines. Prolonged exposure of the cornea to water will result in a halo effect.
3. Illusions of colored flashing lights, scintillating scotomas. Chromatic sensations can be induced by intermittent achromatic stimuli (Fechner's colors).
   (a) disease conditions–retinal detachment, migraine, Moore's lightning streaks, spasms of vessels, chorioretinitis, epilepsy, hysteria.
   (b) drugs and chemicals–bretylium tosylate, caffeine, clomiphene, chloroquine, digitalis, alkaloids, diphenylhydantoins, ergot, guanethidine, hydralazine, mecamylamine, nalidixic acid, pentylenetetrazol, piperazine citrate, propantheline, quinine, sulthiame. Many of the abused drugs, the hallucinogens or psychotomimetics, are said to produce brightly colored illusions which come and go.
4. Intracranial lesions affecting the occipital area may induce sensations of unformed light, fiery globes, circles, teichopsia, rings, blinking light, etc. Migraine, epilepsy and hysteria can also cause similar sensations. Pressure on the eyeball produces transient phosphenes. Other mechanisms cause, for example, blue arcs to be seen.

Reprinted by permission from W. Lyle, "Drugs and conditions which may affect color vision," *J. Am. Opt. Assoc.* **45**: 1974.

7.9. Ocular Diagnostic Agents

Drug	*Route of Administration*	*Dose*	*Response*	*Possible Disadvantage of Test*
Dyes:				
Fluorescein	Topical	0.5 to 2.0%	Stains corneal abrasions or foreign bodies green when viewed with ultraviolet light or a dark blue filtered white light source.	Solutions are susceptible to *Pseudomonas aeruginosa* contamination. This disadvantage could be avoided by using test strips or sterilized fresh solutions.
Rose Bengal	Topical	1%	Similar uses to topical Fluorescein.	More irritating and uncomfortable than Fluorescein but not irritating enough to require local anesthesia.
Mild Silver Protein	Topical		Transfers Circular Disc from Tonomat® Measurement of I.O.P.	
Local Anesthetics:				
Cocaine	Topical	2%	Requires endogenous epinephrine to produce mydriasis and can differentiate Horner's and Raeder's Syndromes.	Cocaine can cause pitting and ulceration of the cornea because of its extreme vasoconstrictor effect. Usually solutions must be made up extemporaneously by a pharmacy and are likely not to be sterile. A narcotic license is required to prescribe cocaine.
Benoxinate	Topical	0.4%	Topical Anesthesia sufficient for tonometry in 60 seconds.	Incidence of side effects is low but superficial corneal edema may occur and caution should be used in patients with cardiac disease, thyroid disease.
Proparacaine (Ophthetic)	Topical	0.5%	Topical Anesthesia for tonometry.	Temporary stinging, burning, and conjunctival redness. Contraindicated in hypersensitive patients.
Tetracaine	Topical	0.5%	Topical Anesthesia for tonometry.	Drug causes a transient smarting of eye in 0.5% concentrations. Rarely produces lacrimation, photophobia, and chemosis.
Water	Oral	1 Liter	Increase I.O.P. in glaucoma-prone individuals.	Could precipitate an acute attack of glaucoma. Glycerin, Mannitol, or Urea should be available to combat the acute glaucoma attack.

(continued)

7.9. Ocular Diagnostic Agents (continued)

Drug	*Route of Administration*	*Dose*	*Response*	*Possible Disadvantage of Test*
Various Steroids: Betamethasone Dexamethasone, etc.	Topical	0.1%	Increase I.O.P. in glaucoma-prone individuals.	Require 4-8 weeks for effect.
Cycloplegics: Homatropine Atropine	Topical	2-5%	Increase I.O.P. in glaucoma-prone individuals.	The hazard is in precipitating an acute attack of glaucoma.
Mydriatics: Mydriaticum®	Topical		Increase I.O.P. in glaucoma-prone individuals.	Better results obtained when combined with dark room testing.
Phenylephrine: (Neosynephrine®)	Topical	10%	Used to diagnose epinephrine maculopathy.	
Epinephrine: (Eppy®)	Topical	0.1%	Mydriasis in patients with acute pancreatitis.	Danger of precipitating glaucoma.
Cholinergics: Methacholine (Mecholyl®)	Topical	2.5%	Differential diagnosis of Argyll Robertson pupil.	
Clinistix® Testape®	Topical		Color change indicates glucose level in tears. Diagnostic for diabetes mellitus.	

Reprinted by permission from M. B. Smith, *Handbook of Ocular Pharmacology*. Acton, Mass., Publishing Sciences Group, 1973.

7.10. Dyes Used in External Ocular Examinations

Dyestuff	*Concentration*	*Synonym*	*Color*	*Specificity*
Fluorescein	1–2%	Uranin	yellow*	epithelial defects
Rose Bengal	1 (–10)%	Bengal rose	red	degenerate, dead cells and mucus
Alcian blue	¼–1%		bluish green	mucus
Tetrazolium	1%	Iodonitro-tetrazolium	unstained red	enzyme-containing degenerate cells and inflamed mucous thread
Trypan blue	(0.1)–1%		blue	dead cells and mucus
Lissamine green	1%	Wool green	green	degenerate, dead cells and mucus
Bromothymol blue	0.2%		pH ⩽ 6.8 yellow pH ⩾ 7.6 blue	degenerate, dead cells and mucus
Fluorexon Fluoresoft	2%		yellow* brown	epithelial defects*, degenerate, dead cells and mucus

***Fluoresces in cobalt-filtered blue light.**

Reprinted from Mogen S. Norn, *External methods of examination*. Copenhagen: Scripto

7.11. Visual Effects of Drug Abuse

	Hallucinogens (LSD, psilocybins, mescaline, STP, DMT, PCP, ololiuqui)	*Cannabinols (marijuana, hashish, THC, hash oil)*	*Narcotics (codeine, heroin, opium, meperidine, morphine, pentazocine, propoxyphene)*	*CNS Stimulants (amphetamines, cocaine, anti-obesity drugs, methylphenidate)*	*CNS Sedatives (barbiturates, diazepam, chlordiazepoxide, meprobamate, methaqualone, glutethimide)*	*Anticholinergic (atropine, belladonna, scopolamine [cyclopentolate is not an abused drug])*
Pupil size	↑	if any change ↓	↓	↑	no change, or ↓	↑ and fixed
Accommodation	↓	slightly ↓	↑	↓ slightly	↓	↓
EMO activity	ACA ↑	nystagmus or diplopia if dose is large	convergence impaired, some get nystagmus	convergence enhanced and ACA ↑	convergence weakened ACA ↓ and nystagmus	near phoria and esophoric
Other	Anxiety or panic, depersonalization, confusion, flashbacks, colored illusions, sometimes blurred vision, macropsia	Conjunctival redness, hunger, thirst, nausea, illusions, dreamy fantasy state. A few get unpleasant reactions, others lose inhibitions.	Constipation pulmonary edema, nausea, myopia, coughing is inhibited, indifference to pain, lower IOP	Arrhythmias, termors, anorexia, dry mouth hyperactivity, can raise IOP if angle narrow	Confusion, ataxia, slurred speech, delirium, amnesia	Amnesia, ataxia, blurred vision, can raise IOP

Reprinted from Lyle, W.: *Drug Abuse*, Optometric Monthly (March 1978, pp 139-141) published by Professional Press, Inc., 101 East Ontario Street, Chicago, IL 60611.

7.12. Systemic Drugs with Ocular Side Effects

Drug Name	*Main Use*	*Side Effects*
Achromycin	Antibiotic	Myopia, blurred vision, ptosis, disturbed color vision
Acrequine	Antimalarial, quinine related	Yellowing of sclera, edema, corneal opacities, xanthopsia, blur, halo
Actest	*See* Acthar	
Acthar	Anti-inflammatory	Transient myopia, cataract, glaucoma, potentiation of infection
Adalin		Cataracts
Adapin	Antidepressant	Disturbance EOM, Acc ↓, mydriasis, flashes, disturbed color vision
Adrenalin		Corneal deposits, macular edema, reactive hyperemia, sensitivity to green
Aerosporin	Antibiotic	Vertigo, blur
Afaxin	*See* vitamin A	
Akineton	Anti-Parkinsonian	IOP↑, Acc↓, mydriasis
Aldemol	Diuretic	Xanthopsia
Aldomet	Antihypertensive	Myopia, ptosis, blur, smarting conjunctiva
Alphalin	*See* vitamin A	
Altafur	Antibiotic	Permanent CV defect
Alupent	Bronchodilator	Blur, mydriasis, IOP↓
Amytal	Sedative	Chloropsia, xanthopsia, Y-G vision changes
Ancobon	Antifungal	Hallucinations, vertigo
Anectine	Neuromuscular blocker	Diplopia, IOP↑, Contraction EOM
Ansolysen		Mydriasis, Acc↓, IOP↓
Antabuse	Antialcohol	Optic neuritis, R-G defect
Antepar	Antihelmintic	
Antistine	Antihistamine	Drowsiness, diplopia, ptosis, mydriasis
Antivert	Antihistamine	Blurred vision
Antrenyl		ACC↓, mydriasis
Aplacote	*See* Argyrol	
Apresoline	Antihypertension	Conjunctival congestion, myopia, blurred vision, lid chemosis, vertigo, edema, flashes
Aquamox	Diuretic	Xanthopsia
Aralen	Antimalarial	Central scotoma for red
Areomycin	Antibiotic	Myopia, ptosis, toxic amblyopia, altered color vision
Argyrol	Antiseptic, silver comp.	Yellowish vision, metallic deposits in conjunctiva
Aristocort	Anti-inflammatory	Edema of lid and face, ptosis, cataract
Arlidin	Blood flow	IOP↑

7.12. Systemic Drugs with Ocular Side Effects (continued)

Drug	*Main Use*	*Side Effects*
Artane	Anti-Parkinsonian	Blur, mydriasis, IOP↑
ASA	*See* aspirin	
Ascorbic Acid	Vitamin C	IOP↓
Aspirin	Analgesic	Xanthopsia, R-G defects, field contraction
Atabrine	*See* Acrequine	
Atarax	Tranquilizer	ACC↓, mydriasis, nystagmus
Atropine	Antispasmodic, cholingeric	Mydriasis, Acc↓, color flashes
Aureomycin	*See* Achromycin	
Aventyl	Antidepressant	Blurred vision, mydriasis
Bactrin	Antibacterial	Stevens-Johnson syndrome, retinal edema, hemorrhage, toxic amblyopia, injection of the conjunctiva
Banthine	*See* Atropine	
Benadryl	Antihistamine	Impaired Acc, ptosis, IOP↑
Bentyl	Anticholingeric	Mydriasis, Acc↓.
Benzadrine	CNS stimulant	Cynaopsia, cyclpegia, IOP↑, widening of palpebral appearance
Benzedrex	Decongestant	Mydriasis
Bonine	Antivertigo	Blurred vision
Boric Acid	Antiseptic	Rash, edema
Bromo Seltzer	Analgesic	Xanthopsia
Brufen	Analgesic	Cataract, blur, motion of lights, color vision disturbances, toxic amblyopia
Butagesic	Analgesic	Chromotopsia, vertigo
Butazolidin	*See* Butagesic	
Cafergot	Vasoconstrictor, migraine	Erythopsia, chromatopsia
Camoquin	Antimalarial	Corneal deposits, retinopathy
Campain	Analgesic	Xanthopsia
Cardiazol	CNS stimulant	Transient xanthopsia, scintillating scotoma
Cardiquin	Cardiac arrythmia	Poor color perception, scotoma, constricted field
Catapres	Antihypertensive	Dry, burning, itchy eyes
Catron	MAO inhibitor Antidepressent	Toxic amblyopia, blurred vision, cycloplegia, poor color vision, extraocular motor palsy, mydriasis, nystagmus
Celestone	Anti-inflammatory steroid	Optic nerve changes, IOP↑, cataract, myopia, papilledema, potentiation of infection

7.12 Systemic Drugs with Ocular Side Effects (continued)

Drug	*Main Use*	*Side Effects*
Celontin	Anorexiant	Transient myopia, blur, diplopia, photophobia
Chloromycetin	Antibiotic	Nystagmus, color, vision defects, toxic amblyopia, optic neuritis
Chlor-promanyl	Tranquilizer	Xanthopsia, erythopsia, brown vision
Choloxin	Hypercholesterolemia	Scintillating lights, flashes
Clomid	*See* Choloxin	
Cocaine	Anesthetic	Mydriasis, cycloplegia
Cogentin	*See* Akineton	
Combi-press	*See* Catapres	
Compazine	Tranquilizer	Vertigo
Cordarone	Cardiovascular	Corneal ulcers, yellow deposits
Cortef	*See* Celestone	
Cortogen	*See* Celestone	
Cortone	*See* Celestone	
Cortril	*See* Celestone	
C-Quens	Oral contraceptive	IOP↓, optic neuritis, photophobia, diplopia, proptosis, retinal edema, blue haloes, hemianopia
Crystodigin	Cardiotonic (digitalis derivative)	Xanthopsia, cyanopsia, central scotoma, IOP↓ chloropsia, paralysis extraocular muscles, snow or frost, toxic amblyopia
Cyclospasmol	Vasodilator	IOP↑
Dactil		Flashing lights, mydriasis, Acc↓
Dalmane	Sedative	Blurring, burning
Damine	Anticholingeric	Mydriasis, Acc↓
Dantrium	Skeletal muscle relaxant	Diploplia, hyperlacrimation
Daranide	Diuretic	Thyopia, retinal edema, Acc↓
Darbid	Antispasmodic	IOP↑, Acc↓, photophobia, mydriasis
Darenthin	Antihypertension	Diplopia, ptosis, myopia, occlusion of CRA
Davorcet N	Analegesic	Miosis
Decadron	*See* Celestone	
Declomycin	Antibiotic	Transient tetartan defect
Delysid	Lysergic acid	Mydriasis, chromatopsia, and others
Desoxyn	CNS stimulant	Cyanopsia
Diabinese	Diabetes	Conjunctival hyperemia, toxic amblyopia, central scotoma, changes in refraction
Diafen	Allergic rhinitis	IOP↑, Acc↓, diplopia, ptosis

7.12 Systemic Drugs with Ocular Side Effects (continued)

Drug	*Main Use*	*Side Effects*
Diamox	Diuretic	Myopia, Acc$\downarrow$, hypotony, retinal edema, Stevens-Johnson syndrome
Dibenzyline	Sympatholytic	Conjunctival hyperemia, ptosis, IOP$\downarrow$
Dibuline		Acc$\downarrow$, mydriasis
Digitaline	*See* Crystodigin	
Digitoxin	*See* Crystodigin	
Digitoxoside	*See* Crystodigin	
Digoxin	*See* Crystodigin	
Dilantin	Epilipsy	Conjunctival hyperemia, ptosis, diplopia, nystagmus, oculogyric crisis, Stevens-Johnson syndrome, haloes, vertigo, headache, hallucination
Dilaudid	Analgesic	Pinpoint pupils
Dimecamine	Cardiovascular	Colored flashes
Dimetane	Antihistamine	Hallucinations, IOP$\uparrow$
Diodquin	Antimalarial	Optic atrophy
Disipal	*See* Akineton	
Diucardin	Diuretic	Xanthopsia
Diuril	Diuretic	Xanthopsia
Donnatol	Vagus inhibitor	Transient erythopsia, IOP$\uparrow$, mydriasis, chromatopsia
Dopar	Anti-Parkinsonian	Blurred vision, diplopia, mydriasis, blepharospasm, miosis
Doriden	Sedative	Mydriasis, blurring
Dorsacaine	Topical anesthetic	Edema
DPF	Parasympathomimetic	Iris cysts, retinal detachment, ciliary spasm myopia, ocular pain, impaired day vision, miosis, low IOP
DXY-11	Antibiotic	Myopia, blurred vision, ptosis
Ecolide	Ganglionic blocker	IOP$\uparrow$, amblyopia, Acc$\downarrow$, cycloplegia
Ecotrin	*See* aspirin	
Elavil	Antidepressant	Mydriasis, Acc$\downarrow$, blur, transient color vision disturbances
Enduron	Diuretic	Xanthopsia
Enovid	*See* C-quens	
Entero-vioform	Antidiarrheal, amoebic	Color vision disturbances
Entrophen	*See* aspirin	
Equanil	Tranquilizer	Acc$\downarrow$
Ergotrate	Oxytocic	Blurring, optic edema, bilateral papillitis
Eroldin	Cardiomuscular	Corneal ulcers, keratoconjunctivitis sicca

7.12 Systemic Drugs with Ocular Side Effects (continued)

Drug	*Main Use*	*Side Effects*
Erythrocin	Antibiotic	Tritan-type color defects
Eserine	Parasympathomimetic	Vertigo, miosis, IOP↓, spasm, pain, myopia
Eskabarb	Sedative (barbiturate)	Lid chemosis, diplopia, nystagmus, xanthopsia
Eskalith	Manic psychoses	Blurring, scotomas
Eutonyl	*See* Catron	
Exna	Anti hypertensive	Xanthopsia, IOP↑
Fastin	Appetite suppresant	Headache, IOP↑
Flavoquin	Antimalarial	Corneal deposits, retinopathy
Floropryl	*See* Eserine	
Fluoracil	Antineoplastic	Hyperlacrimation
Furadantin	Antineoplastic	Itching, burning, tearing, blurring, xanthopsia, diplopia, mac degeneration
Gantanol	*See* Bactrin	
Gantrisin	*See* Bactrin	
Grisactin	Fungustatic agent	Mac degeneration, VI nerve palsy, color vision disturbance
Gynergen	*See* Cafergot	
Haldol	Tranquilizer	Blurring
Harmine	*See* Catron	
Harmonyl	Tranquilizer, hypertension	Color vision disturbance, IOP↑
Hashish	Cannabinolis	Light flashes, color vision disturbance
Herplex	Antiviral	Injection of lid, cornea, or conjunctiva
Hydrazid	Antitubercular	Vertigo, optic neuritis
Hydrazide	Diuretic	Xanthopsia
Hydrodiuril	*See* Hydrazide	
Hydromox	*See* Hydrazide	
Hydrosalunet	*See* Hydrazide	
Hygroton	*See* Hydrazide	
Hypergine	Antihypertensive	Hallucinations
Hyperstat	Antihypertensive	Cataracts
Hyzyd	*See* Hydrazid	

Drug	*Main Use*	*Side Effects*
IDU	*See* Herplex	
Inapsine	Tranquilizer	Oculogyric crisis
Inderal	Antiarrythmic	Mydriasis, blurring
Indocin	Antiinflammatory	B-Y defect, Acc↓, visual field loss
INH	Antitubercular	Toxic amblyopia, vertigo
Inversine	Cardiovascular	Colored flashes
Ismelin	Antihypertensive	Ptosis, flashes, blurring
Isordil	Vasodilator	IOP↑, see nitrates
IUDR	*See* Herplex	
Kemadrin	Anti-Parkinsonian	IOP↑
Kenacort	*See* Celestone	
Kynex	*See* Bactrin	
Lanoxin	*See* Crystodigin	
Largactil	*See* Atarax	
Larodopa	*See* Dopar	
Lasix	Diuretic	Color vision disturbances
Leritine	Analgesic	IOP↑
Levate	Antidepressant	Disturbances EOM, Acc↓, mydriasis, light flashes, intermittant color vision disturbances
Librium	Tranquilizer	Decreased saccadics, blurring
Lithane	*See* Eskalith	
Loestrin	*See* C-quens	
LSD	*See* Delysid	
Luminal	*See* Eskabarb	
Madribon	*See* Bactrin	
Marezine	Motion sickness, antihistamine	Drowsiness, diplopia, ptosis, Acc↓
Marijuana	*See* Hashish	
Marplan	*See* Catron	
Matulane	Antineoplastic	Retinal hemorrhages
Maxidex	*See* Celestone	
Mecholyl	Parasypathomimetic	Miosis, IOP↓, pain, myopia, spasm

7.12 Systemic Drugs with Ocular Side Effects (continued)

Drug	*Main Use*	*Side Effects*
Mederol	Vasodilator	R-G defect, central scotoma
Medrol	*See* Celestone	
Mellaril	Tranquilizer	Amblyopia, blurring, nictolopia, central scotoma, Acc↓, opacities, miosis
Mepacrine	Antimalarial	Yellow sclera, edema, corneal opacities, xanthopsia, blue halo
MER 29	Anticholesterol	Cataracts
Mertcortelone	*See* Celestone	
Mesantoin	*See* Dilantin	
Mestonin		Miosis, Acc↓, spasm, myopia
Metahydrin	Diuretic	Xanthopsia
Methadrine	CNS stimulant	Possible cyanopsia
Methium		
Meticortelone	*See* Celestone	
Metrazol	CNS stimulant	Transient xanthopsia, scintillating scotomas
Miaradon	Anticoagulant	Blurring, Acc↓
Miconor	*See* C-quens	
Midicel	*See* Bactrin	
Miltown	*See* Equanil	
Minocin	*See* Achromycin	
Minocycline	*See* Achromycin	
Mintezol	Antihelmintic	Xanthopsia
Moderil	Antihypertension, Tranquilizer	Xanthopsia, optic atrophy, IOP↑
Moditen	Tranquilizer	Xanthopsia, erythropsia
Monase	*See* Elavil	
Motrin	*See* Brufen	
Mysoline	Anorexiant	Nystagmus, mydriasis, diplopia
Mysteclin	*See* Achromycin	
Naclex	Diuretic	Xanthopsia
Nardil	*See* Catron	
Naturetin	Diuretic	Blurred vision, xanthopsia
Navane	Tranquilizer	R-G defect
NegGram	Anti-infective	Acc↓, photophobia, mydriasis, diplopia, papilledema
Nembutal	*See* Eskabarb	
Neodrine	CNS stimulant	Cyanopsia

Drug	*Main Use*	*Side Effects*
Neoserp	Tranquilizer, Hypertension	Glaucoma, uveitis
Neosynephrine	Sympathomimetic	Whitens conjunctiva
Neptazane	Carbonic anhydrase inhibitor	IOP↓, changes in color vision
Neuleptil	Tranquilizer	Subconjunctival hemorrhage
Niamid	*See* Catron	
Niamol	*See* Catron	
Niconyl	*See* INH	
Nicotinic Acid	Vasodilator	Amblyopia, mydriasis, hyperlacrimation
Nitroglycerine	Vasodilator	IOP↑, yellow and blue haloes
Nivaquine	*See* Aralen	
Noctec	CNS depressant, somnifacient	Diplopia, miosis, transient amaurosis
Noludar		Miosis
Nopramin	*See* Harmonyl	
Norinyl	*See* C-quens	
Norlestrin	*See* C-quens	
Norquen	*See* C-quens	
Novahydrazine	Diuretic	Xanthopsia
Novopramine	Antidepressant	Disturbances in EOM, Acc↓, mydriasis, flashes
Novothalidone	Diuretic	Xanthopsia
Nozinan	*See* Chlor-promanyl	
Nydrazid	*See* INH	
Oracon	*See* C-quens	
Orinase	Antidiabetic	Conjunctival hyperemia, refractive changes, toxic amblyopia, central scotoma
Ortho-novum	*See* C-quens	
Ovral	*See* C-quens	
Ovulen	*See* C-quens	
Oxymetracycline	*See* Achromycin	
Pagitane	Tranquilizer	Mydriasis, Acc↓
Panmycin	*See* Achromycin	
Paradione	Anorexiant	Photophobia, headache, diplopia, impaired dark adaptation
Paredrine	Vasoconstrictor	Mydriasis
Parnate	*See* Catron	

7.12 Systemic Drugs with Ocular Side Effects (continued)

Drug	*Main Use*	*Side Effects*
Parsidol	Anticholinergic	Mydriasis, Acc↓
Periactin	Antihistamine	Headache, diplopia, vertigo
Peritrate	Vasodilator, angina	IOP↓
Permitil	*See* Chlor-promanyl	
Phenazine	*See* Chlor-promanyl	
Phenergan	Antihistamine, tranquilizer	Amblyopia, nictolopia, central scotoma, vertigo opacities, miosis
Phenobarbital	*See* Eskabarb	
Phenurone	Anorexiant	Nystagmus, mydriasis, diplopia
Phinazone	Antipyrine	Urticaria of lids, toxic ambliopia, keratoconjunctivitis
Phospholine	Parasympathomimetic	Miosis, IOP↓, pain, vertigo, myopia, spasm
Placidyl	Sedative	Convergence defect, hallucinations, color and Acc disturbance caeco–central scotoma
Plaquenil	*See* Acrequine	
Polophine	Analgesic	Miosis
Pondimin	Antiobesity	Nystagmus, burning, blurring, IOP↑
Ponstan	Analgesic	Loss of color vision
Ponstel	*See* Ponstan	
Prantal	Antispasmodic, ulcers	Mydriasis, Acc↓, IOP↑, photophobia
Preludin	Antiobesity	IOP↑, change in corneal curvature
Pre-sate	Antiobesity	Photophobia, Acc↓, IOP↑
Priscoline	Vasodilator	IOP↑
Privine	Vasoconstrictor	Puncture keratitis, negative hyperemia
Proaqua	Diuretic	Xanthopsia
Pro-banthine	*See* Atropine	
Prolixin	*See* Moditen	
Promanyl	See Chlor-promanyl	
Propadrine	Sympathomimetic	Mydriasis
Prostigmin	Parasympathomimetic	Miosis, IOP↓, pain, myopia, spasm, vertigo
Provest	*See* C-quens	
Purodigin	*See* Crystodigin	
Pyrobenzamine	Antihistamine	Drowsiness, diplopeia, mydriasis
Pyrmal	Antibiotic	Retinal edema, toxic amblyopic, transient myopia, narrowed fields

Drug	*Main Use*	*Side Effects*
Questran	Antilipemic	Arcus juvenitis, uveitis
Quide	*See* mellaril	
Quinaglute	Arrythmias	Scotoma, color perception disturbances, amblyopia
Quinate	Antimalarial	Scotoma, color perception disturbances
Quincardine	*See* Quinate	
Quinine	*See* Quinate	
Raudixin	Tranquilizer	IOP↑, rare color vision abnorm.
Rautabs	*See* Raudixin	
Rautrax-N	Diuretic	Blurring, xanthopia
Rauwiloid	*See* Raudixin	
Rauzide	*See* Rautrax-N	
Renese	Diuretic	Xanthopsia
Resepoid	*See* Neoserp	
Resorcinol		Toxic amblyopia, allergic conjunctivitis, nystagmus, hallucinations, hypotony
Rifadin	Antitubercular	Transient color vision defects
Rimactane	*See* Rifadin	
Ritalin	Stimulant, antidepressant	Mydriasis
Robaxin	Skeletal muscle relaxant	Conjunctival hypermia, blurring, EOM disturbances
Roniacol	Vasodilator	Amblyopia, hyperlacrimation, mydriasis, toxic maculopthy
Saluron	Diuretic	Xanthopsia
Sansert	Migraine prophylactic	Acc↓, scotoma
Scopolamine	*See* Atropine	
Secogen	Sedative	Chloropsia, Y-G defect, field loss
Seconal	*See* Secogen	
Septra	*See* Bactrin	
Serentil	*See* Mellaril	
Serpasil	*See* Neoserp	
Sinequan	*See* Adapin	
Singoserp	Tranquilizer	Rare color vision disturbances
Slo-tedrin	Asthma relief	Corneal deposits, Mac degeneration, reactive hypermia, sensitivity to green
Softran	Motion sickness	Acc↓, blurring, drowsiness, mydriasis

7.12 Systemic Drugs with Ocular Side Effects (continued)

Drug	*Main Use*	*Side Effects*
Solazine	Tranquilizer	Blurred vision, mydriasis, IOP↑
Somnos	*See* Noctec	
Sparine	*See* Mellaril	
Staphylomycine	Antibiotic	Color vision disturbances
Stelazine	*See* Mellaril	
Stemetil	*See* Compazine	
Stigmonene	Parasympathomimetic	Miosis, myopia, tearing, Acc↓, spasm
Stoxil	*See* Herplex	
Streptomycin	Antibacterial	Optic neuritis, atrophy, toxic amblyopia, scotoma
Streptosol	*See* Streptomycin	
Sulfazuxidine	*See* Bactrin	
Sullamyd	*See* Bactrin	
Sumycin	*See* Achromycin	
Surmontil	*See* Elavil	
Symatrel	Anti-Parkinsonian	Acc↓, mydriasis
Syntropan	Antispasmodic	Glaucoma, mydriasis, widening of palpebral aperture
Talwin	Analgesic	Hallucinations, blurring, Acc↓, vertigo
Tandearil	Analgesic	Conjunctivitis, toxic amblyopia, Stevens-Johnson syndrome, lid scarring, corneal ulcer
Tapiazole	Hyperthyroidism	B-Y defect
Tensilon	Parasympathomimetic	Miosis, Acc↓, spasm
Teracyn	*See* Achromycin	
Terramycin	*See* Achromycin	
Teyretol	Anorexiant	Nystagmus, diplopia
Thallium	Tranquilizer	Cataracts, ptosis, palsies, central scotoma mydriasis
Thiazamine	Antibacterial	Xanthopsia, narrowed field
Thioril	*See* Mellaril	
Thorazine	*See* Chlor-promanyl	
Tofranil	*See* Novopramine	
Tolserol	Skeletal muscle relaxant	Diplopia, nystagmus
Tranxene	*See* Librium	
Trecator	Anti-tubercular	Increased brightness, color vision disturbances
Trest	Anti-spasmodic	Blurred vision, IOP↑

7.12 Systemic Drugs with Ocular Side Effects (continued)

Drug	*Main Use*	*Side Effects*
Tridione	Anticonvulsant, anorexiant	Photophobia, headache, diplopia, impaired dark adaptation, "snow storm effect," color disturbances
Trilafon	*See* Chlor-promanyl	
Triparonol	Anticholesterol	Cataracts
Triptil	*See* Elavil	
Tyvid	*See* INH	
Urecholine	*See* Eserine	
Urispas	Antispasmodic	Blurring
Urozide	Diuretic	Xanthopsia
Valium	*See* Librium	
Vaporole	Vasodilator	Colored rings, xanthopsia
Vasculat	Vasodilator	IOP$\uparrow$, increased blood flow through eye
Vasodilan	Vasodilator	IOP$\uparrow$
Vasopan	Vasodilator	IOP$\uparrow$
Vectrin	*See* Achromycin	
Vesprin	Tranquilizer	Blurring
Vibramycin	*See* Achromycin	
Vioform	*See* Entero-vioform	
Vitamin A		Excess=xanthopsia, deficiency=erythopsia
Visine	Vasoconstrictor	Allergic reactions
Vivactil	*See* Elavil	
Voranil	Anorexiant	Euphoria, dysphoria, glaucoma, IOP$\uparrow$
Winoxin	*See* Digoxin	
Zarontin	Anorexiant	Transient myopia, blurring, diplopia, photophobia
Zaroxolyn	Diuretic	Xanthopsia, color vision disturbances
Zyloprin	Uricorsuric	Allergic conjunctivitis, cataracts, macular changes

7.13. Pharmaceuticals Used in Contact Lens Practice

Table A. Decongestants

Brand Name	*Mfr.*
Allerest	P
Buf opto efrical	PPF
Collyrium	W
Degest	BH
Eye cool	MR
Eye gene	SCH
Eye lo	RE
Eye mo	W
Iso-lo	AM
Isopto-frin	AL
Neozine	PPF
Op-isophrin	R
Ocusol	N
Oph	W
Phenylzin	TY
Prefrin (z)	AP
Soothe	BP
Tear efrin	TY
Ultra clear	MA
Vasi-zinc	AY
Visine	PF
Zinc frin	AL
Zo Zo	SSS

Table B. Artificial Tears

Brand Name	*Mfr.*
Adsorbotear	BP
Hypotears	CV
Isopto Tears	AL
Lacril	AP
Liquifilm Tears	AP
Liquifilm Forte	AP
Lyteers	BH
Methulose	AO
Neo Tears	BH
Tearisol	SM
Tears Naturale	AL
Ultra Tears	
Visculose	AO

Table C. Soft Lens Products

Brand Name	*Mfr.*
Cleaners	
Daily Cleaner	BL
Enzymatic cleaner	A-P
Pliagel	SM
Preflex	BP
Soft mate	BH
Weekly cleaner	BH
Chemical Storage	
Cleaning and Disinfecting	AP
Flexol	BP
Thermal storage/rinsing	
Boil-n-soak	BP
Hydrocare	AP
Lensrins	A-P
Permasol	CV
Preserved saline	BL
Soft therm	BH
Soft Mate Rinsing	BH
Nonpreserved saline	
Blairex System	B
Non Preserved Saline	BP
Sterile Saline	BL
Unisol	SM
Disinfecting/rinsing	
Flex-Care	BP
Normol	BP
Soft Care Disinfectant	BH
Lubricant	
Adapettes	BP
Clerz	CV
Lens Lubricant	BL

Table D. Hard Lens Products

Brand Name	*Mfr.*
Irrigating Solutions	
Blinx	BX
Dacriose	TY
Mirasol	M
M/rinse	MR
Ocurins	WL
Ocusol	N
Soaking Solutions	
Contique	AL
Hydrofil	MO
Ova-nite	MR
Soaclens	BP
Soakare	AP
Soak-tone	R
Soquette	BH
Stericidial	BM
Vistex	TY
Comfort drops	
Adapt	BP
Clerz	SM
Comfort drops	BH
Penavel	SH
Pre-sert	AP
Cleaners	
Blink-n-clean	PL
Clens	BP
Consure	OK
Contique	
Obrite	D
d-film	FP
Gel-clean	BH
Hydrofil	MO
Lensline X	AB
LC-65	AP
Lobob	LO
Milroy Prof	D
Staybrite	SH

Brand Name	*Mfg.*
Sereine	OK
Titan	BH
Vision clear	AX
Wetting Solutions	
Aquafilm	M
Contactisol	TY
Contique	AL
Hydrofil	MO
Hy-flow	CV
I-septic	M
Liquifilm	AP
Micon	ML
O-3	D
Obrig	OB
Ows Blue	D
Sereine	OK
Stay Wet	SH
Visalens	PF
Wetting Solution	BH
Wet-cote	D
Wet tone	PF
Multifunctional	
Clean-n-soak	BH
Clerz	SM
Dual clean	SH
Duo flow	SM
Lensine	CV
Lensmate	AL
One solution	BH
Ova-nite	MR
PCL	WJ
Steri-lens	M
W/J Trifunctional	WJ
Soaclens	BP
Stericidal	BM
Total	AP
Visalens	PF
Wet-n-Soak	AP

Table E. Manufacturers

Name	*Abbrev.*
Abbott Labs	AB
Alcon Labs	AL
Allegan Ph.	AP
American Optical	AO
American Ph.	AM
Ayerest Labs	AY
Automated Optics	AX
Barnes-Hind	BH
Bausch & Lomb	BL
Blairex	B
Breger-Mueller Welt	BM
Burton Parsons	BP
Cooper Vision	CV
Danker	D
Lobob	LO
Maybelline	M
Mi-con	MI
Milton Roy	MR
Morrison Labs	MO
Opti-kem	N
Obrig	OB
Pharmcraft	P
Pfizer	PF
Professional Ph.	PP
Riker	R
Rexall	RE
Santa	S
Schieffelin	SC
Schmid	SD
Sherman	SH
Smith Miller Patch	SM
Tama	T
Tilden-Yates	TY
Warner Lambert	WL
Wesley/Jessen	WJ
Winthrop	W
WTS Ph.	WT
Wyeth	WY

Pathology 8

8.1. Ocular Manifestations of Systemic Diseases

Table A. Infections

Systemic disease	*Ocular disease*
Viral	
Pharyngitis	None
Children: fever, pharyngitis, gastroenteritis	Conjunctivitis
Adults: No systemic disease	Epidemic keratoconjunctivitis
Encephalitis	Secondary to cranial nerve involvement
Fever sores, stomatitis, Kaposi's eruption	Dendritic keratitis
Chickenpox	Uveitis
Meningoencephalitis	Cranial nerves
Zoster	Keratitis, uveitis with invasion of first branch of NV
Adults: mononucleosis-like	Retinitis
Multiple warts	Chronic conjunctivitis, keratitis
Parotitis, orchitis, encephalitis	Interstitial keratitis
Postnatal: skin eruption, fever, pharyngitis	Conjunctivitis
Congenital: microcephaly, deafness, cardiopathy, visceral disease	Cataract, microphalmia, retinitis, glaucoma
Cytomegalic inclusion disease	Uveitis
Smallpox	Vaccinia of lid, keratitis
Measles (rubeola)	Kophk's spots on the caruncle and semilunar fold; conjunctival injection and mucoid discharge; punctate staining of cornea with photophobia; (rare) metastatic uveitis, optic neuritis, esotropia
Congenital rubella	Microphthalmos, glaucoma, corneal edema, aniridia and iris atrophy, cataract, retinopathy, optic atrophy, nystagmus
Postnatal rubella	Mild catarrahal conjunctivitis
Mumps	Dacryoadenitis, conjunctivitis, keratitis; (rare): episcleritis, uveitus, optic neuritis, retrobulbar neuritis, thrombosis of the central retinal artery, paresis of the internal and external ocular muscles
Verrucae (warts)	Cutaneous lesions, conjunctivitis, keratitis (secondary to mechanical irritation from lesions at lid margin)
Bacterial	
Malignant pustule, hemorrhagic mediastinitis, gastrointestinal inflammation, disseminated disease with meningitis	Necrotic ulcer of lids
Acute and chronic febrile disease, encephalitis, meningitis	Keratitis (nummular–coins), uveitis (granulomatous), retrobulbar neuritis and papillitis
diphtheriae	Membranous conjunctivitis with necrosis, postdiptheritic paralysis (N VI and accommodation [N III])
Tetanus	Miosis, orbicularis oculi spasm
Acute poisoning	Paralysis of intraocular and extraocular muscles
Whooping cough	Lid, orbit, and conjunctival hemorrhage
gonorrhoeae	Purulent conjunctivitis, ophthalmia neonatorum, nongranulomatous irdocyclitis
Meningitis	Petechiae and ecchymoses during bacteremia, bilateral panophthalmitis
tuberculosis	Any part of the eye involved: lupus vulgaris, phlyctenular disease, uveitis, periphlebitis
Lepromatous (cutaneous)	Anterior ocular inflammation
Tuberculoid (neural)	Rarely anterior ocular inflammation

(continued)

Table A. Infections (continued)

Systemic disease	*Ocular disease*
Generalized febrile illness	Necrotic conjunctival ulcer (Parinaud's syndrome) Severe conjunctival edema
Pneumococci	Hypopyon keratitis, purulent conjunctivitis
Staphylococci	Sty, blepharitis, conjunctivitis
Streptococci	Pseudomembranous conjunctivitis, keratitis with hypopyon, nongranulomatous uveitis

Table B. Endocrine

Diabetes Mellitus

Visual acuity
- Transient variations in refraction
- Photopsia and diplopia in cerebral hypoglycemia
- Decreased accommodation
- Depressed in cataract, vitreous hemorrhage, macular edema, and macular detachment
- Blindness from proliferative retinopathy
- Diplopia in ophthalmoplegia

Intraocular pressure
- Decreased in acidosis
- Increased in rubeosis of iris

Lids	Xanthelasma	Cosmetic
Conjunctivae	Microcirculatory alteration	May reflect generalized microvascular disorder
Extraocular muscles	Third and sixth nerve palsy	Diplopia; may be mistaken for intracranial neoplasm or aneurysm
Orbit	Mucormycosis	Lethal if untreated
Cornea	Descemet's wrinkles	Unknown, may be an early clinical sign
Iris	Ectropion uveae (without rubeosis)	Unknown, may be an early clinical sign
	Rubeosis iridis	Neovascular glaucoma
	Pigment epithelium vacuolization	Increased pigment of anterior segment
Lens	Refractive changes	Fluctuating vision
	Cataract	Impaired vision
Ciliary body	Basement membrane thickening	Unknown
Vitreous	Asteroid hyalosis	Unknown
Optic nerve	Optic atrophy	May be part of a syndrome

Ocular fundi

Background retinopathy
1. Microaneurysms
2. Deep and superficial hemorrhages
3. Hard exudates
4. Cotton-wool patches
5. Venous dilation and venous beading
6. Dilated, tortuous, kinked intraretinal vessels

Proliferative retinopathy
1. New blood vessels solely (rete mirabile)
2. Fibrous proliferation

Vitreous hemorrhage
1. Fundus can be seen
2. Fundus completely obscured

(continued)

Table B. Endocrine (continued)

Lipemia retinalis
Oculomotor nerves
Neuropathy with muscle paralysis (pupil frequently spared in N III involvement)

Thyroid Dysfunction
Exophthalmos
Bilateral or unilateral
1. Lid retraction exaggerates or simulates appearance
Compressible
1. Common type in thyrotoxicosis
Solid (noncompressible)
1. Common type following medical or surgical ablation of thyroid
Eyelids
Lid retraction (Dalrymple)
1. Indreased by attentive gaze (Kocher) or by conjunctival instillation of epinephrine; decreased by adrenergic blockade (Guanethidine locally or block of superior cervical ganglion); forehead does not wrinkle on upward gaze (Joffrey)
Lid lag (von Graefe)
1. Upper lid delays before following globe in downward gaze
2. Common in thyrotoxicosis
Infrequent blinking (Stellwag)
Miscellaneous
1. Globe lags behind upper eyelid on upward gaze (Means)
2. Lower lid lags behind on upward gaze (Griffith)
3. Increased pigmentation of skin (Jellinek)
Orbital congestion
May be associated with fullness of eyelids (Enroth) and prevent eversion of upper eyelid (Gifford)
Extraocular muscles
Contracture of ocular muscle usually
1. Inferior rectus preventing upward gaze
2. Most common following thyroid ablation
Weakness of convergence (Möbius)
Optic nerve
Most common following thyroid ablation
Papillitis or retrobulbar neuritis
Papilledema
1. Neuroretinal edema

8.2. Symptomology and Classification of Vascular Headaches

	Temporal Arteritis	*Chronic Hypertension*	*Hypertensive Crises*	*Migraine*	*Increased intracranial pressure*	*Diabetic ophthalmoplegia*	*Carotid aneurysm*
Frequency	Relatively high among elderly	Common in moderate to severe hypertension	With virtually every attack				
Onset	Gradual	On awakening	Abrupt				
Duration	May be recurrent	Usually intermittant but may occur daily over prolonged periods (mos–yrs); Attacks last several hours	Varies from minutes to hours				
Location	Follows Temporal Artery and radiates to forehead and back of head Usually Unilateral	Usually occipital but may radiate	Diffuse May be occipital and unilateral from vertex to nape of neck	On one side of head at a time	Variable	Forehead and eye	Supraorbital area
Character	Severe and deep Throbbing	Throbbing, pounding developing into dull, deep ache	Severe Unbearable	Variable severity preceded by visual aura on opposite side	Severe "bursting" or "boring"	Severe	Severe
Cause	Chronic granulomatous inflammatory process	Chronic severe hypertension	Sudden dramatic rise in blood pressure				
Clinical Signs	Temporal artery pulsates and becomes firm, photophobia, lacrimation, retrobulbar pain, transient or permanent visual loss	Classic fundus anomalies -tortuosity, nicking (av), exudates, hemorrhages, increased light reflex, etc., headache worse with bending, better with sitting	Flush, sweats, pallor, dizzy, weak, nausea, exhaustion, etc. Hypertensive history, ie, fundus anomalies	Made worse with bright light and better lying down in dark room	Made worse with bending, sneezing, straining at stool Presence of papilledema	Older age group, diabetes, third nerve palsy with sparing of pupil	Complete third nerve palsy with ptosis and dilated pupil on same side

8.3. Neurological Syndromes Involving the Visual System

Syndrome	*Signs and Symptoms*	*Tests*	*Neurological Involvement*	*Anatomical Site of the Lesion*
Adie's Tonic Pupil	1. The affected pupil is usually dilated 2. Pupil reacts to light and dark slowly 3. Pupil reacts to accommodation-convergence after a delay 4. Unilateral in 80% of the cases 5. Pupil reacts normally to mydriatics 6. Tendon reflexes are absent 7. Usually occurs in 20–30 year old females	1. Direct and indirect pupillary reflexes 2. Accommodation-convergence task 3. Knee jerk and ankle jerk 4. Methacholine (2.5%) will contract an Adie's pupil and not a normal pupil (a)	1. Hypothalamus —autonomic center ? (b) 2. Postganglionic fibers from the ciliary ganglion	Not definitely known
Argyll Robertson Pupil	1. Loss of direct and indirect pupillary reflexes 2. Pupillary constriction on convergence retained 3. Usually bilateral 4. Dilation of the pupil, after pinching the neck is lost 5. Iris atrophy (in some cases) 6. Mioptic pupil is indicative of syphilis	1. Direct and indirect pupillary reflexes 2. Accommodation-convergence task 3. Sensory relfex (neck-pupil) 4. Miotic pupil dilates with atropine (c) 5. No pupil change with cocaine (d)	1. Peripheral III Nerve ? (b) 2. Intercalated neuron of the tectum ? (b) 3. Along path of afferent visual fibers after they have left the optic track and entered the pretectal area. At this point, lateral to the aqueduct of sylvius, they are in proximity to the supranuclear sympathetic fibers of the pupil's dilator apparatus.	Not definitely known
Bell's Phenomenon	1. Normally present: upward and outward rotation of the eye upon forcible lid closure 2. Presence provides evidence that connecting fibers between N. III and N. VIII nuclei are intact	1. Forcible lid closure 2. If there is a normal Bell's phenomenon in a person who cannot voluntarily elevate his eyes, there is an indication of a supranuclear lesion	VII Cranial Nerve Nucleus and the III Cranial Nerve Nucleus, the oblcularis oculus and superior rectus, respectively	(b)

(continued)

8.3. Neurological Syndromes Involving the Visual System (continued)

Syndrome	*Signs and Symptoms*	*Tests*	*Neurological Involvement*	*Anatomical Site of the Lesion*
Bell's Paralysis or Palsy	1. Paralysis of the upper and lower facial muscles 2. The eyelid on the affected side cannot close and has a wider palpebral aperture 3. The cheek on the affected side appears puffed on expiration and sucked in on inspiration 4. There may be epiphora due to sagging of the lower lid on the affected side 5. Exposure keratitis	1. Slit lamp examination of the cornea with fluoroscein 2. Facial motility (e)	VIII Cranial Nerve	Stylomastoid foramen at the exit of the VII Cranial Nerve
Benedict's Sign	1. Homolateral, III Cranial Nerve paralysis 2. Contralateral arm tremor	1. Ptosis due to levator palpebrum superioris 2. Fixed, dilated pupil 3. Exo–Hypotropia	III Cranial Nerve and the Red Nucleus	III Cranial Nerve fibers passing through the Red Nucleus
Foster-Kennedy Syndrome	1. Ipsilateral asnomia 2. Ipsilateral amaurosis 3. Contralateral papilledema	1. Binocular ophthalmoscopy 2. Light perception is absent	I and II Cranial Nerves	Olfactory Trigone, where the Olfactory Tract forms a triangular structure in the rhinencephalon at the anterior perforated substance
Foville's Syndrome (Anterior Inferior Cerebellar Syndrome)	1. Ipsilateral lateral rectus paralysis 2. Ipsilateral absence of conjugate gaze 3. Ipsilateral facial paralysis 4. Contralateral tongue and extremities paralysis	1. Ocular motility 2. Esotropia 3. Facial motility (e)	Pons, VI and VII Cranial Nerves	Caudal portion of the pons, to include the center for conjugate lateral gaze

(continued)

8.3. Neurological Syndromes Involving the Visual System (continued)

Syndrome	*Signs and Symptoms*	*Tests*	*Neurological Involvement*	*Anatomical Site of the Lesion*
Gradenigo's Syndrome	1. VI Cranial Nerve paresis or paralysis 2. Associated facial pain 3. Photophobia and lacrimation 4. Reduced corneal sensitivity 5. Diplopia of recent origin 6. Occipital pain (occasionally)	1. Ocular molity 2. Esotropia	VI and VII Cranial Nerves and the Gasserian Ganglion	Petro-sphenoid ligament which occupies the petro-sphenoid fissure
Horner's Syndrome	1. Miosis 2. Partial ptosis 3. Enophthalmos 4. Hypotony (occasionally) 5. Heterochromia (if in eary life) (f) 6. Transitory increase in facial temperature 7. Alteration of tear secreation; an increase or decrease 8. Loss of sweating	1. Pupillary relfexes 2. Lid examination 3. Epinephrine (1:1000) will dilate a Horner's pupil and not a normal pupil (g)	Descending fibers from the brain stem to the nucleus inter-medialateralis or a lesion at any point in the sympathetic pathway in the brain stem, cervical spinal cord, sympathetic ganglion and post ganglionic fibers	Neck, spinal cord, and/or the hypothalamus (h)
Internuclear Ophthalmoplegia (anterior)	1. Paralysis of one or both medial recti during lateral gaze 2. Nystagmus of the abducting eye (usually) 3. Convergence (usually present)	1. Ocular motility 2. Caloric nystagmus (occasionally will cause contraction of affected medial rectus) 3. Convergence task	Medial longitudinal fasciculus	Medial longitudinal fasciculus at the level of the pons. If convergence is absent, the medial longitudinal fasciculus is affected at the level of the midbrain
Lateral Gaze Syndrome	1. Forceful conjugate deviation of both eyes to the contralateral side of the lesion when attempting to gaze ipsilaterally 2. Convergence is not affected (usually)	1. Ocular motility 2. Convergence task	VII Cranial Nerve Nucleus	Dorsal medial portion of the pons

(continued)

8.3. Neurological Syndromes Involving the Visual System (continued)

Syndrome	*Signs and Symptoms*	*Tests*	*Neurological Involvement*	*Anatomical Site of the Lesion*
Meniere's Syndrome	1. Severe vertigo 2. Tinnitus 3. Unilateral or bilateral deafness 4. Diplopia 5. Contralateral light flashes 6. Nystagmus during an attack 7. Headache	1. Nystagmus evaluation 2. Hearing test	1. Labyrinth VIII Cranial Nerve ? (b) 2. Internal otitis? (b) 3. Abnormal metabolism ? (b)	Not definitely known
Millard-Gubler Syndrome	1. Ipsilateral VI Cranial Nerve palsy 2. Ipsilateral VII Cranial Nerve palsy 3. Contralateral hemiplegia	1. Ocular motility 2. Facial motility 3. Limb motility	Pyramidal fibers in the Pons, the VI, and the VII Cranial Nerves	Fascicular involvement of the VI Cranial Nerve at the ventral para-median portion of the pons
Moebius' Syndrome	1. Bilateral lateral rectus paralysis 2. Bilateral facial paralysis 3. Deafness 4. Webbed fingers or toes 5. Supernumerary toes 6. Supernumerary digits 7. Incomplete eyelid closure 8. Congenital, usually affecting males	1. Ocular motility 2. Convergence (usually present) 3. Nystagmus (caloric and vestibular absent)	VI and VII Cranial Nerves	Supranuclear congenital aplasia
Parinaud's Syndrome (Sylvian Aqueduct Syndrome)	1. Paralysis of conjugate vertical gaze; elevation depression, or both 2. Pupillary dila-tion with failure to react to light or normal and miotic 3. Ptosis or a wide palpebral aperture 4. Diplopia 5. Corectopia 6. Convergence spasm 7. Nystagmus	1. Ocular motility 2. Pupillary relfexes 3. Nystagmus evaluation 4. Lid Evaluation	Supranuclear pathways	Supranuclear near afferent pupil fibers (tumors in the epithalamic area including the pineal pretectal area, the superior colliculus and the aqueduct of sylvius

(continued)

8.3. **Neurological Syndromes Involving the Visual System (continued)**

Syndrome	*Signs and Symptoms*	*Tests*	*Neurological Involvement*	*Anatomical Site of the Lesion*
Pseudo-tumor Cerebri	1. Bilateral papilledema 2. Headache 3. Evidence of increased intra-cranial pressure 4. Normal ventriculography 5. Normal vision except for an enlarged blind spot	1. Binocular ophthalmoscopy 2. Visual fields	II Cranial Nerve	Completely obscure
Raymond's Syndrome (Middle Alternating Hemiplegia)	1. Ipsilateral VI Cranial Nerve palsy 2. Contralateral hemiplegia	1. Ocular motility 2. Esotropia 3. Limb motility	Pyramidal fibers in the Pons and the VI Cranial Nerve	Fascicular involvement of the VI Cranial Nerve at the ventral para-median portion of the pons
Transient VI Nerve Paralysis or Paresis	1. Paralysis or paresis of the lateral rectus muscle 2. Mid-aged or elderly individuals 3. Diplopia of recent onset	1. Ocular motility 2. Esotropia	VI Cranial Nerve	Lesions along the course of the VI Nerve–tumor, otistis
Weber's Syndrome (Alternating Superior Hemiplegia)	1. Homolateral III Cranial Nerve paralysis 2. Contralateral hemiplegia with paralysis of the face and tongue	1. Ptosis due to levator palpebrum superioris 2. Fixed, dilated pupil 3. Exo-Hypotropia 4. Face, tongue and limb motility	III Cranial Nerve	At the III Cranial Nerve before it emerges from the peduncle and the pyramidal fibers above the level of the III Cranial Nerve Nuclei
Wernicke's Hemiopic Pupil	Hemiopic pupil	Pupillary relfexes	II Cranial Nerve	Post-chiasm fibers for the light reflex
Wernicke's Syndrome (Cerebral beriberi)	1. Nystagmus, horizontal and vertical 2. Lateral rectus paralysis 3. Paralysis of conjugate gaze 4. Ptosis 5. Slow pupillary reaction 6. Diplopia 7. Ataxia	1. Ocular motility 2. Esotropia 3. Pupillary reflexes 4. Walking–ataxic gait	III and I Cranial Nerves and the Thalamus	Third and fourth ventricles, Aque-duct Sylvius, mammalary bodies, posterior corpora quadrigemini, and thalamus

Reprinted from J.N. Trachtman and V. Giambalvo, Neurological syndromes involving the visual system, *J. of the American Optometric Assn.*, June, 1976.

8.4. Classifications

Table A. Glaucomas

A. Primary Glaucoma
  1. Open-Angle Glaucoma: Also called simple glaucoma, wide-angle glaucoma, chronic simple glaucoma. The most common form.
  2. Angle-closure glaucoma–Also called narrow-angle glaucoma, closed-angle glaucoma, acute congestive glaucoma
     a. Acute
     b. Subacute or chronic

B. Congential Glaucoma
  1. Primary congenital or infantile glaucoma–Also called buphthalmos or hydrophthalmos
  2. Glaucoma associated with congenital anomalies
     a. Pigmentary glaucoma
     b. Aniridia
     c. Axenfeld's syndrome
     d. Sturge-Weber syndrome
     e. Infantile glaucoma developing late
     f. Marfan's syndrome
     g. Neurofibromatosis
     h. Lowe's syndrome
     i. Microcornea and megalocornea

C. Secondary Glaucoma
  1. Uveitis and postinflammatory glaucoma
     a. Pupillary occlusion
  2. Heterochromia of iris with uveitis
  3. Postoperative glaucoma
     a. Pupillary block in aphakic glaucoma
  4. Phacolytic glaucoma
     a. Swelling of lens
     b. Subluxation of lens
     c. Hypermaturity of lens
     d. Rupture of lens capsule
  5. Epithelial downgrowth
  6. Glaucoma capsulare
  7. Glaucoma secondary to hemorrhage
  8. Glaucoma and venous closure
     a. Extraocular
     b. Central
  9. Traumatic glaucoma
  10. Essential progressive atrophy of iris
  11. Rubeosis iridis
  12. Thyrotropic exophthalmos
  13. Intraocular tumors

D. Absolute Glaucoma: The end result of any uncontrolled glaucoma

Table B. Cataracts

A. *Classification A*

1. *Developmental Cataract And Lenticular Anomalies*
    a. Anterior axial embryonal or fetal cataract: The opacity consists of fine white dots outlining, to varying degrees, the erect (anterior) Y suture and rarely affects vision.
    b. Stellate or sutural cataract: may involve the anterior or posterior Y sutures or both. Their appearance is much more solid than that of the anterior axial variety and it may have some effect on vision. Its presence may be detected in conjunction with other types of developmental cataracts (i.e. embryonal punctate, zonular, etc.).
    c. Congenital punctate cataract (may be embryonal or postnatal): consists of a discoid region of small white dots in the central area of the lens with involvement usually bilateral. It rarely interferes with vision and is frequently seen to contain a stellate cataract with the Y suture easily discernable.
    d. Anterior polar or pyramidal cataract: appears as a sharply circumscribed opacity at the pole of the anterior lens capsule. It usually takes the form of a pyramidal projection protruding into the anterior chamber.
    e. Mittendorf's dot: a commonly seen opacity appearing with the slit lamp as a white dot at the posterior lens capsule and with the ophthalmoscope, in retro illumination, as a distinct black dot against the red reflex of the fundus. In both cases it is located nasally and slightly superior to the posterior pole of the lens. It is simply the remnant of the attachment of the hyaloid artery in the formation of the tunica vasculosa lentis.
    f. Persistent pupillary membrane: involves complete or incomplete persistence of the vascular pupillary membrane, a common congenital anomaly. They may arise from the lesser iris circle and may not adhere to anything (often seen floating into the anterior chamber from their iris attachment) or they may adhere to the lens capsule.
    g. Epicapsular Stars: pigmented remnants of the pupillary membrane, with no visible attachment of the iris, which are frequently found residing on the anterior lens capsule. They are usually star-shaped and are peppered, apparently without any orderly arrangement, on the capsule in the pupillary area. They vary in size and number (from one or two isolated stars to dozens).
    h. Ectopia Lentis: refers to a condition of malposition of the lens secondary to a zonular defect. The lenticular displacement is in a direction away from the defective zonule. It is a hereditary phenomenon and usually occurs bilaterally.

2. *Senescent Cataract*
    a. Senescent cortical cataracts: primarily the result of imbibition of water by the cortex coupled with degeneration of lens fibers. These have the appearance of small globules of petroleum jelly on a piece of glass.
    b. Water vacuoles and water clefts: appear as dark spaces which usually position themselves radially following the sutural system of the lens.
    c. Spokes: basically a descriptive term for the appearance of the radially oriented water clefts as they become opacified.
    d. Lamellar separation: parallel circumferential streaks very similar in nature to water clefts, only running in concentric fashion corresponding to the onion-skin-like layers of the cortex.
    e. Cuneform opacities: flat and amorphous in shape, usually found in the peripheral portions of the lens; may represent coalescence of lamellar separations.
    f. Punctate cortical opacities: commonly found as dotlike flecks of varying sizes scattered at various levels of the cortex; depending on their size and density they may appear white or polychromatic, displaying vivid reds, blues, and greens. If relatively dense in number, they may present a striking contrast to the clear nucleus.

(continued)

Table B. Cataracts (continued)

g. Posterior subcapsular cataract: perhaps the most significant form of cortical involvement. A central area of opacification occurs in the outermost posterior cortical layers. It can be extremely deleterious to vision. It has the appearance of ground glass or "sand on a beach" coupled with a characteristic yellow tinge.
h. Senescent nuclear cataract: primarily the result of lenticular sclerosis. Along with the nuclear sclerosis is the observable color change of the region, in the form of a gradient yellowing.

3. *Senescent Changes Affecting the Entire Lens*
   a. Mature cataract: cataract is said to have reached maturity when it is totally opaque.
   b. Morganian cataract: the combination of a still-intact solid nucleus that has settled to the bottom of a liquid cortex and that yields the clinical picture of Morganian cataract. With a liquid cortex, one may see against its milky opaque appearance a tremulous iris.
   c. Hypermature cataract: may evolve from either the mature cataract or from the Morganian state. In hypermaturity, cortical material leaks out through the capsule, and the lens itself will thus display a marked shriveled or wrinkled appearance.

4. *Traumatic Cataract*
   a. Contusion without rupture:

      Extracapsular (Vossius Ring): with a relatively direct blow to the eye, the posterior pigmented surface of the iris is forced back into contact with the anterior lens capsule. When the iris rebounds forward it has deposited a ring of pigment on the capsule running concentrically with the pupillary margin.

      Intracapsular (rosette cataract): the permanent effects usually follow the sutural arrangement of the lens fibers involving opacification, thus displaying a rosette figure.

   b. Contusion with rupture of the capsule: the entire lens may become opacified and atrophied with a shrunken or shriveled appearance.
   c. Dislocation of the lens: as a result of contusion (either penetrating or nonpenetrating)

5. *Various Etiologies*
   a. Cataract formation induced by metals: Iron induced (Siderosis) cataract begins with subcapsular brown dots over the anterior expanse of the lens, with eventual yellowing and opacification of the entire lens. Copper induced (Chalerosis) cataract presents with a greenish to red brown discoloration following the sutural pattern of the lens giving rise to a "sunflower" cataract.
   b. Cataract formation as the result of various etiologies: cataracts can also be induced by medications (topical and systemic), laser radiation, X-ray, and various toxins.

B. *Classification B*

1. *According to the age of onset*
   a. Congenital
   b. Infantile
   c. Juvenile
   d. Adult
   e. Senile
2. *According to the location of the opacity in the lens*
   a. Nuclear
   b. Cortical
   c. Capsular
   d. Subcapsular

(continued)

Table B. Cataracts (continued)

3. *According to the degree of opacity present*
   a. Immature when transparent lens fibers are present
   b. Mature when the entire lens has become opaque
   c. Hypermature when liquification of the opaque lens fibers occurs
4. *According to the rate of development*
   a. Stationary
   b. Progressive
5. *On the basis of biomicroscopic appearance*
   a. Lamellar
   b. Coralliform
   c. Punctate and others
6. *On the basis of the etiology*
   a. Hereditary
   b. Traumatic
   c. Metabolic
   d. Rare types often occurring with specific syndromes

Reprinted by permission of the publisher from Greenberg, D, and Leslie, W, "Cataract: Current Concepts, Signs, and Symptomology," Journal of the American Optical Association, February 1977.

Table C. Hypertension

Stage	Scheie's Criteria*		Classification of Hypertensive Retinopathy**	
	Sclerotic Changes	*"Hypertense" Changes*	*Ophthalmoscopic Appearance*	*Clinical Classification*
O.	1. only 1 or 2 A-V nicks at the first crossing	1. None; arteriolar venular ratio about 2:3		
I.	1. Scattered slight A-V nicks *or* 2. Definite increase in arteriolar light reflex	1. Probable decrease in arteriolar caliber; A-V ratio about 1:2 (Patient not in congestive failure)	Minimal narrowing or sclerosis of arterioles	"Essential" hypertension (chronic, benign, "arteriosclerotic"
II.	1. Scattered prominent A-V nicks *or* 2. Assymetrical irregularity or angular (not sinuous) tortuosity	1. Definite decrease in vessel caliber, ranging down from less than 1:2 to thread-like arterioles	Thickening and dulling of vessel reflection (copper-wire appearance); localized and generalized narrowing of arterioles; changes at arteriovenous crossings (A-V nicking); scattered round or flame-shaped hemorrhages; vascular occlusion may be present; very small exudates	

(continued)

See also Table 8.6.
**After Keith and Wagener

Table C. Hypertension (continued)

Stage	*Scheie's Criteria**		*Classification of Hypertensive Retinopathy***	
	Sclerotic Changes	*"Hypertense" Changes*	*Ophthalmoscopic Appearance*	*Clinical Classification*
III.	1. A-V nicks profound in 2 or more instances with veins invisible at the crossing, *or* 2. an unequivocal "copper-wire" color of the arterioles	1. any cotton-wool exudates 2. more than one flame-shaped hemorrhage, *or* 3. Round hemorrhages occurring in more than one quadrant of the fundus	Sclerotic changes may not be marked; "angiospastic retinopathy": localized arteriolar spasm, hemorrhages, exudates, "cotton wool patches," retinal edema	Angiospastic hypertension (malignant)
IV.	1. Complete arteriolar occlusion with ghost vessel, *or* 2. Venous occlusion by a crossing arteriole	1. Papilledema, varying from definite blurring of the disk margin to measurable elevation of the nerve head	Same as III, plus papilledema (neuroretinopathy)	

*See also Table 8.6
**After Keith and Wagener

Table D. Corneal Ulcers

A. Bacteria
Streptococcus viridans
Streptococcus pneumoniae (pneumococcus)
Pseudomonas aeruginosa (Bacillus pyocyaneus)
Moraxella liquefaciens (diplobacillus of Petit)
Staphylococcus aureus
Staphylococcus epidermidis
Streptococcus pyogenes
Klebsiella pneumoniae (Friedländer's bacillus)
Nocardia sp
Mycobacterium fortuitum

B. Viruses:
Herpes simplex virus (herpesvirus hominis)
Variola virus
Vaccinia virus
Varicella-zoster virus

C. Fungi:
Candida
Fusarium
Aspergillus
Penicillium
Cephalosporium

D. Hypersensitivity Reactions:
To staphylococci (marginal ulcer)
To unknown allergens or toxins (ring ulcer)
To tuberculoprotein and, rarely, other bacterial proteins (phlyctenular keratoconjunctivitis)

E. Avitaminosis A (Xerophthalmia)

F. Fifth Nerve Lesions (Neurotropic Ulcers)

G. Exposure

H. Unknown Cause: Mooren's ulcer, or "chronic serpiginous ulcer"

Table E. Corneal Edema, Staining, Vascularization, Injection

FDA quantification of slit-lamp observations for edema.

Grade	*Edema description and viewing method*
0	None
1	Microepithelial, intercellular; seen by retroillumination, less than 50 percent of cornea
2	Microepithelial, intercellular; seen by retroillumination, more than 50 percent of cornea
3	Moderate epithelial, intercellular; seen by direct illumination, less than 50 percent of cornea
4	Moderate epithelial, intercellular; seen by direct illumination, more than 50 percent of cornea
5	Circumscribed epithelial, cystic, intracellular; seen with naked eye and flashlight without stromal involvement, less than 50 percent of cornea
6	General epitelial, cystic, intracellular; seen with naked eye and flashlight without stromal involvement, more than 50 percent of cornea
7	Same as 5 with stromal involvement
8	Same as 6 with stromal involvement
Staining	
0	None
1	Minimal, variable, peripheral stippling
2	Superficial punctate staining restricted to a peripheral location and consistent in location from examination to examination
3	Superficial punctuate staining, centrally located
4	Diffuse superficial punctate staining
5	Epithelial dimpling associated with gas bubbles
6	Branching furrows on the epithelial surface
7	Abrasions of the epithelium
8	Foreign body track staining
9	Deep corneal abrasions, ulcerations, scars or other severe complications
Vascularization	
0	None
1	Extension of the limbal vessels more than 1.5 mm inside lower limbal area only
2	Extension of the limbal vessels more than 1.5 mm inside upper limbal area only
3	Extension of the limbal vessels more than 1.5 mm inside limbus over entire periphery
4	Severe extensions of the limbal vessels (to within 2 mm of corneal apex) into the clear epithelial tissue of the cornea
Injection	
0	None
1	Mild congestion and dilation of the limbal vessels
2	Severe congestion and dilation of the limbal vessels
3	Conjunctival hyperemia due to excess lacrimation and epiphora

Table F. Corneal Inflammation (Keratitis)

Type	*Etiology*
Infectious	
Bacteria	
Acute hypopyon (pus in anterior chamber) ulcer	Trauma combined with *Diplococcus pneumoniae; Streptococcus hemolyticus*
Indolent ulcer	*Moraxella liquefaciens*
Pseudomonas aeruginosa ulcer	Trauma and contaminated eyedrops
Virus	
Dendritic keratitis	Herpes simplex *(Herpesvirus hominis)*
Epidemic keratoconjunctivitis	APC (adenopharyngoconjunctival) type 8
Pharyngoconjunctival fever	Exogenous APC types 3, 7, and 18
Trachoma	Psittacosis–lymphogranuloma venereum–*TR*achoma *I*nclusion Conjunctivitis group (Bedsoniae or TRIC group)
Superificial punctate keratitis	Probably virus
Herpes zoster ophthalmicus	Varicella virus involving ophthalmic branch of N V
Keratitis vaccinia and variola	Vaccination or smallpox
Fungi	
Keratomycosis	Injury by plant material; prolonged local antibiotic and corticosteroid therapy
Treponema pallidum	
Interstitial keratitis	Congenital syphilis (rare in acquired type)
Hypersensitivity	
Marginal catarrhal ulcer	Staphylococcic conjunctivitis and blepharitis
Phlyctenular keratoconjunctivitis	Delayed hypersensitivity to tuberculoproteins and other bacterial proteins
Vascular disease	
Ring-type ulcer	Failure of corneal nutrition secondary to disease involving the corneal capillaries: lupus erythematosus, periarteritis nodosa, etc.
Interstitial keratitis with vertigo, tinnitus, and deafness (Cogan's)	Vascular inflammatory disease?
Nutritional deficiency	
Keratomalacia (xerophthalmia)	Vitamin A deficiency
Acne rosacea	Nutritional?
Chronic serpiginous ulcer (Mooren's)	Nutritional? Elderly
Interruption of fifth cranial nerve	
Neurotrophic keratitis	Usually surgical section of trigeminal nerve
Exposure of cornea	
Keratitis e lagophthalmos	Failure of lids to cover eye: (1) proptosis, (2) facial nerve paralysis, (3) severe ectropion, and (4) absence of blinking
Decreased lacrimation	
Keratoconjunctivitis sicca	Conjunctival scarring in erythema multiforme, ocular pemphigoid, and Sjögren's disease

Reprinted from F. Newell and J.T. Ernest, *Ophthalmology*, St. Louis, C.V. Mosby Co., 1974.

8.5. Single Gene Disorders*

Site	*Autosomal Dominant*	*Autosomal Recessive*	*X-Linked*
Globe	Coloboma/microphthalmos Oculodentodigital dysplasia (microphthalmos)	Anophthalmos	
Eyelids	Blepharophimosis + ptosis + epicanthus inversus		
Extraocular Muscles	Familial ophthalmoplegia		Congenital nystagmus External ophthalmoplegia + myopia
Periorbital Tissues	Crouzon's craniofacial dysostosis (exophthalmos + hypertelorism + exotropia) Collins' mandibulofacial dysostosis (antimongoloid slant + lower eyelid coloboma) Waardenburg's syndrome (lateral displacement of medial canthi and lacrimal puncta)		
Cornea	Corneal dystrophies–many forms	Corneal dystrophies–several forms	Fabry's disease (corneal dystrophy) Megalocornea
Angle of AC	Aniridia Juvenile glaucoma Rieger's syndrome (angle dysgenesis)	Congenital glaucoma (buphthalmos)	
Lens	Congenital cataract–many forms Ectopia lentis Marfan's syndrome (ectopia lentis) Alport's syndrome (anterior lenticonus)	Congenital cataract–several forms Homocystinuria (ectopia lentis) Werner's syndrome (adolescent cataracts) Marinesco-Sjögren syndrome (congenital cataracts) Rothmund-Thomson syndrome (juvenile cataracts) Weill-Marchesani syndrome (spherophakia)	Congenital cataract–few forms Lowe's syndrome (congenital cataract)

*Where a named syndrome is given, the major ocular feature(s) follow in parentheses.

(continued)

8.5. Single Gene Disorders* (continued)

Site	*Autosomal Dominant*	*Autosomal Recessive*	*X-Linked*
Retina	Progressive Arthro-ophthalmopathy (myopia + retinal detachment) Wagner's hyaloideo-retinal degeneration Vitelliform macular dystrophy Congenital night blindness Bilateral retinoblastoma Retinitis pigmentosa Spondyloepiphyseal dysplasia (myopia + retinal detachment)	Albinism type I (complete) and type II (incomplete) Leber's congential amaurosis Stargardt's macular dystrophy Gyrate chorioretinal atrophy Favre's hyaloidoretinal tapeto-retinal degeneration Pseudoxanthoma elasticum (angioid streaks) Retinitis pigmentosa Complete achromatopsia	Ocular albinism Choroideremia Incomplete achromatopsia Partial color blindness (protan and deutan) Myopia + night blindness Norrie's disease (pseudoglioma) Retinitis pigmentosa Juvenilte retinoschisis
Optic Nerve	Optic atrophy—congenital and juvenile	Optic atrophy—congenital and infantile	Leber's optic atrophy
CNS and Eye	Neurofibromatosis (optic nerve glioma, exophthalmos, glaucoma) Olivopontocerebellar atrophy with retinal degeneration (macular or peripheral) Tuberous sclerosis (retinal astrocytomas) von Hippel-Lindau syndrome (retinal angiomatosis)	Cerebral lipofuscinosis/juvenile amaurotic idiocy (maculocerebral degeneration) Retinitis pigmentosa Laurence-Moon-Bardet-Biedl syndrome (retinitis pigmentosa) Cockayne's syndrome (retinitis pigmentosa) Refsum's syndrome (retinitis pigmentosa) Usher's syndrome (retinitis pigmentosa) Abetalipoproteinemia (retinitis pigmentosa)	

*Where a named syndrome is given, the major ocular feature(s) follow in parentheses.

Reprinted from G.C. Crozier, Genetic ocular disorders, *Optical Journal*, Philadelphia: Chilton Publications, February, 1979.

8.6. Signs of Soft Contact Lens-Induced Giant Papillary Conjunctivitis

Stage	*Lens Condition*	*Size and Elevation of Papillae*	*Staining of Tops of Giant Papillae with 2% Fluorescein*	*Hypermia and Edema*	*Method of Diagnosis*	*Mucus on Conjunctiva*	*Corneal Condition*
1. Preclinical		No change from baseline			Symptoms only		
2. Early clinical	Mild coating	Elevation of normal papillae and initial formation of giant papillae	Occasional staining of papillae	None or mild erythema	UV light,* 2% fluorescein, and high power on slit lamp	Usually mild, in sheets over papillae	Rare mild punctate staining superiorly
3. Moderate	Moderate to severe coating	Increased number, size, and elevation of papillae	Staining during exacerbation	Variable erythema and edema	Slit lamp and sometimes naked eye	Heavy sheets, strands, and globs	Like State 2, but less rare
4. Severe or terminal	Severe coating	Flattening of apex of elevation and progression of State 3	More papillae staining	Erythema more constant, edema variable	Naked eye	Severely increased	Occasional white arcuate infiltrate in superior cornea

*UV indicates ultraviolet.

Reprinted from M.R. Allansmith, D.R. Korb, J.V. Greiner, A.S. Henriquez, M.A. Simon, and V.M. Finnemore, "Giant papillary conjunctivitis in contact lens wearers, *American Journal of Ophthalmology*, June 1977.

8.7. Retinal Hemorrhages: Location, Description, Common Causes, and Examples

Hemorrhage Type	*Description*	*Common Causes*
Vitreous	May stain entire vitreous or localized regions; bright red to plum colored; obscures all retinal detail	Any condition causing vaso-proliferation • Diabetes • Central retinal vein occlusion • Trauma • Cataract surgery • Eales' disease
Subhyaloid (preretinal)	Bright red; dense; flat superior border, arcuate inferior border; obscures fundus detail	• Diabetes • Vascular occlusions • Systemic hypertension • Arteriosclerosis Trauma Idiopathic
Flame	Thin light red sheets; follow direction of nerve fibers; irregular striate edges; usually overlie retinal vessels	• Systemic hypertension • Vascular occlusions • Diabetes Ansemia Papilloedema Papillitis Sickle cell disease Thrombocytopenia Polycythaemia
Dot and Blot	Dark red; round discrete deposits below retinal vessels; often associated with microaneurysms; size typically 1–2 major vessel widths	• Diabetes • Vascular occlusions Systemic hypertension Eales' disease
Macular	Dark red-brown; discrete but irregular; often associated with drusen and pigment; may be very small to 0.2–0.5 DD	• Disciform degeneration • Senile macular degeneration Arteriosclerosis Myopia
Choroidal	Hazy outline; brown-red with grayish bloom; usually extend over 1–3 DD beneath fundus features	• Neovascularization • Arteriosclerosis Systemic hypertension Choroiditis Trauma Old glaucoma Angloid streaks Myopia

Reprinted from D. Cockburn, Haemorrhages in the posterior segment of the eye: A guide to the diagnosis and optometric management, *Austral J of Opt*, October, 1979.

8.8. Some Causes of Anisocoria

- I. Local ocular causes
  - A. Drugs topically instilled: mydriasis or miosis
  - B. Injury
    1. Rupture of iris sphincter with contusion (traumatic iridoplegia)
    2. Adhesions between iris and cornea following laceration (adherent leukoma or anterior synechiae)
  - C. Inflammation
    1. Keratitis (miosis)
    2. Acute iridocyclitis (middilation)
    3. Adhesions between iris and lens (posterior synechiae)
  - D. Angle-closure glaucoma (middilation)
  - E. Ischemic anterior ocular segment
    1. Retinal separation surgery
    2. Internal carotid artery insufficiency
  - F. Diseases of iris
    1. Essential atrophy
    2. Aniridia
    3. Congenital variation
- II. Paralysis of sphincter pupillae muscle (pupil dilated)
  - A. Cerebral disease
    1. Neoplasm
    2. Aneurysm
    3. Degenerations
    4. Infectious disease: syphilis, herpes zoster ophthalmicus, encephalitis, botulism, diphtheria
    5. Cavernous sinus thrombosis
    6. Subdural and extradural hemorrhage
  - B. Toxic polyneuritis (alcohol, lead, arsenic, carbon dioxide)
  - C. Diabetes mellitus (pupil spared in 75% of cases of diabetic ophthalmoplegia)
- III. Paralysis of dilatator pupillae muscle (pupil constricted)
  - A. Horner's syndrome
- IV. Lesion of intercalated neuron
  - A. Argyll Robertson pupil (tabes dorsalis, pupil constricted)
  - B. Midbrain lesions (pupil dilated)

8.9. Common Ocular Diseases Amenable to Glucocorticoid Therapy

Nonspecific keratitis
Certain chemical burns of the cornea
Superficial punctatate keratitis
Juvenile xanthogranuloma
Marginal (sensitivity) corneal ulcers
Disciform keratitis
Iritis and iridocyclitis
Most forms of posterior uveitis
Optic neuritis (various acute forms and dysthyroid types)
Immune reaction after keratoplasty
Progressive thyroid (malignant) exophthalmos
Neonatal hemangioma of eyelids
Contact dermatitis of the eyelids and conjunctiva
Allergic blepharitis and conjunctivitis
Vernal conjunctivitis
Phlyctenular conjunctivitis and keratitis
Ocular pemphigus
Mucocutaneous conjunctival lesions
Acne rosacea keratitis
Insterstitial keratitis
Sympathetic ophthalmia
Herpes zoster
Episcleritis and scleritis
Pseudotumor of the orbit
Temporal arteritis (giant cell arteritis)
Sclerosing keratitis

Reprinted from Ellis, E.R.: Ocular Therapeutics and Pharmacology, 5th Ed., published by C.V. Mosby Co., St. Louis, Missouri.

8.10. Tearing and Dry Eye

- I. Lacrimation (excessive tear production)
  - A. Psychic stimulation
  - B. Parasympathetic stimulation
    - 1. Cholinergic drugs (Mecholyl)
    - 2. Anticholinesterase drugs
  - C. Lacrimal gland inflammations and neoplasms
  - D. Trigeminal irritation
    - 1. Lesions of the lids, conjunctiva, cornea, iris
    - 2. Glaucoma
  - E. Retinal simulation by glare and excessive light
  - F. Facial nerve
    - 1. Sphenopalatine ganglion stimulation by inflammation and neoplasms
    - 2. Misdirected regeneration following seventh nerve paralysis (crocodile tears)
- II. Epiphora (defective tear drainage)
  - A. Abnormalities of puncta
    - 1. Ectropion, orbicularis oculi muscle weakness, cicatrization, occlusion
  - B. Lacrimal obstruction
    - 1. Canaliculi–inflammation, cicatrix
    - 2. Lacrimal sac and duct
      - a. Congenital abnormalities, inflammation, neoplasms
    - 3. Meatus
      - a. Congenital stenosis, acquired, or local nasal disease
- III. Dry eyes
  - A. Conjunctival cicatrization
    - 1. Erythema multiforme (Stevens-Johnson disease)
    - 2. Trachoma
    - 3. Ocular pemphigoid
    - 4. Thermal, chemical, and radiation burns
  - B. Sjögrens's syndrome
  - C. Lagophthalmos
  - D. Riley-Day syndrome
  - E. Absence of lacrimal gland
  - F. Paralytic
    - 1. Facial nerve (between facial lacrimal nucleus and geniculate ganglion), greater superficial petrosal nerve, sphenopalatine ganglion
    - 2. Trigeminal nerve (decrease in reflex lacrimation)
  - G. Toxic
    - 1. Cholinergic blockade (atropine)
    - 2. Deep anesthesia
    - 3. Debilitating disease

Reprinted from F. Newll and J.T. Ernest, *Ophthalmology*, St. Louis: C.V. Mosby Co., 1974.

8.11. Etiology and Characteristics of Conjunctivitis

Agent	*Clinical Characteristics*
Bacterial	
Diplococcus pneumoniae	Acute catarrhal conjunctivitis with subconjunctival hemorrhages; occurs most frequently during winter months; may cause epidemics; usually does not become chronic
Staphylococcus aureus	Acute catarrhal conjunctivitis often associated with blepharitis and punctate keratitis (with staining most prominent over lower half of cornea); often occurs with chronic blepharoconjunctivitis; an important cause of angular conjunctivitis
Neisseria meningitidis	Causes both purulent conjunctivitis (closely resembling that due to *N. gonorrhoeae*) and catarrhal conjunctivitis
Neisseria gonorrhoeae	Hyperacute, purulent conjunctivitis
Neisseria catarrhalis	Acute catarrhal conjunctivitis
Hemophilus aegyptius (Koch-Weeks bacillus)	Causes acute, purulent conjunctivitis with subconjunctival hemorrhages; also acute catarrhal conjunctivitis; corneal complications occur; epidemic usually in the spring, and endemic in regions with a warm climate; incidence greatest in preschool children
Hemophilus influenzae	Subacute conjunctivitis frequently with a mucopurulent exudate; often occurs in association with upper respiratory infections; may be associated with corneal ulceration; rarely becomes chronic
Streptococcus viridans	May produce membranous, pseudomembranous, or acute catarrhal conjunctivitis
Pseudomonas aeruginosa	Primarily produces corneal ulcers; occasionally causes conjunctivitis in absence of corneal involvement
Corynebacterium diphtheriae	Causes membranous and pseudomembranous conjunctivitis
Moraxella lacunata (Morax-Axenfeld bacillus)	Inflammation affecting the canthi and lid margins; marginal ulcers may occur; zinc as well as antibiotics are effective in treatment
Pasteurella tularensis	Single or multiple necrotic papules usually on lower cul-de-sac, followed by generalized conjunctivtis and ipsilateral preauricular lymph node enlargement
Mycobacterium tuberculosis	Ulcers, nodules and phlyctenular keratoconjunctivitis
Spirochetal	
Treponema palliaum (syphilis)	Primary syphilitic lesions; gumma of conjunctiva can occur in tertiary syphilis
Viral	
Trachoma	Keratoconjunctivitis characterized by follicle formation, papillary hyperplasia, and pannus
Adenovirus	
Types 3 and 7	Pharyngoconjunctival fever
Type 8	Epidemic keratoconjunctivitis
Inclusion conjunctivitis	Acute follicular conjunctivitis in infants (important type of ophthalmia neonatorum) children, and adults caused by a virus that is indistinguishable from that causing trachoma; response to sulfonamides or antibiotics

(continued)

Agent	*Clinical Characteristics*
Herpes simplex	Keratoconjunctivitis; corneal lesion is of paramount importance
Molluscum contagiosum and verrucosum	Follicular or papillary conjunctivitis may occur secondary to lesions on the lid margins; rarely primary lesions may occur on conjunctiva
Variola and vaccinia	Conjunctivitis may occur in association with cutaneous eruption on eyelids, hypopyon ulcers of cornea, uveitis, and vitreous opacities
Others: infectious mononucleosis, lymphogranuloma venereum, cat-scratch fever, rubeola, rubella, and Newcastle disease	Discussed in section on ocular manifestations in systemic viral infections
Fungal (rare cause of conjunctivitis)	
Candida albicans	
Actinomyces israelii (Streptothrix)	
Sporotrichum schenckii	
Leptotrichiae (questionable cause of conjunctivitis)	

8 12. Differential Diagnosis: Diseases of the Lids and Lacrimal Apparatus

Table A. Lids and Lacrimal Apparatus

	Hordeolum Externum	*Hordeolum Internum*	*Chalazion*	*Prelacrimal Abscess*	*Acute Dacryocystitis*	*Ethmoiditis*
Pain	Present	Intense	Discomfort	Present	Acute pain	Pain may or may not be present
Edema	Of eyelid with pointing externally	Marked pointing on conjunctival surface	Localized swelling and cyst formation	Near medial canthus	Of lower eyelid near medial canthus	Present; eye may be displaced temporally
Redness	Of eyelid	Of eyelid	Localized grayish area in conjunctiva	Of skin	Localized to sac and surrounding area	Of eyelid and conjunctiva
Tenderness	Marked and localized	Marked and localized	Absent or slight	Marked and localized	Localized to area of redness	Localized to upper inner part of orbit
Location of lesion	In Zeis's gland	In a meibomian gland	In a meibomian gland	In subcataneous tissue	In lacrimal sac	In sinus
Course and result	Acute–may rupture or subside	Yellow spot seen in tarsus through tarsal conjunctiva; may rupture through conjunctival surface or empty through natural orifice, seldom through skin	Chronic or subacute –may rupture through conjunctivia	Acute–may rupture through skin or subside	May rupture through skin	May result in mucocele of orbit
Secretion	After pointing, thick pus may exude from sty	On conjunctival surface after rupture or at orifice on edge of eyelid when expressed	After rupturing, liquefied contents may exude	None until breaks through the skin	From puncta or may break through skin	From nose and postnasally

Reprinted from Joshua Zuckerman, *Diagnostic examination of the eye.* Philadelphia: J.B. Lippincott Company, 1964.

Table B. Bumps, Lumps

1. **Sudoriferous Cysts**
Frequently at the margins of the eyelids (greater towards the inner canthi) are found small, rounded, elevated masses caused by a blockage of the excretory ducts of the glands of Moll. They may range in size from as small as 1 to 2 mm in diameter, to greater than 2 centimeters widths. They are covered by a thin membrane of epithelial cells and contain a fluid or casseous material. They are frequently multiple in presentation and are almost always benign and painless.

2. **Chalazion**
Meibomian glands, and glands of Zeis frequently produce a granulomatous mass secondary to mechanical and/or infectious stimulation. The process may either be of an acute onset or an insidious development. When acute, the patient may present with or report a history of pain and inflammation of the eyelid followed by a resultant nontender mass. The chronic form develops gradually with no history of pain or acute inflammation. The resultant chronic granuloma can range in size, shape, and location within the lid structure, or evulse through to the palpebral conjunctiva or surface skin. Secondary infection and inflammation occasionally aggravate the chalazion, particularly when chronic marginal blepharitis is present and/or was the precipitating cause of the chalazion itself.

3. **Verrucae**
Viral origin is the cause of these small (usually one half centimeter wide, but sometimes larger) warts occuring at or near the lid margins. They may have a reduplicated or cauliflower-like (verruca vulgaris) appearance or may be smooth and flat (verruca plana) with both types varying in their degree of pigmentation. In most cases these growths are benign and the patient is asymptomatic with the patient presenting exclusively due to the cosmetic appearance. However, on occasion, those extremely proximal to the lid margins can produce a chronic keratoconjunctivitis (with superficial punctate keratitis) which proves unrelenting and requires indefinite heavy lubrication of the eye or surgical removal of the insulting wart.

4. **Papilloma**
These common, benign epithelial tumors occur most frequently on or near the lid margins. They vary considerably in size, shape, and pigmentation, and a very large percentage of them become keratinized with aging (cutaneous horns) into long fingerlike projections.

5. **Sebaceous Cysts**
These cysts can be present in any area of the body, particularly when hair follicles are abundant (axillary regions), and are found in the eyelid region with their greatest propensity towards the eyebrows. They tend to be painless, round, firm, rubbery masses, usually covered by dermis (textured skin) and varying dramatically in size. The cysts themselves are always benign but when presenting in multiples may have a staphylococcal nature to them and hence, would warrant a medical evaluation for systemic antibiosis.

6. **Hordeolum**
This bump is a relatively tender and painful mass, which is almost invaribly a staphylococcal infection of a Meibomian gland (internal hordeolum) or a gland of Zeis or Moll (external hordeolum or style). The abscessed gland usually produces dramatic redness and swelling (edema) of the lid itself. When the lid is heavily edematous, the bump of the hordeolum itself may be buried and inobservable. Careful palpation of the entire lid for a focal area of tenderness is required for definitive diagnosis.

7. **Xanthelasma**
These bilateral symmetrical yellowish placques consist of lipoid material and may present either insidiously, over many years, or relatively rapidly reaching a subsequent static state. They present most frequently in the medial aspect of the upper lids and are relatively flat with a slightly granulated surface. In that as many as 50

(continued)

Table B. **(continued)**

7. **Xanthelasma (continued)**
percent of the individuals with Xanthelasma may show hyperlipemia, referral for medical evaluation and blood work is indicated. However, many cases are idiopathic or familial in nature. These well demarcated lesions are totally benign in themselves.

8. **Dermoid**
These benign congenital, collagenous tumors are found most frequently on the conjunctiva and cornea (particularly at the limbus), but may also present as subdermal lid and brow lumps or bumps. They are found in numerous parts of the body and are believed to be misplaced tissue masses secondary to associated defects or colobomas of the surrounding structures. They are invariably smooth, firm, immovable, rounded masses that overlying skin slides easily over. They tend to remain basically the same size and historically are present for as long as the patient can recall.

9. **Molluscum Contagiosum**
This is a small umbilicated nodule of definite viral origin found at or near the lid margin. It tends to have a contagious nature particularly when the central area of the mass produces a yellow, cheesy material upon expression. These small tumors can occur on other parts of the body and when in close proximity to the lid margin occasionally produce a superficial punctate keratitis. When the lesion is dry and quiet, no particular treatment is necessarily indicated and occasionally spontaneous regression may be observed.

10. **Hemangioma**
While there are numerous forms of hemangiomas, the most common seen are the congenital capillary type. They are slightly elevated and range in size from small circumscribed areas to covering the full lid and even one half the face (as in the Sturge-Weber syndrome). The smaller hemangiomas may either increase or decrease in size during infancy with the possibility of spontaneous regression (not predictable) by adolescence. Frequently, crying, straining, etc., may cause a dramatic change in coloration and size of these vascular lesions. The general coloration varies from a faint blue or red to the classic "portwine stain" color. The elevation of the lesion will vary according to its type (capillary versus cavernous or mixed), depth within the tissue, shape, etc. If relatively superficial, the lesions may blanch to pressure, thus differentiating them from a raised pigmented nevus. Treatment of any kind should be discouraged in favor of careful management and observation. While sequalae to hemangioma may be found in the choroid of the eye, the optometrist should also consider the potential for systemic implications and refer appropriately for pediatric or medical evaluation.
Beyond these ten most common lumps and bumps of the eyelids, differential diagnosis must begin to include the more dramatic possibilities of:
    a. Basal cell carcinoma
    b. Squamous cell carcinoma
    c. Granulomatous diseases
    d. Adenocarcinomas of the Meibomian glands
    e. Lymphosarcoma
    f. Metastatic carcinoma

Reprinted from L.J. Catania, Lumps and Bumps of the Eyelids, *Southern Journal of Opt,* May, 1979.

Table C. Etiology of Punctal and/or Canalicular Occlusion

I. Infections
   A. Chlamydial: Trachoma
   B. Fungal: Aspergillus
   C. Bacterial: Actinomyces, Diptheria, Streptococci
   D. Viral: Herpes zoster, Herpes simplex
II. Injuries
   A. Trauma: Lacerations
   B. Chemical Burns: Alkali
   C. Irradiation
III. Cicatrizing Diseases
   A. Ocular Pemphigoid (BMMP)
   B. Stevens-Johnson Syndrome
   C. Ligneous
IV. Tumors of the Conjunctiva
V. Iatrogenic
   A. Cautery
   B. Chemicals: Conc. $AgNO_3$
   C. Drugs: IDU, phospholine iodide, epinephrine, prolonged use of eye drops
VI. Idiopathic, Congenital

8.13. Differential Diagnosis: Papilledema, Papillitis, Pseudoneuritis

	Papilledema	*Papillitis*	*Pseudoneuritis*
Media	Clear	Vitreous opacities common	Clear
Color of disk	Red and cloudy	Red and cloudy	Red but not cloudy
Swelling of disk	Marked and progressive	Usually slight and temporary	Usually slightly elevated
Margins of opic disk	Fairly well-defined	Indistinct in relation to amount of swelling	Somewhat indistinct
Vessels and hemorrhages	Marked disproportion between veins and arteries. Veins enlarged and tortuous. Arteries small. Hemorrhages may be present.	Arteries unchanged. Veins broad and tortuous. Hemorrhages usually present	Veins broad and tortuous. No hemorrhages
Peripapillary edema	Present	Present	Absent
Vision	Often unaffected. Gradual loss of vision usually observed after edema is present for some time. Transistory attacks of blurred vision are common	Rapid loss of vision; more marked than ophthalmoscopic appearance might suggest	Usually normal with correction
Refraction	Not characteristic	Not characteristic	Usually high hyperopia and astigmatism
Visual fields	Concentric contraction but slight in relation to amount of swelling. Enlargement of the blindspot. Colors only slightly affected. Central scotomas rare.	Central scotoma. Peripheral fields may or may not be affected. Peripheral contraction. Enlargement of the blindspot marked in relation to degree of swelling. Color field affected more than in papilledema	Blindspot may be smaller than the normal avergage

Reprinted from Joshua Zuckerman, *Diagnostic examination of the eye,* Philadelphia: J.B. Lippincott Company, 1964.

Table 8.14. Differential Diagnosis: Iris Nodules

	Unpigmented				*Pigmented*	
	Tuberculous Nodule	*Syphilitic Nodule*	*Unpigmented Sarcoma*	*Granulation Tumor Surrounding Foreign Body*	*Pigmented Sarcoma*	*Melanoma*
Age	Usually under 20 years	Older than 20	Older than 20	Any age	Older	Any age
Site	Not characteristic	At pupillary or cilary margin of iris	Not characteristic	Not characteristic	Not characteristic	Not characteristic
Color	Gray	Papule: yellowish-red	Unpigmented	Reddish	Brown or black	Brown or black
Rate or growth	Appears and disappears	Disappears under anti-syphilitic treatment	Usually slow	Slow	Variable	Stationary or slow growth
Vascularity	Avascular	Not very vascular	Variable, usually vascular	Very vascular	Variable, usually vascular	Avascular in early cases
Associated with	Adjacent, small gray nodules; iritis early	Iritis in early stage	Iritis at later stage	Other foreign bodies suggest injury; corneal scars	Iritis in later stages	
General examination	Tuberculin test; roentgen rays of chest	Wassermann test	Exclusion of tuberculosis, Boeck's sarcoid and syphilis	(History of foreign body in iris) Roentgen ray	(History of nodule) Melanomas in other parts of body. Melanin may be found in urine.	

Reprinted from Joshua Zuckerman, *Diagnostic examination of the eye*. Philadelphia: J.B. Lippincott Company, 1964.

8.15. Differential Diagnosis: Conjunctivitis

Table A. Causes

		Bacterial				
	Viral	*Purulent*	*Nonpurlent*	*Fungal and Parasitic*	*Allergic*	*Chlamydial*
Discharge	Minimal	Profuse	Minimal	Minimal	Minimal	Profuse
Tearing	Profuse	Moderate	Moderate	Minimal	Moderate	Moderate
Itching	Minimal	Minimal	None	None	Marked	Minimal
Injection	Generalized	Generalized	Localized	Localized	Generalized	Generalized
Localized conjunctival lesions	None	None	Frequent	Frequent	None	None
Preauricular node	Common	Uncommon	Common	Common	None	Common in inclusion conjunctivitis only
Stained smear	Monocytes	Bacteria, PMNs*	Bacteria, PMNs*	Usually negative	Eosinophils	PMNs, plasma cells, inclusion bodies
Associated sore throat and fever	Occasionally	Seldom	None	None	None	None

*Polymorphonuclear cells

Table B. Types of Chronic Allergic Conjunctivitis

	Chronic Atopic Conjunctivitis	*Microbiallergic Conjunctivitis Due to the* Staphylococcus
History	Familial allergy frequent	Familial allergy infrequent
	Other associated allergies	No associated allergies
Allergens	Pollens, danders, inhalants, foods	Bacterial products, mainly *Staphylococcus* toxin
Allergic response	Immediate	Delayed
Symptoms	Burning, irritation, and often severe itching	Burning, irritation, and often marked dryness
Discharge	May be mucopurulent	Watery, no pus
Lid margins	Usually uninvolved	May be swollen; possible blepharitis
Conjunctiva	May appear same in both types	May appear same in both types
	Often little objectively noted	Papillary, but scattered follicles may appear
	Sometimes edematous	Dry, no chemosis
Cornea	Generally not involved	May have superficial punctate keratitis involving inferior portion of cornea
Epithelial scrapings	Eosinophils almost always found sooner or later	No eosinophils
Cultures	Normal flora	Toxin-producing staphylococci found, or normal flora
Intracutaneous *Staphylococcus* toxin or toxoid	Moderate delayed response	Marked delayed response, at least 3 × 3 cm, usually more; may have marked immediate response also; may get systemic reactions (arthritis)

8.16. Differential Diagnosis: Spontaneous Nystagmus

Type of Nystagmus	*Etiology*
I. Fixation Nystagmus	
1. Congenital–primary position a. pendular b. none c. uniocular jerk both jerk on lateral gaze	Insufficiently developed fixation mechanism
2. Aquired pendular jerks in lateral gaze, pendular near the midline	Disseminated sclerosis
3. Latent on occlusion of one eye, nystagmus of both (towards the open eye)	Unknown
4. Miner's pendular or irregular often in upper gaze only	Failing fixation mechanism due to insufficient use
II. Vestibular Nystagmus	
1. Peripheral horizontal rotary jerks toward one side gradually decreases	Lesion of inner ear
2. Central a. horizontal rotary jerks b. pure vertical or pure rotary jerks (neither a or b decrease with time)	Lesion of vestibular nucleus
3. Periodically alternating jerky with reversal of direction in regular periods (Vestibulars are always horizontal, rotary and jerky)	Unknown
III. Gaze Nystagmus*	
1. Muscle paretic jerks in gaze toward the paretic side, stronger in the now paretic eye	Muscle palsy
2. End position (with latent period) jerks in extreme lateral gaze to R & L after a latency period	Inability to maintain maximum innervation
3. End position (abrupt) jerks in extreme lateral gaze to R & L with no latency period	Nervousness
4. Symmetric gaze jerks start equidistant from midline and are equal in intensity (less on upward gaze)	Disseminate sclerosis
5. Asymmetric gaze jerks start nearer to midline on one side and are stronger on this side	Lesion of gaze center
6. Vertical gaze vertical jerks	Lesion on collicular region
IV. Convergence Nystagmus	
1. Retraction Clonic retractions of the eye especially on convergence or upward movements	Lesion in Sylvan aqueduct
2. Voluntary and hysterical enormously frequent jerks in convergence and divergence	Not pathological

***(In gaze nystagmus, the jerks start before the motion is completed and have no rotary component)**
Reprinted from Kestenbaum, *Clinical methods of neuro-ophthalmological examination*, New York: Grune & Stratton, 1954.

8.17. Differential Diagnosis: Torticollis

	Congenital	*Ocular*
Age	Onset at birth or shortly thereafter	Onset rarely before 18 months
Head position	Passive or voluntary straightening of head is difficult or impossible	Head can easily be straightened passively or voluntarily or tipped to opposite side
Neck muscles	Palpation reveals hardening of sternocleidomastoid muscle	Palpation negative
Vision	No visual disturbances	Frequently diplopia on straightening of head or tilting it to opposite side
Effect of occlusion	Torticollis not influenced by occlusion of either eye	Head straightens on occluding the paretic eye except when secondary skeletal changes have occurred

Reprinted by permission from vonNoorden, Gunter K: ***Burian-von Noorden's Binocular Vision and Ocular Motility*****, 2nd ed., St. Louis: The C.V. Mosby Co., 1980.**

8.18. Differential Diagnosis: Deniform Keratis

Disease	*Epithelium*	*Location*	*Stroma*	*Tear Film*	*Staining*	*Debridement*	*Cutaneous Manifestations*	*Corneal Sensitivity*
Herpes Simplex	Fine, lacy dendrites (possibly with terminal end bulbs	Central	Variable involvement	Usually normal	Edges stain with rose bengal; denuded ulcer stains with fluorescein	Removed only with epithelium	Current or past history of fever blisters	Anesthesia
Herpes Zoster Acute	Smaller lesions, often stellate; raised contour	Usually peripheral	None	Mucoid discharge	Stains only sparingly with with both rose bengal and fluorescein	Removed only with epithelium	Typical zoster rash and lid vesicles	Anesthesia only rarely
Delayed	Coarse, elevated gray-white plaques	Movable	Diffuse haze	Unstable with rapid break-up time	Rose bengal stains whole lesion; moderately with alcian blue and and sparingly with fluorescein	Removed with minimal damage to underlying epithelium	Typical zoster scarring on same side	Anesthesia
Keratitis sicca	Blotchy, amorphous lesion (possibly with filaments); could assume dendridritic "drying" pattern	Lower one-third to one-half	Minimum haze	Mucoid discharge, rapid break-up time, thin tear film	Triangular inter palpebral staining with rose bengal; fine superficial punctate staining with fluorescein; plaques vividly stain with rose bengal, faintly with florescein	Removed only with epithelium; plaques easily removed	Dryness of mouth or other nonocular mucous membranes; joint pain and swelling	Normal
Epithelial Healing Dendriform	Flat, fine dendrite; superficial	Paracentral inferior to visual axis	Haze, infiltrate	Normal	No staining with rose bengal or alcian blue; only moderate to minimal fluorescein staining	Removal only with epithelium	None; history of resolving large corneal abrasion	None

Reprinted from J.E. Terry, Dendriform keratitis, ***J. of the American Optometric Assn.*****, April 1979.**

8.19. Differential Diagnosis: Abnormal Pupillary Reflexes

Type	*At Rest*	*Reaction to Light*	*Reaction to Convergence*	*Etiology*
Marcus-Gunn	Often unequal	Affected pupil dilates when normal eye is closed. When light is directed into the normal eye there is constriction OU; when then directed into the affected eye, there is dilation OU.	Normal	Retrobulbar neuritis, vascular accident, tumor.
Wernicke	Usually equal	Poor reaction to light directed from the hemianopic fields	Normal	Tumor, infection, vascular accident
Argyl-Robertson	Miotic, unequal	No reaction to direct light, no consensual, poor dilation in dark	Normal	Syphillitic (90% of cases)
Tonic (Adie's)	Involved pupil usually larger	None or slow initial reaction to direct or indirect; overreacts to prolonged light and overdilates after a while in dark	Overreacts at prolonged near fixation (30 sec)	Benign disease, viral (?)
Fixed	Involved pupil is larger	None	None	Demyelinating tumors, trauma, vascular accident
Horner's	Ptosis and miosis	Slight consensual, slight direct, no dilation in dark (also anhidrosis)	Slight	Arterial occlusion, metastatic and mediastinal tumors, Hodgkins' disease
Claude Bernard's	Lid retraction and mydriasis usually unilateral	Slight direct, slight consensual	Slight	Apical lung lesions, hemorrhages
Amaurotic	Involved pupil is larger if no other lesion is present	None	Normal	Lesion in retina or in the optic nerve before the chiasm
Aberrent regeneration of the III nerve	Dilated, fixed	Constricts only on conjugate gaze		Nerve fibers growing into the pupillary pathway
Anisocoria	Normal (1 mm or less diff. occur 30% of time)	Normal	Normal	If not physiological, may be serious. Aneurism, neoplasm, inflammation, infectious

8.20. Differential Diagnosis: Extraocular Muscles: Paresis and Spasms

Table A. Cyclovertical

Hyper eye in primary position	*Hyper greater on lateral gaze to:*	*Hyper more noticeable on head-tilt toward*	*Affected extraocular muscle*
R	R	R	L10
R	R	L	R1R
R	L	R	R50
R	L	L	L5R
L	R	R	R5R
L	R	L	L50
L	L	R	L1R
L	L	L	R10

Table B. Three Step Method

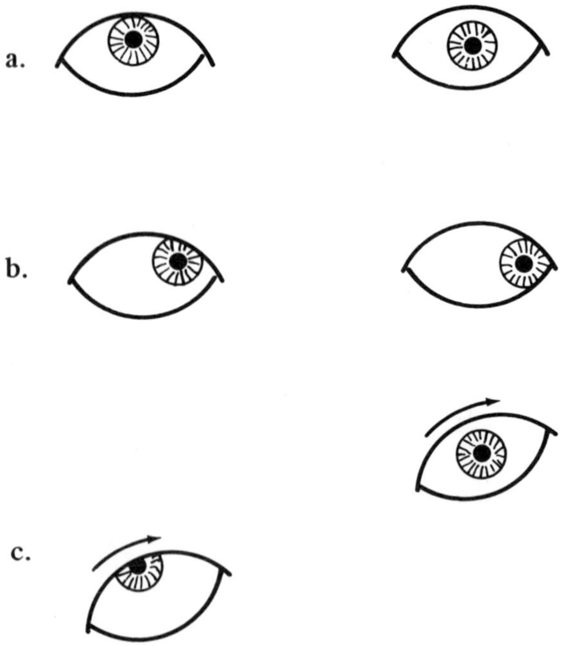

The Three-Step Method for diagnosing an isolated paretic cyclovertical muscle. The right superior oblique is affected in this example. (a) Right hypertropia in the primary position; (b) Hyperdeviation increases on levoversion; (c) Further increase of right hyper on right head tilt. Arrows indicate the direction of compensatory torsional movements. The examiner must make this measurement by tilting his or her head the same amount as the patient's.

Adapted from John Griffin, *Binocular anomalies, procedures for vision therapy*, Chicago: Professional Press, 1976.

Table C. Direction of Deviation and Limitation of Movement

	Paresis			*Spasm*
	Deviation			
	Primary *(sound eye fixing; palsied eye moves:–)*	Secondary *(paretic eye fixing, sound eye moves:–)*	*Limitation of movement of paretic eye and direction of greatest diplopia*	*Direction of increased movement of spastic eye and of increased diplopia*
Lat. Rectus	inwards	inwards	outwards	outwards
Med. Rectus	outwards	outwards	inwards	inwards
Sup. Rectus	down	up	up and out to paretic side	up and out to spastic side
Inf. Rectus	up	down	down and out to paretic side	down and out to spastic side
Sup. Oblique	up	down	down and in to sound side	down and in to sound side
Inf. Oblique	down	up	up and in to sound side	up and in to sound side

Reprinted from Sir Stewart Duke-Elder and Kenneth Wybar, *Ocular motility and strabismus, Vol. VI of System of ophthalmology.* St. Louis: C.V. Mosby Co., 1973.

8.21. Differential Diagnosis: Inflammatory Diseases of the External Eye

Disease	*Incidence*	*Pain*	*Discharge*	*Injection*	*Intraouclar Pressure*	*Lacrimation*	*Photophobia*
Acute conjunctivitis	Extremely common	Little	Moderate–copious	Palpebral and fornical conjunctiva inflamed	Normal		Some
Acute glaucoma	Uncommon	Severe	None; may tear	Entire eye inflamed; deep reddish appearance, conjunctiva and ciliary injection	Elevated	Mild	Moderate
Acute iritis	Common	Moderate	None; much tearing	Ciliary injection	May be lower than normal	Tearing	Severe
Blepharitis a. external hordeolum		None Some pain	None, but matting of lashes	None except at lid margin		None	None
b. charlazion		Some pain	b. discharge when breaks	b. localized over affected gland			
Acute dacryocystitis		Severe	None; may tear	Inflammation of nasal half of lid, none of eyeball		Tearing	None
Episcleritis		Little	None	Two types: localized nodule and Episcleritis Fugax (fine haze, entire globe)		Mild	Moderate
Scleritis		Moderate	None	Deep yellowish-brown inflammation, very tender eyeball		Tearing	Moderate
Keratitis or corneal trauma	common	Moderate	Watery or purulent	May be circumcorneal injection	Normal	Much tearing	Severe

(continued)

8.21. Differential Diagnosis in Inflammatory Diseases of External Eye (continued)

Disease	*Corneal Lustre*	*Visual Acuity*	*Lid Swelling*	*Tenderness of Eye*	*Chemosis, Swelling of Conjunctivia*	*Pupil Size*	*Pupillary Light Response*
Acute conjunctivitis	Normal	Normal	None*	None	Not much;* movable	Normal	Normal
Acute glaucoma	Dull, "steamy"	Blurred (rainbow)	Swollen	None	Swelling; immovable	Moderately dilated and fixed	None
Acute iritis	Normal	Diminished slightly	Usually no	Tender	Moderate; immovable	Small	Poor
Blepharitis	Normal	Normal	None; margin reddened	None	None		
a. hordeolum			localized				
b. chalazion			localized				
Acute dacryocystitis	Normal	Normal	Inner 2/3 lower, 1/3 upper swollen	None	None		
Episcleritis	Normal	Normal	None	Some	May be some around nodule	Normal	
Scleritis	Normal	Normal	May be some	Severe	Marked chemosis	Normal (small if secondary iritis)	
Keratitis or corneal trauma	Loss of lustre	Diminished unless localized in periphery	Moderate	None	May be in severe cases; immovable	Normal (small if secondary iritis)	Normal

*except in purulent conjunctivitis

8.22. Differential Diagnosis: Visual Field Defects

Table A. Generalized Diagrams

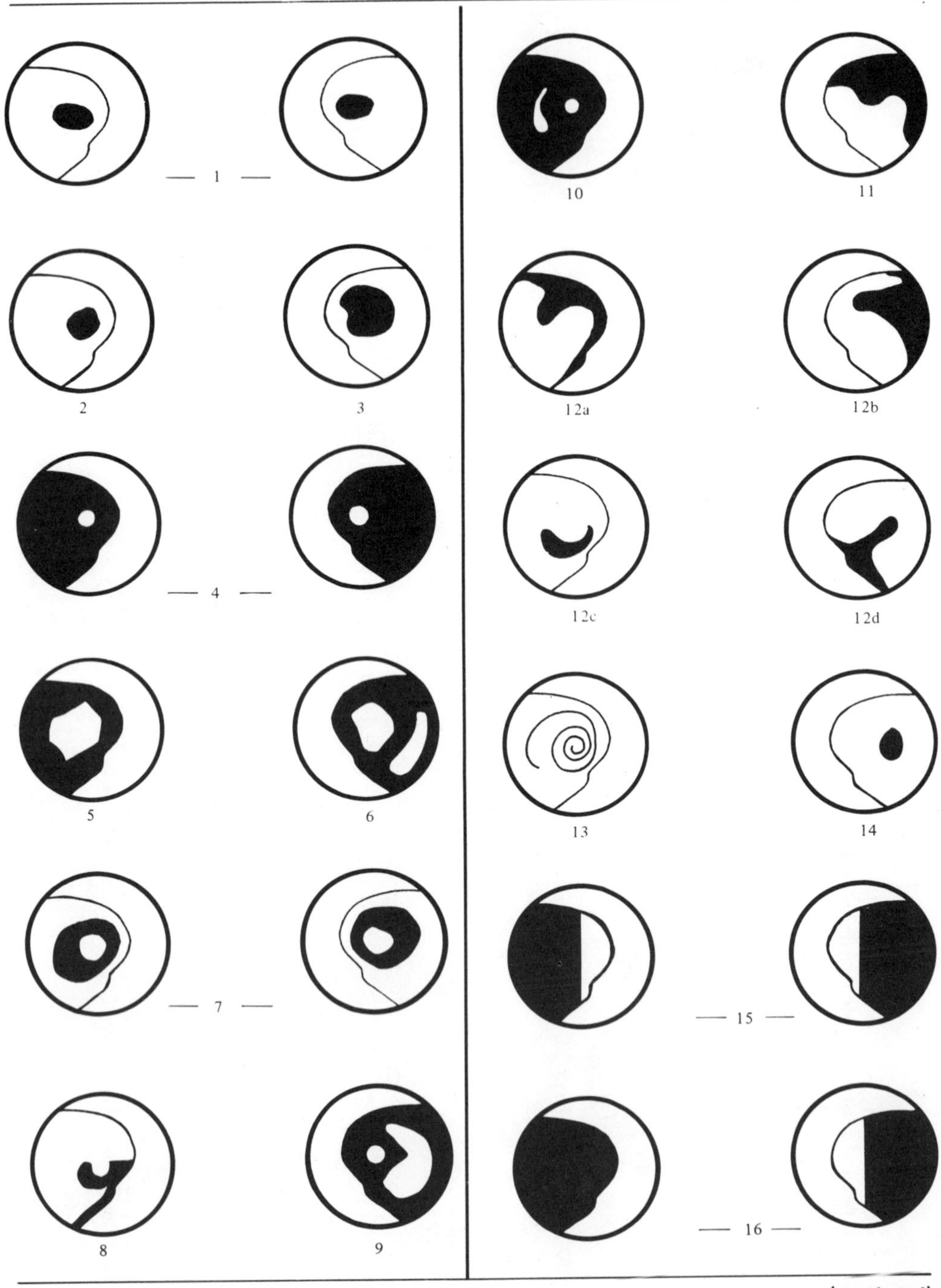

(continued)

Table A. Generalized Diagrams (continued)

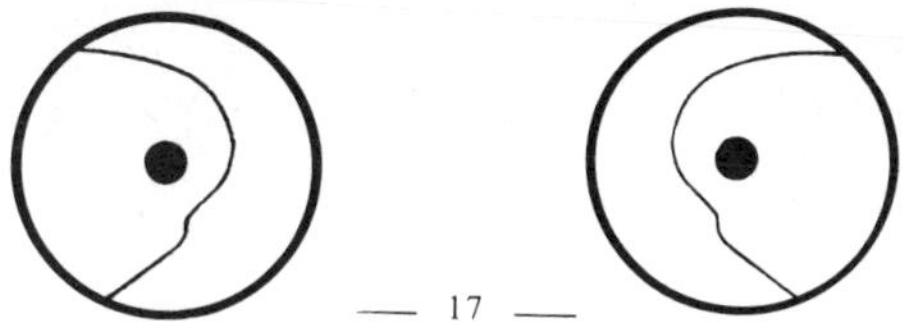

17

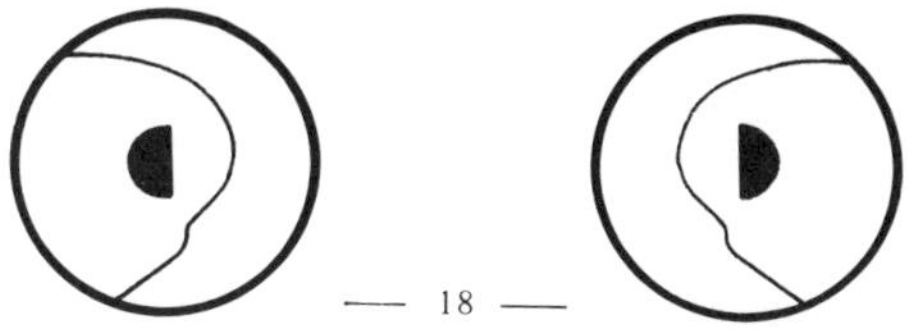

18

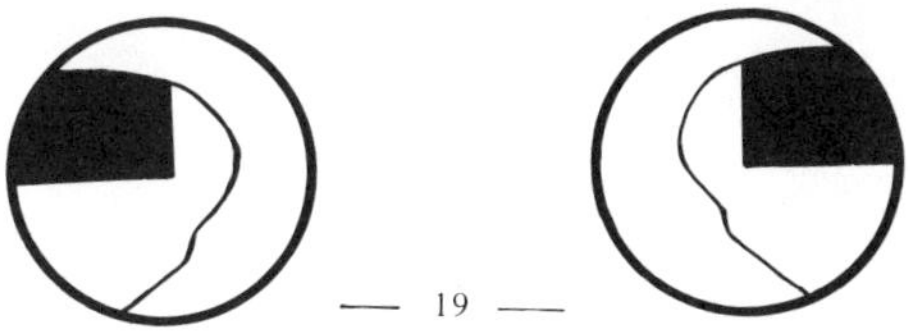

19

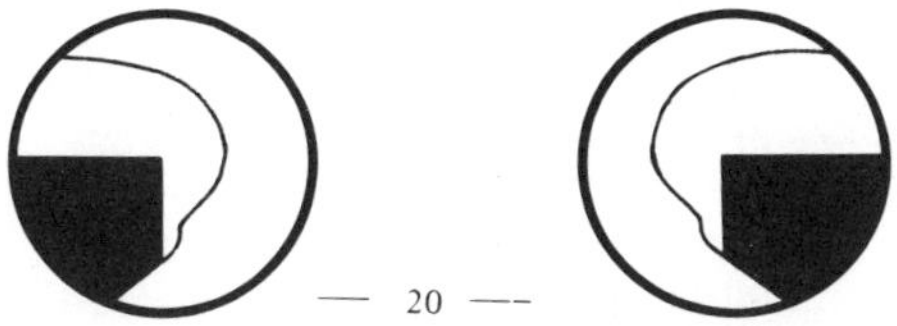

20

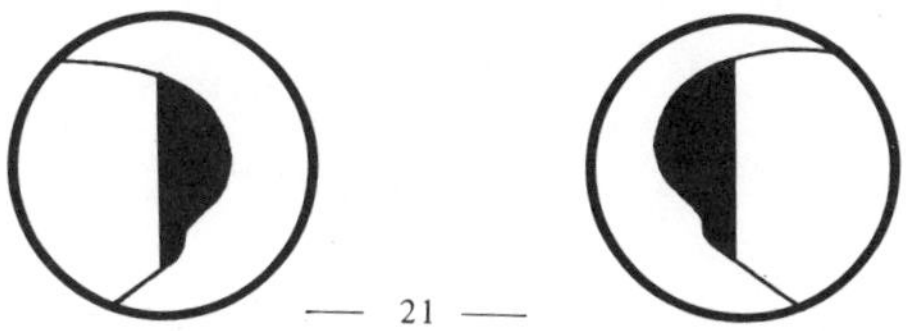

21

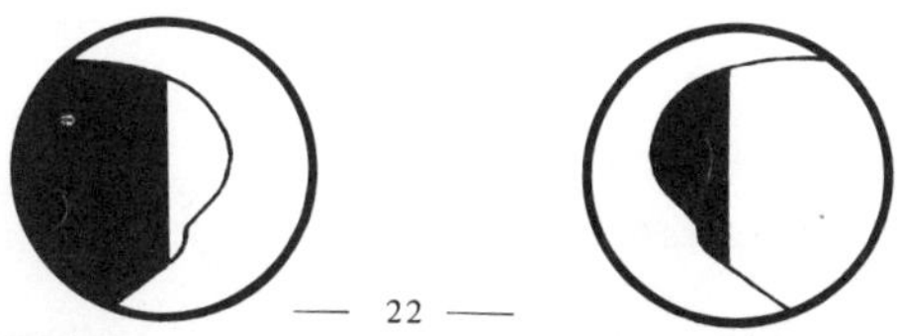

22

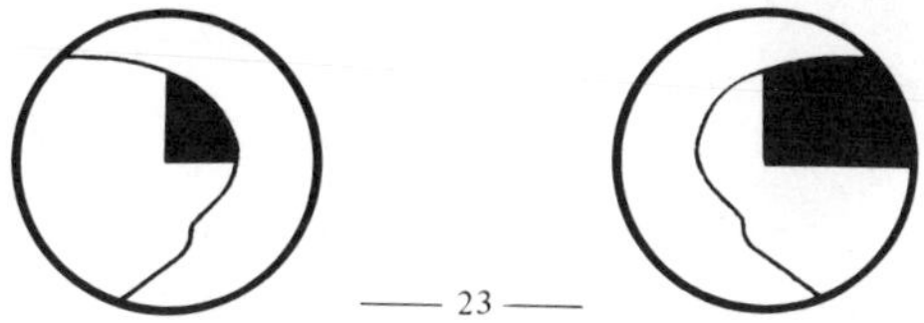

23

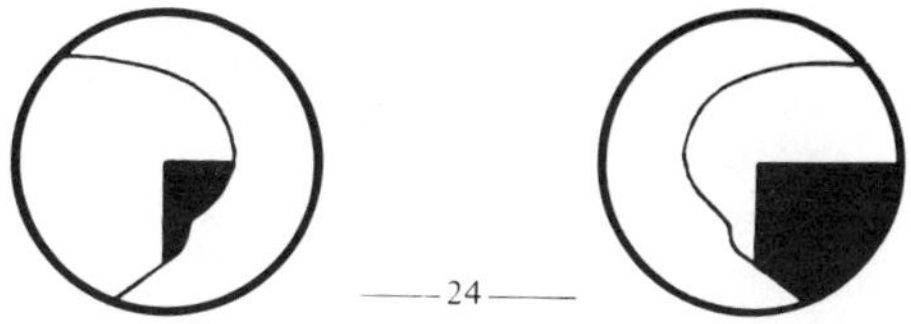

24

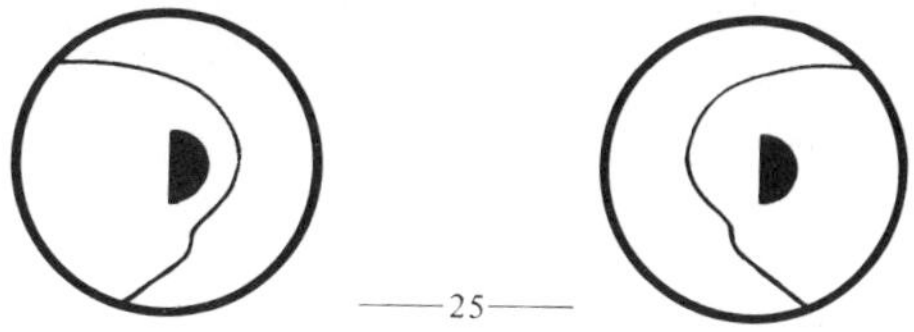

25

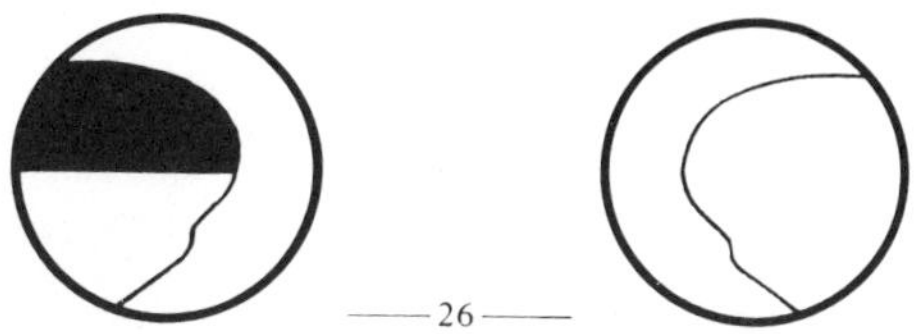

26

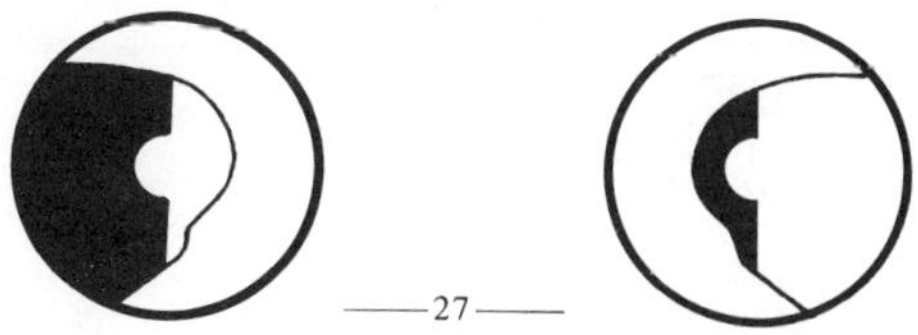

27

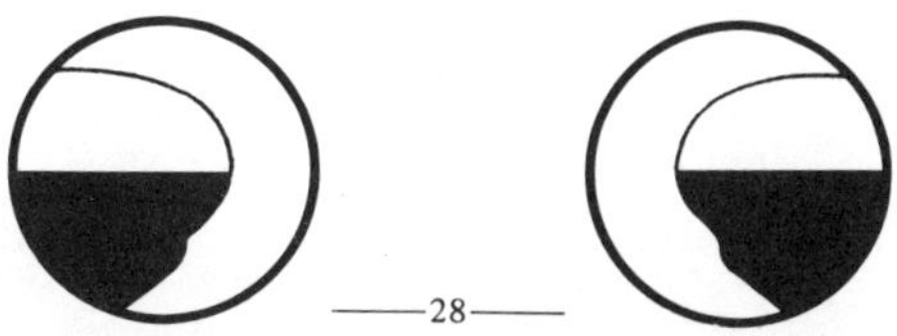

28

(continued)

Table A. Generalized Diagrams (continued)

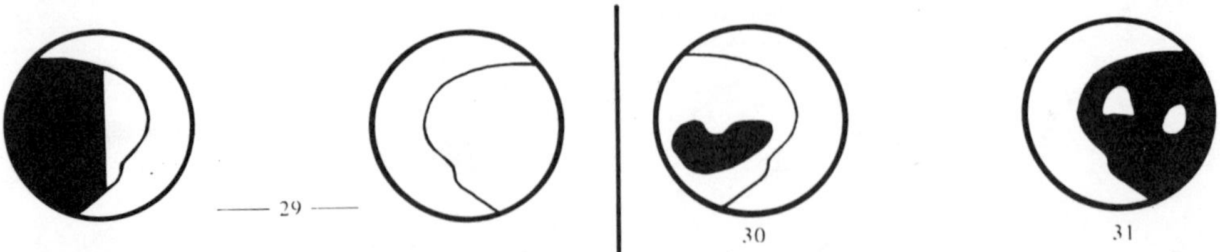

1. Bilateral central scotomas
2. Central scotoma in retrobulbar neuritis
3. Large central scotoma in retrobulbar neuritis
4. Concentric constriction of the visual field in tapetoretinal degeneration
5. Concentric visual field loss in long standing papilledema leading to optic atrophy
6. Refraction, ring scotoma, caused by strong convex lenses
7. Ring scotoma in tapetoretinal degeneration
8. Glaucoma, Bjerrum scotoma, nasal step
9. Glaucoma, nasal step and Bjerrum scotoma, both inferiorly and superiorly
10. Glaucoma, central and peripheral islands of vision
11. Inferior retinal detachment
12. Crescent-shaped visual field loss in juxtapapillary chorioretinitis
    a. lesion inferior temporal to the disk
    b. lesion inferior nasal and peripheral to the disk
    c. lesion superior temporal to the disk
    d. lesion superior temporal to the disk
13. Enlarged blind spot in papilledema
14. Spiraling on a functional basis
15. Heteronymous-bitemporal hemianopia due to a pituitary tumor
16. Chiasmatic lesion with destruction of crossed and uncrossed fibers from the left eye: amauroses left and temporal hemianopia right
17. Lesion pressing on the anterior angle of the chiasm = anterior = bitemporal central scotoma
18. Lesion pressing on the posterior angle of the chiasm = posterior = bitemporal, paracentral scotoma
19. Pressure on the chiasm from above = superior = bitemporal inferior quadrantanopsia
20. Pressure on the chiasm from below resulting in bitemporal upper quadrantanopsia
21. Bilateral external pressure on the chiasm resulting in binasal hemianopia*
22. Left homonymous hemianopsia
23. Damage to the temporal loop (Meyer's) of the optic radiations = contralateral homonymous superior quadrantanopsia
24. Damage to the inner portion of the optic radiations = contralateral homonymous inferior quadrantanopsia
25. Damage to the macular portion of the occipital cortex of one hemisphere = contralateral macular homonymous hemianopia
26. Left homonymous hemianopsia with macular sparing
27. Altitudinal hemianopia with superior field loss due to occlusion of the inferior branch of the central retinal artery
28. Inferior altitudinal homonymous hemianopia following repeated blood loss
29. Temporal field loss, left eye only, from damage to crossing fibers from the nasal retina in the region of the chiasm
30. Caeco-central scotoma
31. Bitemporal hemianopia – late states – pituitary tumor

***A field, with perfect binasal hemianopia bisecting fixation bilaterally is anatomically almost impossible and speaks strongly in favor of a hysterical etiology.**

***Binasal field loss* is generally due to retinal disease when the defects are incongruous and do not bisect the fixation point.**

Adapted with permission from Pau, Hans. *Differential Diagnosis of Eye Diseases.* (Stuttgart: Georg Thieme Verlag, 1978).

Table B. The Typical Field Defects Caused by Lesions

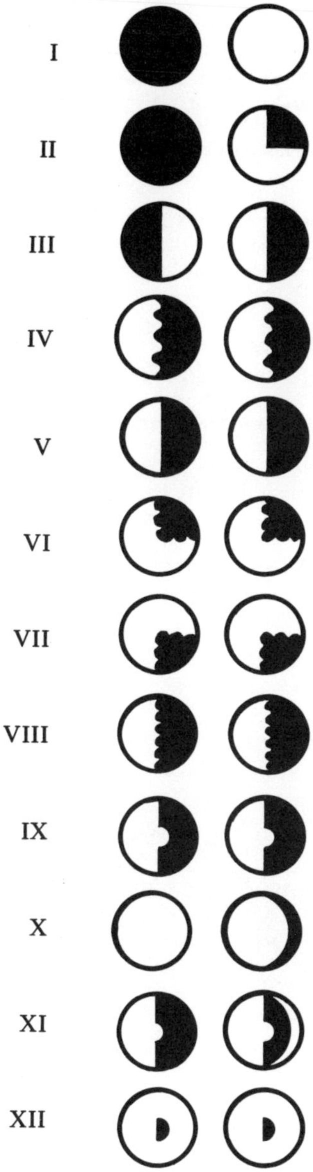

I. Optic nerve–ipsilateral blindness
II. Commencement of optic nerve–ipsilateral blindness with contralateral temporal upper quadrantanopia
III. Median chiasma–bitemporal hemianopia
IV. Optic tract–markedly incongruous homonymous hemianopia
V. Proximal part of optic tract, lateral geniculate body or lower part of radiations–clear-cut homonymous hemianopia without macular sparing
VI. Anterior loop of optic radiations–incongruous superior quandrantanopia
VII. Upper part of optic radiations–slightly incongruous inferior quadrantanopia
VIII. Middle of optic radiations–slightly incongruous homonymous hemianopia without macular sparing
IX. Posterior part of optic radiations–congruous homonymous hemianopia with macular sparing
X. Anterior part of calcarine cortex–contralateral blindness in temporal crescent
XI. Middle part of calcarine cortex–congruous homonymous hemianopia with sparing of the macula and contralateral sparing of temporal crescent
XIII. Posterior part of occipital cortex–congruous homonymous hemianopic central scotoma.

Reprinted from Sir Stewart Duke-Elder and Kenneth Wybar, Neurophthalmology, Vol. XII of System of ophthalmology. St. Louis: C.V. Mosby Co., 1971.

8.23. Differential Diagnosis: Acute and Chronic Uveitis

	Chronic (Granulomatous)	*Acute (Nongranulomatous)*
Anterior uvea		
Pain, photophobia	Minimal or absent	Severe
Vision	Gradual reduction	Abrupt reduction
Course	Protracted, remissions, and exacerbations	Self-limited (1-6 weeks), often recurrent
Keratic deposits	Heavy, coalesce, often "mutton fat," crenated margins, macrophages, phagocytized pigment	Pinpoint, lymphocytes, and plasma cells
Aqueous humor	Few cells, often large, little aqueous flare	Many cells, monocytes, intense aqueous flare, sometimes coagulation
Iris nodules and precipitates	Frequent	None
Posterior uvea		
Retinal and subretinal edema	Usually slight or moderate and localized around exudates	Marked and generalized, with blurring of neuroretinal margins and retinal vascular bed
Choroidal exudates	Heavy massive exudates, edges possibly blurred by surrounding retinal and subretinal edema	No heavy massive exudates, occasionally localized areas of deeper infiltration
Secondary retinal involvement	Almost invariable, with retinal destruction	None or limited to pigment epithelium and rods and cones
Residual organic	Heavy glial scars with massive pigment surrounding the lesion	None or fine granular changes in pigment epithelium with damage to neuroepithelium and superficial gliosis
Anterior segment changes	Sometimes epithelioid or mutton-fat keratic deposits	Usually none
Vitreous changes	Usually heavy vitreous blurring, heavy, veil-like opacities frequent	Slight to intense general blurring, fine muscae or string-like, fibrinous opacities

Reprinted from F. Newll and J.T. Ernest, *Ophthalmology*, St. Louis: C.V. Mosby Co., 1974

8.24. Differential Diagnosis: Ocular Headaches

	Refractive Error: Hyperopia, Astigmatism, Presbyopia	*Muscle Imbalance: Convergence and Divergence Insufficiencies*	*Glaucoma: Open Angle*	*Glaucoma: Closed Angle, Chronic/Acute*	*Uveitis: Anterior*	*Optic Neuritis*	*Minute Foreign Bodies*	*Inflammation of the External Eye and Adnexa*
Onset	With prolonged demand on visual system	With prolonged demand on visual system	Gradual	Chronic: basically gradual Acute: abrupt	Gradual	Usually abrupt	Relatively sudden	Varies with each condition
Duration	Chronic	Chronic	Chronic	Usually chronic with occasional attacks (severe)	May be chronic	May be recurrent	Depends on when treatment began	Variable
Location	Starts about eyes, radiates to frontal and temporal region	From eyes radiates to frontal and temporal regions; also occipital pain	Follows ophthalmic nerve to eye, forehead, temple	Follows distribution of ophthalmic nerve to eye, forehead, temple	Orbit, nose, temple, frontal	Orbit, frontal	Around eyes; radiates frontal	Pain above eye; involves ophthalmic branch of the 5th CN
Character	Dull, low grade	Dull, low grade	Dull, low grade throbbing	Chronic: dull, low grade Acute: severe, unbearable	Acute throbbing pain; eye painful and and tender	Pain behind eye aggravated by movement of eye	Pain in front of eye	Chronic throbbing
Cause	Sustained contraction of ciliary muscle and resulting demand on EOM system	Excessive and sustained effort by EOM's	Low grade insidious rise in intraocular pressure	Congestion of aqeous outflow pathway causing increased IOP, rapid in acute or attack phase	Inflammation of anterior uveal tract	Inflammation of optic nerve	Variable	Meibomitis; hordeolum; orbital cellulitis; conjunctivitis; episcleritis; keratitis; etc.
Clinical Signs	Not in AM; sandy feeling; blurring of print; worse at end of day; reading makes presbyope drowsy	Not in AM; aggravated by fatigue; worse at end of day	Hazy vision; pupils sluggish; lacrimation; haloes around lights; conjunctival injection	Early: haloes Attack: blurred vision, nausea, hazy cornea, chemosis, ciliary injection, fixed oval dilated pupil	Flare; miotic pupil; photophobia; lacrimation; ciliary injection; blurred vision	Flare; pupils sluggish; possible sudden vision loss	Photophobia; lacrimation	Inflammatory reactions usually aid in the diagnosis

Reprinted from W.J. Leslie and D.R. Greenburg, Headache: Discussion classification, differential diagnosis for optometrist. ***J. of the American Optometric Assn., July/August, 1974.***

8.25. Differential Diagnosis: Follicular Conjunctivitis and Vernal Catarrh

	Vernal Catarrh	*Follicular Conjunctivitis*
Appearance of lesions	Flat broad nodules in cobblestone arrangement on upper and lower tarsal conjunctiva, covered by a milky film	Pale-pink elevations arranged like rows of beads
Size of lesions	Large elevations	Small elevations
Location of lesions	Tarsal or palpebral type: tarsal conjunctiva involved, fornix free Limbal or bulbar type: limbus involved, fornix free, tarsal conjunctiva free (mixed types common) Tarsus-not involved Stringy, thready, milky	Mainly on lower tarsal conjunctiva and in lower fornix Tarsus-not involved Mucoid or mucopurulent
Type of secretion	Eosinophiles characteristic and constant in secretion	Scrapings not characteristic (Koch-Weeks: Morax-Axenfeld, micrococcus catarrhalis, staphylococcus, pneumococcus)
Smears	Corneal infiltrations (in limbal type)	Ulcer of the cornea
Complications or sequelae	Pseudoptosis (in tarsal type)	Blepharitis Ectropion (in chronic cases)

Reprinted from Joshua Zuckerman, *Diagnostic examination of the eye*, Philadelphia: J.B. Lippincott Company, 1964.

8.26. Differential Diagnosis: Strabismus

Table A. Paralytic vs. Nonparalytic Strabismus

	Paralytic	*Nonparalytic*
Type of onset	Often sudden but may be gradual or congenital	Usually gradual or congenital; rarely sudden
Age of onset	Any age	Usually during childhood
History of head trauma	Frequent	Infrequent
Difference between primary and secondary deviation	Characteristic finding	Absent
Diplopia	Frequent	Infrequent
ARC or severe amblyopia or both	Infrequent	Frequent
Comitance	Only in late stages	Frequent
Head posture	Frequently abnormal	Rarely abnormal
Cyclotropia	Frequent with cyclovertical paresis	Infrequent except in A and V patterns
Neurologic findings or systemic disease	May be present	Usually absent
Past-pointing	Frequent with recent paresis	Rare

Reprinted by permission from von Noorden, Gunter K: *Burian-von Noorden's Binocular Vision and Ocular Motility*, 2nd ed., St. Louis: The C.V. Mosby Co., 1980.

Table B. Congenital ET vs. Acquired ET

Congenital ET	*Acquired ET*
Alternating deviation (often a midline switch)	Unilateral deviation
Lack of correspondence (neither N.R.C. nor A.R.C.)	Presence of correspondence (either N.R.C. or A.R.C.)
No awareness of diplopia (only alternate perceptions)	Diplopia awareness possible (true simultaneous perception)
Double hyper deviations (may also have excyclo rotation of covered eye)	No double hyper deviation
Insignificant refractive errors	Significant refractive errors (either hyperopia or anisometropia)
Normal or low AC/A	High AC/A
Little or no functional amblyopia	Unilateral amblyopia (non-organic)
History of neurological defects (including organic amblyopia)	Absence of associated neurological signs or symptoms

Reprinted by permission from Griffin, John: *Binocular Anomalies: Procedures for Vision Therapy*, published by Professional Press, Inc., 101 East Ontario Street, Chicago, Illinois 60611, 1976.

8.27. Differential Diagnosis: Asteriod Hyalosis and Synchysis Scintillans

	Asteriod Hyalosis	*Synchysis Scintillans*
Age of patient	Elderly	Usually young
Bilaterality	Usually unilateral	May be bilateral more often
Incidence	Rare	Extremely rare
Appearance	Spherical white bodies	Flat, angular crystals
Motility	Moves with vitreous structure and returns to original position	Moves freely and falls to floor of vitreous cavity
Chemistry	Calcium soaps	Cholesterol crystals
Associated ocular disease	None: diabetes mellitus?	Secondary to other ocular disease or trauma

8.28. Differential Diagnosis: Optic Disc Typography

Feature	*Differential Diagnostic Criteria in Glaucoma*
Disc cupping	extensive, particularly significant in small (hypermetropic) eyes; asymmetry of cup to disc ratio of >0.2 between fellow eyes; vertical elongation within a round disc; volume >1 mm^3; asymmetry of volume >0.1 mm^3 between fellow eyes; depth $>5D$; large depth in discs which show a small cup to disc ratio
Visual configuration	"kinking" of vessels at the cup margin; nasal displacement (angulation) in a small cup; arterial pulsation on slight digital pressure; vessel engorgement; ischemia of nerve head capillaries
Pallor of disc	central; greater than anticipated for the age of the patient; pale area $<$ area of cupping; asymmetry of pale area between discs of fellow eyes
Rim of nerve tissue at the cup edge	below the level of the retina; shelving; overhang particularly significant in the inferior temporal quadrant
General appearance of disc (disc type)	Temporal changes, even of apparently normal features

Reprinted from A. Tomlinson, Optic disc topography in glaucoma, *Journal of the AOA*, February, 1977.

8.29. Differential Diagnosis: Retinal Venous Stasis/Occlusive Disease*

Incidence	*VSR (common) stasis retinopathy*	*Acute CRVO (rare)*	*BRVO (common)*	*Papillophlebitis (uncommon)*	*Papilledema*	*Hypertension*
Age	Young adult and past middle age	Past middle age	Past middle age	Young adults	Any age	Usually middle/age past
Symptoms	None; progressive loss of central	Acute; marked loss red out	Relative to absolute VF defect or central loss if macular venule involved	Often minimal central loss	TOV; slow progressive	None; slow central and and VF depression
Fundus:						
Retinal veins	Early: markedly engorged, turgid, and tortuous Late†: possible sheathing	Late: sheathing	Early: engorgement limited to 1 to 3 vessels		Maybe engorged	Pseudoengorgement from narrow arteriole
Retinal hemorrhages	Posterior pole Few to many flame-shaped and punctate periphery: punctate	Gross hemorrhage; posterior pole decreasing as reach periphery	Limited to drainage area of vessels occluded: flame and punctate		Flame; variable no.; posterior pole	Distribution similar to CRVO but variable no.
Cotton wool spots	Rare	Common	Variable	Common	Rare	Common when more severe
Optic disc	Often hyperemic and edematous Late†: WNL	Plethoric; late: palor frequent	Variable—often late: WNL	Mild edema; late: WNL	Marked to mild edema; late: often polar	Variable, depending on severity; Late: ?

*VSR = venous stasis retinopathy; CRVO = central retinal vein obstruction; BRVO = branch retinal vein occlusion; VF= visual field; TOV = transient obstruction of vision; WNL = within normal limits; CME = cystoid macular edema; NVE = neovascularization elsewhere; A-V = arteriovenous.

† Late: 6 to 9 months.

(continued)

8.29. Differential Diagnosis: Retinal Venous Stasis/Occlusive Disease* (continued)

Incidence	*VSR (common) stasis retinopathy*	*Acute CRVO (rare)*	*BRVO (common)*	*Papillophlebitis (uncommon)*	*Papilledema*	*Hypertension*
Macula	Normal to mild hemorrhages/ edema Late: WNL to CME	Gross hemorrhages and edema; Late: often mottled	Variable – if macular BRVO, edema, and hemorrhages; Late: variable	Variable	WNL	Macular star in severe cases
Retinal arterioles	WNL or arteriolo-sclerotic	Arteriolo-sclerotic		WNL	WNL	Frequently arteriolo-sclerotic
Fluorescein angiography early	Venous stasis; retinal staining and macular edema; retinal ciliary vessels	And retinal cap. obliteration; NVE‡ and A-V shunts; and disk staining	Delayed/absent filling and emptying; Late: collaterals; macular edema		Variable; disk staining and hyper-fluorescence	
Prognosis	Good	Poor	Good	Good	Variable but guarded	Poor for life
Course	Self-limited	Progressive	Variable, often self-limited	Self-limited	Variable	Progressive
Sequelae	CME, may proceed to hemorrhagic retropathy	Macular degen-eration; vitreous hemorrhages; retinitis proli-ferans; primary or neovascular glaucoma	Macular degenera-tion; neovasculari-zation collaterals	Few CME	Optic atrophy	

*VSR = venous stasis retinopathy; CRVO = central retinal vein obstruction; BRVO = branch retinal vein occlusion; VF = visual field; TOV = transient obstruction of vision; WNL = within normal limits; CME = cystoid macular edema; NVE = neovascularization elsewhere; A-V = arteriovenous.

†Late: 6 to 9 months.

‡Neovascularization elsewhere from disk.

Reprinted from T.R. Stelmack, W. Jones, and J. Maino, Retinal venous stasis and occlusive disease, *Opt Monthly*, March, 1980, pp 64-73. With the special permission of the Professional Press, Inc., 101 East Ontario Street, Chicago, Illinois 60611.

8.30. Differential Diagnosis: Inflammations of the Lids and Sclera

	Lid Inflammation					*Scleral Inflammation*	
	Local		*Diffuse*			*Superficial*	*Deep*
	Pain	*No Pain*	*Burning, Itching*		*Dull Pain*		
	Hordeolum	*Chalazion*	*Blepharitis*	*Dermatitis*	*Cellulitis*	*Episcleritis*	*Scleritis*
Onset and Distinguishing Feature	Days; localized red swollen area; tenderness, external and internal types	Weeks; localized red lump; usually upper lid	Days; red-rimmed eyes; usually confined to lid margin; crusty lids	Hours to days	Days to weeks; swollen orbit	Hours to days; superficial injection	Days to weeks; deep injection
Incidence	Common	Common	Common	Common	Rare	Common	Rare
Etiology	Staphylococcal infection of of glands of Zeis and Moll	Inflammation due to blockage of Meibomian gland	Staphylococcus or Pityrosporum ovale	Entire range of allergins	Cell inflammation due to adjacent infection	Unknown; history of allergies or arthritis	Unknown; usually systemic disorder
Prognosis	Good; usually resolve within one week	Chronic	Chronic	Rapid resolution if remove offending allergin	Good, if treated promptly	Good, but tends to recur	Poor; difficult to treat
Treatment	Topical antibiotics; warm compresses, incision, and evacuation of pus	Documentation; excision if becomes large	Local and scalp hygiene; topical sulfonamides	Removal of allergin; topical corticosteroids	Hospitalization; removal of abcess; systemic antibiotics	Removal of inflammatory stimulus; local cortiosteroids	Treatment of systemic problem; local corticosteroids
Complications	Possible blepharitis; orbital cellulitis (rare)	Induced astigmatism; problems with lid apposition	Conjunctivitis, hordeola, chalazia	Secondary staphylococcal infection	Spread of infection to deeper sinuses	May lead to scleritis or thinning of sclera	Sclerosing keratitis; uveitis; rupture of globe

Reprinted from K.L. Alexander, Some inflamations of the external eye and adnexa, *J Am Opt Assn*, February, 1980.

8.31. Differential Diagnosis: Vascular Signs of Ocular Diseases

Ocular signs	*Clinical Entity Examples (workers)*	*Fluorescein Angiography*	*Direct Ophthalmoscopy*
Microaneurysms	Diabetic retinopathy (Scott *et al.* 1963)	(+) fluorescent, differentiating from spots hemorrhage	(–) if small, (+) ? if large
Hemorrhages	Diabetic and/or hypertensive retinopathy (Dollery *et al.* 1963)	(–) nonfluorescent, differentiating from microaneurysms (in a negative sense)	(+) if large
Vascular attenuation	Arteriolar sclerosis (Oosterhuis *et al.* 1965, Kato *et al.* 1971	(+) irregular column of dye in vessel lumen	(+) advanced stage (–) early stage
Focal opacities around retinal vessel	Normal or arteriolar sclerosis (Kato *et al.* 1971)	(+) irregular column of dye in vessel lumen	(+) advanced stage (–) early stage
Tortuous vessels	Papilloedema, hypertensive retinopathy (Foulds 1973)	(+) delayed flow, (leakage of dye around optic disc	(+) moderate and advanced stage
Neovascularization	Diabetes mellitus (Little 1974)	(+) fluorescein shows early sign and extent of neovascularization	(+) moderate and advanced stage (–) early stage
Increased capillary permeability	Diabetes (Scott *et al.* 1963); Hypersion (Dollery *et al.* 1963)	(+) fluoresce in early stage, showing leakage of dye	(–) early stage
Increased vascular permeability at optic disc	Papilloedema (Haining 1969)	(+) fluorescent dye leakage spread beyond disc margins (normal disc fluoresce confined within disc margin)	(–) early stage (+) morderate stage
	Temporal arteritis (Haining 1969)	(+) excess leakage of dye beyond disc margins in late venous phase	(–) ?
Decreased vascular permeability at optic disc	Optic atrophy, multiple sclerosis, Leber's disease, retinitis pigmentosa (Haining 1969)	(–) no fluorescent indicating decreased circulation (normal disc fluoresce confined within disc margins)	(–) early stage (+) advanced stage
Local occlusion of arteriole circulation, in experimental pigs	Retinal vascular embolism (Dollery *et al.* 1965)	(+) local dark areas of nonfluorescent, suggesting nonperfused capillaries, static column of fluorescent blood in arterioles	(–) ?

(continued)

8.31. Differential Diagnosis: Vascular Signs of Ocular Diseases (continued)

Ocular signs	*Clinical Entity Examples (workers)*	*Fluorescein Angiography*	*Direct Ophthalmoscopy*
Delayed and slow arteriovenous filling	Central retinal artery occlusion (David *et al.* 1967)	(+) delayed fluorescent arterial phase 33 sec (normal arterial at 10.9 sec); granular appearance to fluorescent column, because R.B.C. absorb dye	(+)
	Carotid occlusion (David *et al.* 1966)	(+) delayed appearance of fluorescein and slowing of sequence of retinal circulatory cycles	(–) ?
	Partial carotid occlusion (Hisatomi 1974)	(+) asymmetric circulatory dynamics in the two optic discs (simultaneous comparison of bilateral F.A.)	(–)
Arteriolar plaque	Hypertension (Linhart *et al.* 1964)	(+) delayed flow	(–) if small
A-V nippings	Arterio-sclerosis (Oosterhuls *et al.* 1964, Kottow *et al.* 1971)	(+) turbulent flow, as compared with normal laminal flow	(+) if marked (–) if subtle
White round deposits	Drusen (Trevor-Roper 1974)	(–) no residual fluorescence	(±) depending on other clinical data
Hard exudates in macular star or local lesion	Malignant hypertension (Chester 1973)	(–) no fluorescent indicating neural lesion at outer plexiform layer, not serous exudates from retinal vessels	(–) if small (+) if large, depends on other signs to differentiate from drusens
Soft exudates or cotton wool patches	Diabetes (Scott *et al.* 1963); hypertension (Dollery *et al.* 1963)	(+) fluorescent of the involved area, indicating increased vascular permeability	(–) in early stage (+) in late stage
Retinal edema, e.g. macular edema	Retinitis and vitritis and Behcet's (Gass 1970)	(+) fluorescent, dye leakage	(–) in early stage
Macular pigment epithelium degeneration	Stargardt's disease (Francois *et al.* 1971)	(+) early phase: annular fluoresce of macular area; late phase: irregular fluorescent disc in macular showing the choroidal vessels, because pigment epithelium disappears	(±) depends on the stage of pathology

(continued)

8.31. Differential Diagnosis: Vascular Signs of Ocular Diseases (continued)

Ocular signs	*Clinical Entity Examples (workers)*	*Fluorescein Angiography*	*Direct Ophthalmoscopy*
Pigment epithelium detachment	Serous detachment of the retinal pigment epithelium (Maumenee 1971)	(+) fluorescent in detached areas	(–) in early stage
Neuroepithelium detachment	Cystic macular degeneration (Francois *et al.* 1971)	(+) early confluent fluorescent spots around central lesion, and late phase shows localized areas of detachment as bright fluorescent	(–) in early stage
Retinal detachment from Bruch's membrane	Junius-Kuhnt disease or disciform macular degeneration (Francois *et al.* 1971, Norton *et al.* 1964)	(+) progressively increasing fluorescent in the affected area	(–) in early stage
Macular atrophy	Senile abiotrophy of macula (Maumenee 1971)	(–) characteristic absence of fluorescent in macular area (discrete outlines) confirming the absence of choriocapillaris	(–) in early stage
Epithelial pigmentary changes	Benign nevi (Norton *et al.* 1964)	(–) nonfluorescent	(±) need other clinical data, and frequent reviews
Pigmentary lesions	Malignant melanoma (Norton *et al.* 1964, Alezzandrini 1971)	(+) fluorescent in early arterial phase, and persists for several minutes	(+) an needs additional confirmation tests
		(+) fluorescent choroidal vessels (use infrared spectral reflectance)	
Elevated lesion	Metastatic tumor (Norton *et al.* 1964)	(–) nonfluorescent	(±) nondifferential; need additional tests
Elevated lesion	Choroidal hemangioma (Norton *et al.* 1964)	(+) fluorescent in early arterial phase and persists, similar pattern as melanoma	(±) need additional tests
Raised I.O.P. induced in experimental pig	Raised intra ocular press (Dollerey *et al.* 1968, Kohner 1969)	(+) reduced flow speed in retinal arterioles	(–)

(continued)

8.31. Differential Diagnosis: Vascular Signs of Ocular Diseases (continued)

Ocular signs	*Clinical Entity Examples (workers)*	*Fluorescein Angiography*	*Direct Ophthalmoscopy*
Reduction of vascular supply to optic disc	Glaucoma (Hayreh and Perkins 1969)	(–) reduced fluorescent at optic disc due to raised I.O.P.	(–) at early stage
Vasoconstriction of retinal vessels and decreased blood flow	Hyperoxia induced in experimental monkeys (Eperon *et al.* 1975)	(+) detected by reduction in fluorescein densitometry; vascular feedback sensitive to changes in Po	(–) if subtle
Vasodilation of retinal vessels and increased blood flow	Hypoxia induced in experimental monkeys (Eperon *et al.* 1975)	(+) detected by increase in fluorescein densitometry; vascular feedback sensitive to changes in Po	(–) if subtle

Reprinted from B. Tan, Fundas photography: Some evolutionary perspectives and some methods of the Zeiss fundus camera, *Australian J. Opt.*, December, 1976.

8.32. Differential Diagnosis: Central Scotomas: Retinal vs. Neurological

Central Scotoma	*Inflammatory*	*Neoplastic*	*Vascular*	*Degenerative*	*Toxic*
Retinal (macular)	Chorioretinitis Histoplasmosis Sarcoid *Toxocara* Toxoplasmosis	Melanoma	Blood dyscrasias Central vein thrombosis Diabetes Hypertension Ischemia	Familial (hereditary) Senile Myopia Trauma	Drugs (chloroquine)
Optic nerve	Demyelinating (multiple sclerosis) Infectious (syphilis, herpes zoster) Optic neuritis Xanthemata	Craniopharyngioma Glioma Orbital (neurofibroma)	Blood dyscrasias Ischemia Hypotension	Metabolic Familial (Leber's)	Nutritional Drugs (digitalis) Ethanol Methanol Lead

After Thomas R. Kuhns, M.D.

8.33. Differential Diagnosis: Retinitis Pigmentosa

	Retinitis Pigmentosis	*Pseudo Retinitis*	*Cone-Rod Dystrophy*	*Foveo-Macular Dystrophies*
Case History	Night blindness tunnel vision, familial involvement	Aging, drug ingestion, trauma, infection	Visual acuity loss, color vision loss, hemeralopia, normal or slightly improved night vision	Visual acuity loss, normal color vision, no hemeralopia, normal night vision
Visual acuity	Normal or near normal	Normal	Reduced, improved under low illumination	Reduced
Color vision (Panel D-15)	Normal or mild tritan defect	Normal	Extensive color loss	Normal or mild color loss
Visual fields	Annular scotopic defect	Normal	Central scotoma	Normal, or mild central scotoma
Adaptometry	Elevated cone and final rod threshold, inverted profile	Normal	Absent cone portion, normal or slightly elevated final rod threshold	Normal
ERG–EOG	Dimished or Absent	Normal or near normal	Selectively diminished	Normal or selectively diminished

Reprinted from L.C. Norden, The diagnosis and management of retintis pigmentosa, *Southern Journal of Opt*, April 1977.

8.34. Color Vision Defects and Possible Etiologies

Disease	*Defect*
Congenital jaundice	Extreme deuteranomaly
Albinism	Extreme deuteranomaly
Peripheral pigmentary dystrophy	Deuteranopia, blue-yellow and red-green defects
Central pigmentary dystrophy	Red-green and blue-yellow
Albipunctate dystrophy	Blue-yellow
Choroideremia	Blue-yellow
Sorsby's dystrophy	Red-green
Choroidal sclerosis	Blue-yellow and red-green
Fuchs's gyrate atrophy	Red-green
Vogt-Spielmeyer's disease	Red-green
Juvenile macular degeneration	Red-green
Senile macular degeneration	Blue-yellow
Grönblad-Strandberg syndrome	Blue-yellow
Cystic macular degeneration	Congenital: deuteranopia
Retinoschisis	Blue-yellow
Malignant myopia	Blue-yellow, red-green
Retinal detachment	Blue-yellow, red-green
Siderosis	Blue-yellow
Chorioretinitis	Blue-yellow
Central serous retinopathy	Blue-yellow
Hypertensive retinopathy	Blue-yellow
Diabetic retinopathy	Blue-yellow
Retinal vascular occlusions	Blue-yellow
Choroidal malignant melanoma	Blue-yellow
Glaucoma	Blue-yellow
Drusen of the optic disc	Red-green, blue-yellow
Optic atrophy (dominant)	Blue-yellow
Optic atrophy (sex-linked)	Red-green
Papilloedema	Red-green, blue-yellow
Retrobulbar neuritis	Red-green
Chiasmal lesions	Red-green
Alcohol-nicotine intoxication	Red-green

Vision Training & Developmental Vision 9

9.1. Optometric Utilization of Objective Standardized Perceptual Tests

Table A. Perceptual Tests

Type of Test	*Name of Test*	*Author*	*Publisher*
Visual Motor Integration	Bender Visual-Motor Gestalt	Bender	Psychological Corp.
	Dennis Visual Perception Scale	Dennis	Western Psychological Services
	Developmental Test of Visual-Motor Integration	Beery	Follett Publishing Co.
	Minnesota Percepto-Diagnostic	Fuller	Clinical Psychology Pub. Co.
	Perceptual Forms	Publication Committee	Winter Haven Lions Research Foundation
	Perceptual-Motor (VKT)	Vane	Clinical Psychology Pub. Co.
	Primary Visual-Motor Test	Hawort	Grune and Stratton
	Rutgers Drawing Test	Starr	Starr
	Simkov Perceptual Organization Inventory	Kovacevich	Antof Educational Supp.
	Slosson Drawing Coordinator	Slosson	Slosson Educational Pub.
	Visual Copying (SLD)	Slingerland	Educators Publishing Service
	Visual Copying (START)	Ahr	Priority Innovations
	Visual-Motor Coordination (CB)	Clymer and Barrett	Personnel Press
Auditory Memory	Auditory Attention Span for Unrelated Words (DTLA)	Baker and Leland	Bobbs-Merrill
	Auditory Attention Span for Related Syllables (DTLA)	Baker and Leland	Bobbs-Merrill
	Auditory Memory (START)	Ahr	Priority Innovations
	Auditory Recall (SLD)	Slingerland	Educators Publishing Service
	Auditory Sequential Memory (ITPA)	Kirk, McCarthy, and Kirk	University of Illinois
Auditory-Visual Integration	Auditory-Visual (RPS)	Rosner et al.	University of Pittsburgh
	Following Directions (G-M)	Gates and MacGinitie	Teachers College Press
	Oral Directions (DTLA)	Baker and Leland	Bobbs-Merrill
Perceptual-Motor	Lincoln-Oseretsky Motor Development Scale	Sloan	Stoelting
	Motor Skills (RPS)	Rosner et al.	University of Pittsburgh
	Oseretsky Tests of Motor Proficiency	Doll	American Guidance Service

(continued)

Table A. Perceptual Tests (continued)

Type of Test	*Name of Test*	*Author*	*Publisher*
	Purdue Perceptual Motor Survey	Roach and Kephart	Merrill
	Southern California Perceptual-Motor Tests	Ayres	Western Psychological Services
Auditory Discrimination	Auditory Closure (ITPA)	Kirk, McCarthy, and Kirk	University of Illinois
	Auditory Discrimination	Wepman	Language Research Assoc.
	Auditory Discrimination (CB)	Clymer and Barrett	Personnel Press
	Auditory Discrimination (GM)	Gates and MacGinitie	Teachers College Press
	Auditory Organization (RPS)	Rosner et al.	University of Pittsburgh
	Screening Test for Auditory Perception	Kimmel and Wahl	Academic Therapy Publications
Eye-Hand Coordination	Coordination (FACT)	Flanagan	Science Research Assoc.
	Dex-Aim (PFD)	Holmes	Psychometric Affiliates
	Dex-Man (PFD)	Holmes	Psychometric Affiliates
	Eye-Motor Coordination (FDTVP)	Frostig	Follett Publishing Co.
	Motor Speed and Precision (DTLA)	Baker and Leland	Bobbs-Merrill
	Precision (FACT)	Flanagan	Science Research Assoc.
	So. California Test of Motor Accuracy	Ayres	Western Psychological Services
	Vision, Hearing and Motor Coordination	Sullivan, Clark, and Tiegs	California Test Bureau
	Visual-Motor Coordination (G-M)	Gates and MacGinitie	Teachers College Press
Visual Form Discrimination	Components (FACT)	Flanagan	Science Research Assoc.
	Embedded Figures	Benton and Spreen	University of Victoria
	Embedded Figures	Witkin	Consulting Psychologists Press
	Figure-Ground (FDTVP)	Frostig	Follett Publishing Co.
	Form Constancy (FDTVP)	Frostig	Follett Publishing Co.
	Size Perception	Schrock	Creative Associates
	So. California Figure-Ground	Ayres	Western Psychological Services
	Space Completion (JTPA)	Jastak	Guidance Associates
	Visual Closure (ITPA)	Kirk and McCarthy	University of Illinois
	Visual Discrimination (G-M)	Gates and McGinitie	Teachers College Press
	Visual Discrimination (START)	Ahr	Priority Innovations
	Visual Organization	Hooper	Western Psychological Services
	Welsh Figure Preference	Welsh	Consulting Psychologists Press

(continued)

Table A. Perceptual Tests (continued)

Type of Test	*Name of Test*	*Author*	*Publisher*
Perceptual Speed	Coding (JTPA)	Jastak	Guidance Associates
	Inspection (FACT)	Flanagan	Science Research Assoc.
	Minnesota Clerical Test	Peterson and Eungstaff	Psychological Corp.
	Perceptual Speed (GZAS)	Guilford and Zimmerman	Sheridan Supply Co.
	Perceptual Speed (MAS)	Segel and Raskin	California Test Bureau
	Perceptual Speed and Accuracy (MTMA)	MacQuarrie	California Test Bureau
	Perceptual Speed (PMA)	Thurstone	Science Research Assoc.
	Per-Verb (PFD)	Holmes	Psychometric Affiliates
	Per-Numb (PFD)	Holmes	Psychometric Affiliates
Visual Memory	Visual Tracing	Groffman	Keystone View Co.
	Benton Visual Retention	Benton	Psychological Corp.
	Memory for Designs	Graham and Kendall	Psychological Test Specialists
	Memory for Designs (DTLA)	Baker and Leland	Bobbs-Merrill
	Memory for Forms (GDK)	Ilg and Ames	Harper
	Visual Attention Span for Letters (DTLA)	Baker and Leland	Bobbs-Merrill
	Visual Attention Span for Objects	Baker and Leland	Bobbs-Merrill
	Visual Memory (GLPE)	Gilliland	Eastern Montana College
	Visual Memory (SLD)	Slingerland	Educators Publishing Service
	Visual Memory (START)	Ahr	Priority Innovations
	Visual Sequential Memory (ITPA)	Kirk, McCarthy and Kirk	University of Illinois
Spatial Orientation	Harris Tests of Lateral Dominance	Harris	Psychological Corp.
	Leavell Hand-Eye Coordinator	Leavell	Keystone View Co.
	Orientatin (DTLA)	Baker and Leland	Bobbs-Merrill
	Right and Left (GDK)	Ilg and Ames	Harper and Row
	Right-Left Discrimination (SCPM)	Ayres	Western Psychological Services
	Right-Left Discrimination and Finger Localization	Benton	Hoeber
	Right-Left Orientation–Victoria Form	Benton and Spreen	University of Victoria
	Road-Map Test of Direction Sense	Money	Johns Hopkins Press
	Spatial Orientation (GZAS)	Guilford and Zimmerman	Sheridan Supply
	Spatial Relationships (CMMT Long Form)	Sullivan, Clark, and Tiegs	California Test Bureau

(continued)

Table A. Perceptual Tests (continued)

Type of Test	*Name of Test*	*Author*	*Publisher*
Spatial Visualization	Assembly (FACT)	Flanagan	Science Research Assoc.
	Ayres Space Test	Ayres	Western Psychological
	Disarranged Pictures (DTLA)	Baker and Leland	Bobbs-Merrill
	Minnesota Spatial Relations	Trabue et al.	American Guidance Corp.
	Object-Completion	Curtis	Psychometric Affiliates
	Orientation of Forms (GDK)	Ilg and Ames	Harper
	Patterns (FACT)	Flanagan	Science Research Assoc.
	Position in Space (FDTVP)	Frostig	Follett Publishing Co.
	Rev. Minnesota Paper Formboard	Likert and Quasha	Psychological Corp.
	Space-Form	Curtis	Psychometric Affiliates
	Space Series (JTPA)	Jastak	Guidance Associates
	Spatial Orientation (GZAS)	Guilford and Zimmerman	Sheridan Supply
	Spatial Relations (ANAT)	Kobol and Wrightstone	Psychometric Affiliates
	Spatial Relationships (CMMT)	Sullivan, Clark, and Tiegs	California Test Bureau
	Spatial Relations (FDTVP)	Frostig	Follett Publishing Co.
	Spatial Relations (PMA)	Thurstone and Thurstone	Science Research Assoc.
	Spatial Visualization (GZAS)	Guilford and Zimmerman	Sheridan Supply
	Spatial Visualization (MAS)	Segel and Raskin	California Test Bureau

Table B. Specific Batteries of Tests that Have Proven Useful for Determining Overall Perceptual Functioning and Specific Perceptual Deficits at Various Grade Levels

Perceptual Ability (Grade)	*Visual Form*	*Perceptual Speed*	*Visual-Motor Integration*	*Visual Memory*	*Auditory Memory*	*Spatial Orientation*	*Spatial Visualization*
K–1	So. California Figure-Ground Visual Closure	Perceptual Speed (PMA) Form K–1	Rutgers Drawing Test Form A	Visual Sequential Memory (ITPA)	Auditory Sequential Memory (ITPA)	Right-Left Discrimination (SCPM)	Spatial Relations (PMA) Form K–1
2–4	So. California Figure-Ground Visual Closure	Perceptual Speed (PMA) Form 2–4	Rutgers Drawing Test Form B	Vis. Seq. Mem. (ITPA) Vis. Att. Span For Objects (DTLA)	Aud. Seq. Mem. (ITPA) Aud. Span for Unrelated Words (DTLA)	Right-Left Discrimination (SCPM)	Spatial Relations (PMA) Form 2–4
4–6	So. California Figure-Ground Visual Closure	Perceptual Speed (PMA) Form 4–6	Developmental Test of Visual-Motor Integration	Vis. Att. Span For Objects (DTLA) Vis. Att. Span For Letters (DTLA)	Aud. Span for Unrelated Words (DTLA)	Road Map Test of Direction Sense	Spatial Relations (PMA) Form 4–6
7–9	So. California Figure-Ground Visual Organization	Perceptual Speed (MAS)	Minnesota Percepto-Diagnostic	Vis. Att. Span For Objects (DTLA) Vis. Att. Span For Letters (DTLA)	Aud. Span for Unrelated Words (DTLA)	Road Map Test of Direction Sense	Spatial Relations (PMA) Form 6-9
10–12	So. California Figure-Ground Visual Organization	Perceptual Speed (MAS)	Minnesota Percepto-Diagnostic	Vis. Att. Span For Objects (DTLA)	Aud. Span for Unrelated Words (DTLA)	Road Map Test of Direction Sense	Spatial Relations (PMA) Form 9–12

Table C. Multiple Test Batteries

Name of Test Battery	*Abbreviation*
Acorn National Aptitude Tests–Non-Verbal	ANAT
California Mental Maturity Test	CMMT
Clymer-Barrett Pre-Reading Battery	CB
Detroit Tests of Learning Aptitude	DTLA
Flanagan Aptitude Classification Tests	FACT
Frostig Developmental Test of Visual Perception	FDTVP
Gates-MacGinitie Readiness Skills	GM
Gesell Development Kit	GDK
Gilliland Learning Potential Examination	GLPE
Guilford-Zimmerman Aptitude Survey	GZAS
Illinois Test of Psycholinguistic Abilities	ITPA
Jastak Test of Potential Ability and Behavior Stability	JTPA
MacQuarrie Test of Mechanical Aptitude	MTMA
Multiple Aptitude Survey	MAS
Perfludex	PFD
Primary Mental Abilities	PMA
Rosner Perceptual Survey	RPS
Screening Test for Assignment of Remedial Treatments	START
Screening Tests for Identifying Children with Specific Language Disability	SLD
Southern California Perceptual-Motor Tests	SCPM
Vane Kindergarten Test	VKT

Table D. Publishers Directory

Academic Therapy Pub.
1539 Fourth St.
San Rafael, Cal. 94901

American Guidance Service
720 Washington Ave. S.E.
Minneapolis, Minn. 55414

Antof Educational Supplies
Medina, Ohio

Bobbs-Merrill Co., Inc.
4300 W. 62nd St.
Indianapolis, Ind. 46206

California Test Bureau
Delmonte Research Park
Monterey, Cal.

Clinical Psychology Pub. Co.
4 Conant Square
Brandon, Vt. 05733

Consulting Psychologist Press
577 College Ave.
Palo Alto, Cal 94306

Creative Associates
P.O. Box 281
Aptos, Cal. 95003

Eastern Montana College
517 Rimrock Rd.
Billings, Mont. 59102

Educators Publishing Service, Inc.
301 Vassar St.
Cambridge, Mass. 02139

Follett Publishing Co.
1010 West Washington Blvd.
Chicago, Ill. 60607

Grune and Stratton
381 Park Avenue South
New York, N.Y. 10016

Guidance Associates
1526 Gilpin Ave.
Wilmington, Del.

Harper & Row
49 E. 33rd St.
New York, N.Y. 10013

Hoeber Medical Division
Harper & Row Pub.
49 East 33rd St.
New York, N.Y. 10013

(continued)

Table D. Publishers Directory (continued)

Johns Hopkins Press
Homewood
Baltimore, Md. 21218

Keystone View Co.
Meadville, Pa. 16335

Language Research Associates
950 E. 59th St., Box 95
Chicago, Ill. 60637

Chas. E. Merrill Pub. Co.
1300 Alum Creek Drive
Columbus, Ohio 43216

Personnel Press, Inc.
20 Nassau St.
Princeton, N.J. 08540

Priority Innovations
P.O. Box 792
Skokie, Ill. 60076

Psychological Corp.
304 E. 45th St.
New York, N.Y. 10017

Psychological Test Specialists
Box 1441
Missoula, Mont. 59801

Psychometric Affiliates
Chicago Plaza
Brookport, Ill. 62910

Science Research Associates
259 E. Erie St.
Chicago, Ill. 60611

Sheridan Supply Co.
P.O. Box 837
Beverly Hills, Cal. 90213

Slosson Educational Publications
140 Pine St.
East Aurora, N.Y. 14052

Anna S. Starr
126 Montgomery St.
Highland Park, N.J. 08904

C. H. Stoelting Co.
424 North Homan Ave.
Chicago, Ill. 60624

Teachers College Press
Teachers College
Columbia University
New York, N.Y. 10027

University of Illinois Press
Urbana, Ill. 61801

University of Pittsburgh
Learning and Research Dev. Center
Pittsburgh, Pa. 15213

University of Victoria
Neuropsychology Lab.
Dept. of Psychology
Victoria, B.C.

Walker Education Book Corp.
720 5th Ave.
New York, N.Y. 10019

Western Psychological Services
12031 Wilshire Blvd.
Los Angeles, Cal. 90025

Winter Haven Lions Research
Foundation, Inc.
Box 111
Winter Haven, Fla. 33880

Reprinted from S. Groffman, Optometric utilization of objective standardized perceptual tests, *American Journal of Optometry*, October, 1971.

9.2. Sequence of Standard Pleoptic Procedures

A. Preparation of patient for pleoptics
   1. Diagnosis of amblyopia and abnormal fixation (history, visual acuity testing, and visuoscopy)
   2. Consultation
   3. Occlusion considerations
      a. direct (if central fixation, possibly if unsteady eccentric)
      b. red filter (worn over amblyopic eye if eccentric fixation with total occlusion of nonamblyopic eye)
      c. inverse (for eccentric fixation, particularly if steady eccentric)

B. Inverse prism therapy
      a. Cüppers
      b. Pigassou

C. Euthyoscopy to protect the fovea and dazzle eccentric fixation point

D. Intermittent photic stimulation of fovea
      a. Bangerter
      b. Allen

E. Afterimages
   1. Euthyoscopic afterimage
      a. perception of positive afterimage
      b. perception of negative afterimage
   2. Transferred afterimage (vertical line transferred from fovea of nonamblyopic eye)
   3. Direct afterimage for home training (e.g., Inouye's disc)

F. Haidinger's brushes
   1. Perception on surface of instrument (e.g., MITT)
   2. Perception in space (e.g., Space Coordinator)

G. Fixation training using combinations of procedures
   1. Afterimage on real object
      a. doughnut on Snellen letter
      b. transferred vertical line on Snellen letter
   2. Afterimage and letter with pointing
   3. Combination of afterimage and Haidinger's brushes
      a. without pointing
      b. with accurate pointing to letter (overlay on MITT)
      c. quick pointing exercises with letter
      d. pointer with A.I. and H.B. on picture for pursuit tracing
      e. saccadic fixations with A.I. and H.B. with Snellen chart
   4. Quick pointing with H.B. and letter
   5. Pointer with H.B. on picture for pursuit tracing
   6. H.B. on picture for pursuit tracing without pointer
   7. Saccadic fixations with H.B. and Snellen chart
   8. H.B. and Snellen letter in space
   9. H.B. on picture for pursuit tracing in space
   10. H.B. on Snellen chart for saccadic fixations in space
   11. Transferred A.I. in space (pursuits and saccades)
   12. Steady, pursuit, and saccadic fixations without A.I. or H.B., but occasional monitoring (to insure central fixation)

H. Monocular training activities with direct occlusion

I. Binocular considerations
      a. Begin binocular training when visual acuity is 20/40.
      b. Continue amblyopia therapy with binocular training and use binocular methods to improve amblyopia.

9.3. Stereopsis

Table A. Titmus Stereotest Limits: Lower Limits of Stereoacuity on Titmus Stereotest, in Subjects with normal Binocular Single Vision

Age Group	*Stereoacuity*
3½–5	3000″
5–5½	140″
5½–6	100″
6–7	80″
7–9	60″
Over 9	40″

Table B. Howard-Dolman: Stereoacuities*

Alignment error (mm)	*Stereoacuity*
5	2″
10	3″
20	7″
30	10″
40	13″
50	16″
60	20″
80	26″
100	33″
200	66″
300	99″
400	132″
500	165″

***Performed at 6 meters; assume I.P.D. of 60 mm**

Table C. Verhoeff: Corresponding Acuities*

Test Distance (cm)	*Stereoacuity (seconds of arc)*
10	3090″
20	772″
30	343″
50	124″
60	86″
80	48″
100	31″
110	26″
130	18″
150	14″
200	8″
300	3″

***All eight targets must be responded to correctly. The stereothreshold values are calculated for an interpupillary distance of 60 mm. The eta value (stereoacuity) are calculated using an alignment error of 2.5 mm.**

Table D. Shephard Percentages and Corresponding Values (approximate)

Seconds of Arc	*Shepard Percentage*
1000	4
400	16
200	31
100	51
50	72
40	78
20	95
15	100
10	106

9.4. Expected Normal Development of the Child According to Age Levels

Primitive reflexes (suck, grasp, blink, etc.)	Newborn
Eyes may move independently	Newborn
Head momentarily lifted up	4 Weeks
Binocular vision may begin	6 Weeks
Laughter	16 Weeks
Rolls–prone to supine	24 Weeks
Holds bottle	24 Weeks
Crawls on abdomen	40 Weeks
Creeps–hands and knees	44 Weeks
Creeps–all fours (bear walk)	52 Weeks
Walks–no help	13 Months
Goes up and down stairs without help	18 Months
Stacks 3 to 4 cubes	18 Months
Runs	2 Years
Turns door knob	2 Years
Rides tricycle	3 Years
Draws, copies a circle	3 Years
Normal speech	3 Years
Skips	4 Years
Copies a cross	4 Years
Copies a triangle	5 Years
Copies a diamond	6 Years

9.5. Classification of Correspondency

Type of Correspondence	*Relationship of angles**
A. Normal (N.R.C.)	H = S and A = zero
B. Anomalous (A.R.C.)	H ≠ S A ≠ Zero
1. Harmonious	H = A and S = O
2. Unharmonious	
a. typical	H > H and S < H
b. atypical	
(1) paradoxical type one	A > H and S < zero
(2) parodoxical type two	S > H and A < zero

***A = H—S; where**

A = Angle of Anomaly,
H = Objective Angle, and
S = Subjective Angle.

Reprinted from Griffin, John: *Binocular Anomalies: Procedures for Vision Therapy*, p. 162, published by Professional Press, Inc., 101 East Ontario Street, Chicago, Illinois 60611.

9.6. Resultant Prism for the Treatment of Two-Axis Strabismus

Vertical Prism Required (in diopters)	*Horizontal Prism Required (in Diopters)*													
	1	2	3	4	5	6	7	8	9	10	11	12	13	14
1	2Δ/30°	2Δ/30°	3Δ/19°	4Δ/14°	5Δ/12°	6Δ/10°	7Δ/8°	8Δ/7°	9Δ/6°	10Δ/6°	12Δ/5°	12Δ/5°	15Δ/4°	15Δ/4°
2	2Δ/84°	3Δ/42°	4Δ/30°	4Δ/30°	5Δ/24°	6Δ/19°	7Δ/17°	8Δ/14°	9Δ/13°	10Δ/12°	12Δ/10°	12Δ/10°	15Δ/8°	15Δ8°
3	3Δ/84°	4Δ/49°	4Δ/49°	5Δ37°	6Δ/30°	7Δ/25°	8Δ/22°	9Δ/19°	9Δ/19°	10Δ/17°	12Δ/14°	12Δ/14°	15Δ/12°	15Δ/12°
4	4Δ/84°	5Δ/53°	5Δ/53°	6Δ/42°	6Δ/42°	7Δ/35°	8Δ/30°	9Δ/26°	10Δ/24°	10Δ/24°	12Δ/19°	12Δ/19°	15Δ/15°	15Δ/15°
5	5Δ/84°	6Δ/56°	6Δ/56°	6Δ/56°	7Δ/46°	8Δ/39°	9Δ/34°	9Δ/34°	10Δ/30°	12Δ/25°	12Δ/25°	12Δ/25°	15Δ19°	15Δ/19°
6	5Δ/84°	7Δ/59°	7Δ/59°	7Δ/59°	8Δ/49°	9Δ/42°	9Δ/42°	10Δ/37°	10Δ/37°	12Δ/30°	12Δ/30°	12Δ/30e	15Δ/24°	15Δ/24°
7	7Δ/84°	7Δ/84°	8Δ/61°	8Δ/61°	9Δ/51°	9Δ/51°	10Δ/44°	10Δ/44°	12Δ/36°	12Δ/36°	12Δ/36°	15Δ/28°	15Δ/28°	15Δ/28°
8	8Δ/84°	8Δ/84°	9Δ/63°	9Δ/63°	9Δ/63°	10Δ/53°	10Δ/53°	12Δ/42°	12Δ/42°	12Δ/42°	15Δ/32°	15Δ/32°	15Δ/32°	15Δ/32°
9	9Δ/84°	9Δ/84°	10Δ/64°	10Δ/64°	10Δ/64°	10Δ/64°	12Δ/49°	12Δ/49°	12Δ/49°	15Δ/37°	15Δ/37°	15Δ/37°	15Δ/37°	15Δ/37°
10	10Δ/84°	10Δ/84°	10Δ/84°	12Δ/56°	12Δ/56°	12Δ/56°	12Δ/56°	12Δ/56°	15Δ/42°	15Δ/42°	15Δ/42°	15Δ/42°	15Δ/42°	15Δ42°
11	12Δ/66°	12Δ/66°	12Δ/66°	12Δ/66°	12Δ/66°	12Δ/66°	12Δ/66°	15Δ/47°	15Δ/47°	15Δ/47°	15Δ/47°	15Δ/47°	15Δ/47°	20Δ/33°
12	12Δ/85°	12Δ/84°	12Δ/84°	12Δ/84°	15Δ/53°	15Δ/53°	15Δ/53°	15Δ/53°	15Δ/53°	15Δ/53°	15Δ/53°	15Δ/33°	20Δ/37°	20Δ/37°
13	15Δ/60°	15Δ/60°	15Δ/60°	15Δ/60°	15Δ/60°	15Δ/60e	15Δ/60°	15Δ/60°	15Δ/60°	15Δ/60°	15Δ/60°	20Δ/41°	20Δ/41°	20Δ/41°
14	15Δ/69°	15Δ/69°	15Δ/69°	15Δ/69°	15Δ/69°	15Δ/69°	15Δ/69°	15Δ/69°	15Δ/69°	20Δ/44°	20Δ/44°	20Δ/44°	20Δ/44°	20Δ/44°
15	15Δ/86°	15Δ/84°	15Δ/84°	15Δ/84e	15Δ/84°	15Δ/84°	20Δ/49°	20Δ/49°	20Δ/49°	20Δ/49°	20Δ/49°	20Δ/49°	20Δ/49°	20Δ/49°

Chart of resultant prism power and angle of orientation for given combinations of horizontal and vertical prism power requirement. For example, a requirement of 10 diopters horizontal prism and 3 diopters vertical indicates "10Δ/17°," i.e., a 10-diopter prism with its base set at an angle of 17°.

Chart is designed for use with the powers available in Fresnel prisms.

Reprinted from Reinecke, Simons, Moss, and Morton, An improved method of fitting resultant prism in treatment of two-axis strabismus, *Archives of Ophthalmology*, July, 1977.

9.7. Referral Recommendations for Binocular and Perceptual Deficiencies

Table A. Symptoms in the Accommodative System

Symptoms of difficulties in the accommodative system:
1. Asthenopia at near associated with excessive rubbing of the eyes
2. Periodic blurring at distance after near point activities or blurring at near
3. Reduced vision at distance
4. A working distance closer than expected when doing near point tasks.
5. Reports of headaches or nausea with near point activities
6. Diplopia periodic at near
7. Excessive general fatigue, towards the end of the day
8. Difficulty or inability to sustain near point work

Findings indicating accommodative difficulties when associated with symptoms are:
1. NRA and PRA of lower than + and −1.75
2. + and −2.00 flipper test monocularly and binocularly showing less than 12 cycles per minute with the patient viewing a 20/30 line at 16 inches, or a difference of more than 2 cycles/minute between the two eyes
3. MEM Retinoscopy – lag greater than 0.75 diopter
4. Net 14B greater than 0.75 diopter
5. Reduced Ampitude of Accommodation of more than 2 diopters below Donders' Age Expecteds, or greater than 0.50 diopter difference between the two eyes

Table B. Symptoms in the Vergence System

Symptoms of difficulties in the vergence system:
1. Asthenopia distance and/or near
2. Intermittent diplopia at either distance or near
3. The patient reports confusion of what is being seen
4. The individual reports closing or covering one eye
5. Repetition of letters within words or difficulty aligning columns of numbers
6. The patient manifests a head tilt
7. Postural changes noted when working at a desk
8. Letters words, or both appear to float or move around

Findings indicating vergence difficulties when associated with symptoms are:
1. A near point of convergence manifesting a break point greater than 5 cm and/or a recovery greater than 8 cm
2. Phoria at distance greater or less than 0–2 exophoria
3. Phoria at near greater or less than 0–6 exophoria
4. Distance vergence ranges:
   Base out to blur - less than 7 prism diopters
   Break of less than 15 diopters
   Recovery of less than 8 prism diopters
   Base in to Break of less than 5 prism diopters
   Recovery of less than 3 prism diopters
5. Near Vergence Ranges:
   Base out to blur less than 14 prism diopters
   Break less than 18 prism diopters
   Recovery less than 7 prism diopters
   Base in blur less than 11 prism diopters
   Break less than 19 prism diopters
   Recovery less than 10 prism diopters
6. Opposing vergence blur should be twice the phoria
7. A manifest fixation disparity of any amount
8. Flipper prisms with 4 Base in and 8 Base out lenses at distance and 8 Base in and 12 Base out at near. The prisms are utilized as in the accommodative flipper test and the patient views a 20/30 line of print. Eight-ten cycles/min. are expected

Table C. Symptoms in the Ocular Motor System

Symptoms of difficulty in the ocular motor system:
1. Excessive head movement when reading
2. Frequent loss of place when reading or copying materials
3. Omission of words when reading or copying materials
4. Skipping of lines when reading
5. Use of the finger or a marker of some kind when reading in order to maintain place
6. Lack of comprehension when reading
7. A short attention span manifest when performing visual tasks

4+ System for evaluating ocular motor abilities:
1. Pursuit ability for either eye:
   4+ smooth/accurate
   3+ one fixation loss
   2+ two fixation losses
   1+ more than two fixation losses
2. Saccadic ability for either eye:
   4+ smooth/accurate
   3+ slight undershoot
   2+ gross undershooting or overshooting or increased latency
   1+ inability to do task or increased latency

Table D. Symptoms in the Sensory System

Anomalies of the sensory system demonstrating the following symptoms:
1. Report of the loss or absence of stereopsis
2. Report of the sensation that both eyes are "not working together"
3. Patient reporting that one eye is not seeing as clearly as the other
4. Report of turning head away from the straight ahead position in order to get the clearest image

Findings indicating deficiencies in the sensory system are:
1. Lack of second or third degree fusion as manifested on the Worth 4 dot or red lens test and tests for stereopsis respectively
2. The patient should manifest better than 60 seconds of arc on tests for stereopsis (It is important that tests for stereopsis be done at appropriate distances or be recalculated to give accurate results.)
3. The patient should be able to manifest far-point simultaneous binocular vision on the 20/30 line of the vectographic slide
4. Any difference of greater than one line visual acuity after correction between the two eyes, or worse than 20/25 corrected acuity in both eyes.

Table E. Symptoms in the Perceptual System

Gross motor and bilateral integration:
1. Lack of coordination and balance between 2 sides of system
2. Lends to fall and bump into objects excessively
3. Does poorly in athletics
4. Tends to play with younger children
5. Has difficulty with rhythmic activities
6. Had difficulty sitting or standing still and generally controlling motor activities
7. Tendency to work with one side of his system while the other side doesn't participate
8. Can't sit still

Directionality:
1. Difficulty learning right and left
2. Reverses letters and words when writing or copying
3. May read in either left to right or right to left direction

Visual perceptual discrimination and attention skills:

Form perception
1. Confusion of likenesses and minor differences
2. Mistakes words with similar beginnings
3. Tends to use other senses to make what should be visual discriminations (tactical, kinesthetic, and verbal)
4. Has difficulty recognizing same word on same page
5. May have difficulty recognizing alphabet or even single forms
6. Tends to over generalize in placing objects into classes

Figure-ground
1. Has difficulty determining what is significant from what is insignificant when doing visual tasks
2. Tends to either stop work before completion or persevere on details when copying, writing, or drawing
3. Tendency to have difficulty completing work
4. Not aware of what he or she should attend to
5. Performs slowly compared to peers
6. Difficulty learning to read

Visual closure
1. Ignores details when doing visual tasks
2. May be able to perform several parts of task but cannot put them together
3. Work is incomplete
4. Performs slowly compared to peers
5. May manifest poor comprehension when doing visual tasks such as reading

Visual sequencing
1. Has difficulty organizing self and materials
2. Poor spelling skills
3. Ignores left to right direction
4. Has difficulty placing visual information into groups
5. Difficulty with tasks that require more than one step

Visualization
1. Has difficulty visualizing what is read
2. Poor comprehension
3. Difficulty learning new materials
4. Difficulty anticipating next step in tasks presented to him or her
5. Poor spelling
6. Poor recall of visually presented materials
7. Tends to whisper to self when reading silently

(continued)

Table E. Symptoms of the Perceptual System (continued)

Visualization (continued)

8. Uses other sensory support when doing visual tasks
9. Difficulty with mathematical concepts
10. Tends to avoid new situations
11. Difficulty with "look and say" method of learning to read

Visual motor integration or eye-hand coordination

1. Sloppy writing or drawing skills
2. Poor spacing and inability to stay on lines
3. Excessive erasures when doing written work
4. Uses hand to keep place when writing or reading
5. Poor in eye-hand coordination tasks that require following directions
6. Poor ability to properly place materials on page when drawing or writing
7. Can respond orally but cannot get answers on paper
8. Seems to know materials but does poorly when tested

Auditory perceptual discrimination and attention:

Auditory memory

1. Poor in rhythmic activities
2. Can't follow verbal directions
3. Poor spelling
4. Poor ability to sequence verbally presented materials
5. Doesn't recall verbally presented materials

Auditory visual integration

1. Difficulty relating what is seen with what is heard
2. Difficulty relating symbols to their sounds
3. Difficulty with phonic method of learning to read
4. Poor spelling

Auditory discrimination

1. Mistakes similar words presented verbally
2. Tendency to ignore auditorially presented materials
3. Poor spelling

Reprinted from L.G. Hoffman and M. Rouge, Referal Recommendations for Binocular Functions and/or Developmental Perceptual Deficiencies, *J. Am. Optom. Assn.*, March, 1980

9.8. Sources of Vision Training Equipment and Accessories

Michigan Tracking Programs
Ann Arbor Publishers, Inc.
P. O. Box 388
Worthington, Ohio 43085

Anaglyphs
Bernell Co.
316 S. Eddy Street
South Bend, Ind. 46617

Tracing Board
Childcare Company
P. O. Box 366
Loveland, Colo. 80537

Magnets; Puzzles
Edmund Scientific Co.
Edscorp Bldg.
Barrington, N. J. 08007

Workbooks; Soma Cubes
Pencil Grips
Efficient Seeing Publ.
P. O. Box 218 A
Aptos, Cal. 95003

Equipment; Anaglyphs
Keystone View Co.
2212 – 12th Street
Davenport, Iowa 52803

Letter Form Recognition
Field Targets
Dr. L. W. Macdonald
471 Washington Street
Newton, Mass. 02158

Translid Binocular Interactor
Manico
P. O. Box 832
Fredericksburg, Va. 22401

Hidden Word Tablet
Materials for Tutors
5808 Ferree Street
Pittsburgh, Pa. 15217

1″ Crayons
National Crayons Co.
Main Street
Easton, Pa. 18042

Colored Twine (Optometric)
New England Twine and Cordage Co.
Pawtucket, R. I. 02862

Workbooks: Visual Memory,
Tracing Persuit, GO Board Patterns,
Visual Fixation Patterns
Per Con Inc.
3483 Path Drive
Akron, Ohio 44319

Near-Far Clear Target
Dr. Everett N. Pierce
21 Park Street
Attleboro, Mass. 12703

Flash Cards, Parquetry
Playskool Mfg. Co.
3720 North Kedzie Avenue
Chicago, Ill. 60618

Peripheral Ring Target
Dr. Irving Shapiro
2722 Sheridan Avenue
Tonawanda, N. Y. 14150

Vectograms; Quoits
Stereo Optical Co.
Chicago, Ill. 60641

Creative Matching Workbook
Dr. J. B. Swartwout
1 Herbert Drive
Latham, New York 12110

9.9. Typical Sequence of Out-of-Office Procedures Recommended for Eso Problems

---

Nearpoint

1. Ductions and versions for motility
2. Bifocals
3. Pencil push-ups
4. Binocular accommodative rock (Van Orden Trainer used with Correct-Eye-Scope or custom-made devices)
5. Pola-Mirror with decreasing fixation distance
6. Orthopic (uncrossed) fusion with acetate rings (Eccentric Circles on transparent acetate)
7. Polachrome Orthoptic Trainer (Vectograms and Tranaglyphs)
8. Titmus Stereo Tests with flip prisms
9. Bar reading
10. Remy Separator (Septum Orthoptic Trainer, Bernell)
11. Supplemental Procedures
12. Combinations

Farpoint

1. Deductions and versions for motility
2. Pencil push-aways
3. Base-out prism in spectacles
4. Peripheral fusion training
   a. Keystone anaglyphs
   b. Root Rings
   c. Wheatstone stereoscopes with para-macular targets (e.g., mirror stereoscope)
5. Hand-held stereoscopes (e.g., Stori-View, G.A.F. Viewmaster or other Brewster stereoscopes)
6. Brock string techniques (e.g., red-green filters, minus lenses, nine positions of gaze, pursuit vergences, saccadic vergences)
7. Prism demand flippers (base-out and base-in; e.g., those using Bausch and Lomb Comparators)
8. T.V. Trainer
   a. Red-green (custom-made or Bernell)
   b. Polaroid (A.O. or Bernell)
9. Fusion walk-aways
   a. Worth lights (viewed through red-green spectacles)
   b. Bagolini striated lenses
10. Reduction of power of base-out prism in spectacles
11. Supplemental procedures (e.g., hole-in-hand game, Tranaglyphs, T.B.I., Eccentric Circles – Keystone Transparent acetate, flannel board training, etc.)
12. Combinations

Reprinted from Griffin John: Binocular anomalies, procedures for vision therapy, p. 294, 308, published by Professional Press, Inc., 101 E. Ontario St., Chicago, Ill. 60611, 1976.

9.10. Recommended Instrumentation and Targets for Training Procedures in Cases of Divergence Insufficiency

A. Stereoscopes
   1. Wheatstone
      a. Office (e.g., Synoptophore)
      b. Out-of-office (e.g., Bernell Mirror Stereoscope)
   2. Brewster
      a. Office (e.g., Telebinocular for "tromboning")
      b. Out-of-office (e.g., Stori-View Stereoscope)

B. Vectographics (in-office or out-of-office)
   1. Pola-Mirror
   2. Vis-A-Vis
   3. Vectograms
   4. Titmus Stereo Tests
   5. A.O. Vectographic Slide
   6. T.V. Trainer

C. Colored Filters (in-office or out-of-office)
   1. Worth lights (4-dot test)
   2. Anaglyphics (e.g., Keystone Basic Binocular Test Set)
   3. Root Rings

D. Septums (Turville Septum or vertical bar on window)

E. Directly Viewed Instruments
   1. Penlight push-aways
   2. Penlight and Bagolini striated lenses
   3. Penlight with flip prisms
   4. Brock String
   5. T.B.I.
      a. Chiastopic (crossed) fusion
      b. Orthopic (uncrossed) fusion
   6. Eccentric Circles (Keystone transparent acetate)
   7. Two thumbs

F. Combinations

Reprinted from Griffin, John: ***Binocular anomalies, prodedures for vision therapy*****, p. 288. Published by Professional Press, Inc., 101 E. Ontario St., Chicago, Ill. 60611, 1976.**

Miscellaneous 10

10.1. Dictionary of Ophthalmic Abbreviations

Abd	Abduction
Abn	Abnormal, abnormality
Acc	Accomodation
Act	Active electrode
ACT	Alternate cover test
Add	Adduction
ALB	Anterior lenticular bevel
Alt	Alternate
Amp	Amplifier, amplitude ampere
ARA	Against the rule astigmatism
A-scan	Amplitude mode
ASCVD	Atherosclerotic cardio-vascular disease
Avg	Averager or averaged
BC	Base curve
BCP	Bipolar cell potential (b-wave)
BCR	Base curve ratio
Bilat	Bilateral
Bl	Blur point
BP	Blood pressure
Br	Break point
B-scan	Brightness mode
BUN	Blood urea nitrogen
$\bar{c}$	With
CAB	Cellulose acetate butyrate
CC	Chief complaint
CCC	Central corneal clouding
CCV	Central color field
C/D	Cup to disc ratio
CEP	Cortically evoked potential
CF	Count fingers (at_____feet)
CFF	Critical flicker frequency
CL	Contact lens
CNAG	Chronic narrow angle glaucoma
CNB	CN bevel
c/o	(with) complaint of
CP	Central pooling
CSG	Chronic simple glaucoma
CT	Cover test
CV	Central vision
CVC	Chief visual complaint
D	Diameter, diopter
DA	Dark adaptometry
dB	Decibels
DD_x	Differential diagnosis
Div	Divergence
DO	Direct ophthalmoscopy
DVER	Difference visual evoked response
D_x	Diagnosis
ECG or EKG	Electrocardiogram (electrocardiography)
EDTA	Disodium edetate
EEG	Electroencephalogram (electroencephalography)
ENG	Electronystagmogram (electronystagmography)
EOG	Electrooculogram (electrooculography
EOM	Extraocular muscles
EP	Evoked potential or esophoria at distance
EP′	Esophoria at near
ERG	Electroretinogram (electroretinography)
ERP	Early receptor potential
ERTG	Electroretinopography
ET	Constant esotrophia at distance
ET′	Constant esotrophia at near
EVR	Evoked visual response
EXOPH	Exophthalmos or exophthalmometry
FB	Foreign body
FD_h	Fixation disparity horizontal at distance
FD_h'	Fixation disparity horizontal at near
FD_v	Fixation disparity vertical at distance
FD_v'	Fixation disparity vertical at near
FFF	Flicker fusion frequency
FH_x	Family history
Fl Ån	Fluorescein analysis
FLP	Full line presentation
FMA	Fine motor adaptive
f/u	Follow-up
F_x	Findings
G	Gonioscopy
GLP	Good light perception
GLP&P	Good light perception and projection
GM	Gross motor
GPC	Giant papillary conjunctivitis
GTT	Drops
Hem	Hemorrhage
HEMA	Hydroxyethylmethacrylate
HM	Hand motion (at______feet)
Hor	Horizontal
HSV	Herpes simplex virus
H_x	History
H_x/o	History of

(continued)

IDO	Indirect ophthalmoscopy
IET	Intermittent esotropia at distance
IET′	Intermittent esotropia at near
Imp	Impression
Inf	Inferior
Int	Intermittent
IOP	Intraocular pressure (measured by manometry)
IOT	Intraocular tension (measured clinically)
IVP	Intravenous pyleogram (radiology)
IXT	Intermittent exotropia at distance
IXT′	Intermittent exotropia at near
K	Keratometry
KCS	Keratoconjunctivitis sicca
KP	Keratic precipitate
Lat	Lateral
LIA	Laser interference acuity
LIO	Left inferior oblique
LIR	Left inferior rectus
LKP	Lamellar keratoplasty
LLP	Lacrimal lens power
LLR	Left lateral rectus
LP/DT	Light peak, dark trough ratio
LR	Laser refraction
LSO	Left superior oblique
LSR	Left superior rectus
M	Mannifest refraction
M_c	Mannifest refraction $\bar{p}$ cycloplegia
MB	Muscle balance
Mot	Motility
MS	Mean spherical equivalent
M-scan	Motion mode
M_x	Management
Myo	Mydriatic
N	Normal
NAG	Narrow angle glaucoma
Neg	Negative
NI	No improvement
NIPH	No improvement with pin hole
NKA	No known allergy
NLP	No light perception
NPC	near point of convergence
NVD	Neovascularization other than at disc
NVE	Neovascularization
$\bar{O}$	None
Ø	Lateral orthophoria at distance
Ø′	Lateral orthophoria at near
OAD	Overall diameter
OAG	Open angle glaucoma
Obl	Oblique
O.D.	Right eye
ODM	Opthalmodynamometry
OFH_x	Ocular family history
OH_x	Ocular history
OKN	Optokinetic nystagmus
ONA	Optic nerve atrophy
OP	Oscillatory potential
O.S.	Left eye
OT	Ocular tension by Schiotz indentation tonometer
O.U.	Both eyes
OZ	Optical zone
PC	Peripheral curve
P.D.	Interpupillary distance
PE	Progress examination, or physical examination
PEE	Punctate epithelial erosions
PEP	Photically evoked potential
Pk to Pk	Peak to peak (trough of a-wave to peak of b-wave)
PMH_x	Past medical history
PMMA	Polymethylmethacrylate
PP	Puntum proximum
PSK	Punctate subepithelial keratitis
PVA	Polyvinyl alcohol
PVP	Polyvinylpyrollidone
P_x	Prognosis
R_c	Retinoscopy $\bar{p}$ cycloplegia
Rec	Recovery
R-G	Red-green
RIO	Right inferior oblique
RIR	Right inferior rectus
RLR	Right lateral rectus
RMR	Right medial rectus
R/O	Rule out
RSO	Right superior oblique
RSR	Right superior rectus
RT	Return
R_x	Prescription
$\bar{s}$	Without
SC	Secondary curve
SC_r	Secondary curve radius
SC_w	Secondary curve width
Sib	Sibling
SLE_x	Split lamp examination biomicroscopy
SLP	Single line presentation
Sn	Snellen
SR_x	Spectacle prescription
STT_1	Schirmer tear test I
STT_2	Schirmer tear test II
STT_b	Basal Schirmer tear test

(continued)

10.1 Dictionary of Ophthalmic Abbreviations (continued)

Sup	Superior
S_x	Symptoms
T_a	Ocular tension by Goldman applanation tonometer
TC	Tertiary curve
TC_r	Tertiary curve radius
TC_w	Tertiary curve width
TD_x	Tentative diagnosis
TF	Trial frame
TFR	Trial frame refraction
T_{mm}	Ocular tension by Mackay-Marg tonometer
T_{nct}	Ocular tension by noncontact tonometer
T_x	Treatment
UDE	Undetermined etiology
USG	Ultrasonography
VA	Visual acuity
VA $\overline{cc}$	Visual acuity with spectacle correction (aided)
VA $\overline{ccl}$	Visual acuity with contact lens correction (aided)
VAokn	Visual acuity by optokinetic nystagmus
VAph	Visual acuity with pin hole
VA $\overline{sc}$	Visual acuity without spectacle correction (unaided)
VA $\overline{tf}$	Visual acuity with trial frame
VECP	Visual evoked cortical potential
VEP	Visual evoked potential
VER	Visual evoked response
VF_c	Visual fields by confrontation
VF_g	Visual fields by Goldman-type perimeter
w/	With
wo	Without
W-4-D	Worth four dot
WRA	With the rule astigmatism
X,	Exophoria at distance
X′	Exophoria at near
XT	Constant exophoria at distance
XT′	Constant exophoria at near

Abstracted chiefly from: Mark Flora, O.D., *Glossary of ocular and general abreviations for clinical use.*

10.2. The Schematic Eye

		Gullstrand No. I (Exact) Eye		
		Relaxed	*Accom.*	*Aphakic*
Refractive Indices	Cornea . .	1.376	1.376	1.376
	Aqueous and Vitreous . .	1.336	1.336	1.336
	Lens: cortex	1.386	1.386	
	core	1.406	1.406	
Positions	Cornea: anterior . .	0	0	
	posterior . .	0.5	0.5	.5
	Lens: anterior . .	3.6	3.2	
	posterior . .	7.2	7.2	
	core, anterior	4.146	3.8725	
	core, posterior	6.565	6.5275	
Radii of Curvature	Cornea: anterior . .	7.7	7.7	7.7
	posterior . .	6.8	6.8	6.8
	Lens: anterior . .	10.0	5.33	
	posterior . .	−6.0	−5.33	
	core, anterior	7.911	2.655	
	core, posterior	−5.76	−2.655	
Powers	Cornea . .	43.05	43.05	43.05
	Lens	19.11	33.06	
	Complete eye	58.64	70.57	43.05
Focal lengths of complete eye.	First	−17.05	−14.17	23.23
	Second . .	+22.78	+18.93	30.89
Positions	Principal, first . .	1.348	1.772	−0.50
	second . .	1.602	2.086	.09
	Nodal: first . .	7.08	6.53	7.75
	second . .	7.33	6.85	7.89
	Focal: first . .	−15.70	−12.40	−23.28
	second . .	−24.38	21.02	30.98
	Fovea . .	24.0	24.0	24.00
Refractive condition	. .	+1	−9.6	+11.63
Position of near point	. .	–	−102.3	

The phakic eye has a hypermetropia of 1.00 D. However, taking spherical aberration into account it is an emmetropic eye.

10.3. Safety Glasses

Table A. Selection Chart for Eye and Face Protectors for Use in Industry, Schools, and Colleges

This selection chart offers general recommendations only. Final selection of eye and face protective devices is the responsibility of management and safety specialists. (For laser protection, refer to American National Standard for Safe Use of Lasers, ANSI Z136.1-1976.)

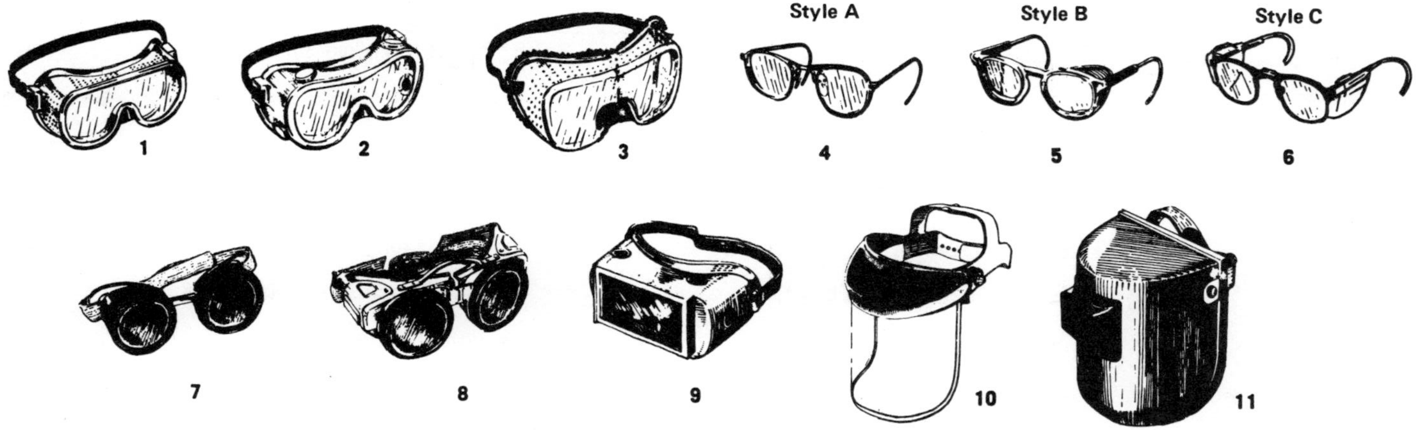

1. GOGGLES, Flexible Fitting, Regular Ventilation
2. GOGGLES, Flexible Fitting, Hooded Ventilation
3. GOGGLES, Cushioned Fitting, Rigid Body
*4. SPECTACLES, without Sideshields
5. SPECTACLES, Eyecup Type Sideshields
6. SPECTACLES, Semi-/Flat-Fold Sideshields
7. WELDING GOGGLES, Eyecup Type, Tinted Lenses (Illustrated)

7A. CHIPPING GOGGLES, Eyecup Type, Clear Safety Lenses (Not Illustrated)
8. WELDING GOGGLES, Coverspec Type, Tinted Lenses (Illustrated)
8A. CHIPPING GOGGLES, Coverspec Type, Clear Safety Lenses (Not Illustrated)
9. WELDING GOGGLES, Coverspec Type, Tinted Plate Lens
10. FACE SHIELD, Plastic or Mesh Window (see caution note)
*11. WELDING HELMET

*Nonsideshield spectacles are available for limited hazard use requiring only frontal protection.

CAUTION:
- Face shields alone do not provide adequate protection.
- Plastic lenses are advised for protection against molten metal splash.
- Contact lenses, of themselves, do not provide eye protection in the industrial sense and shall not be worn in a hazardous environment without appropriate covering safety eyewear.

Table B. Applications

Operation	*Hazards*	*Protectors*
Acetylene–burning Acetylene–cutting Acetylene–welding	Sparks, harmful rays, molten metal, flying particles	7, 8, 9
Chemical handling	Splash, acid burns, fumes	2 (for severe exposure add 10)
Chipping	Flying particles	1, 3, 4, 5, 6, 7A, 8A
Electric (arc) welding	Sparks, intense rays, molten metal	11 (in combination with 4, 5, 6, in tinted lenses, advisable)
Furnace operations	Glare, heat, molten metal	7, 8, 9 (for severe exposure add 10)
Grinding–light	Flying particles	1, 3, 5, 6 (for severe exposure add 10)
Grinding–heavy	Flying particles	1, 3, 7A, 8A (for severe exposure add 10)
Laboratory	Chemical splash, glass breakage	2 (10 when in combination with 5, 6)
Machining	Flying particles	1, 3, 5, 6 (for severe exposure add 10)
Molten metals	Heat, glare, sparks, splash	7, 8 (10 in combination with 5, 6, in tinted lenses)
Spot welding	Flying particles, sparks	1, 3, 4, 5, 6, (tinted lenses advisable; for severe exposure add 10)

CAUTION:
- Face shields alone do not provide adequate protection.
- Plastic lenses are advised for protection against molten metal splash.
- Contact lenses, of themselves, do not provide eye protection in the industrial sense and shall not be worn in a hazardous environment without appropriate covering safety eyewear.

10.4. The Boxing System of Measurement

A unit system of frame and lens measurement, called the Boxing System, was instituted in 1962. Since that time, most products manufactured in the United States conform to this system. The salient features of the system, as it applies to this lens standard, are shown below. Basically, all measurements are made from frame or lens centers and lens bevel apices and are expressed in millimeters.

A: The horizontal box dimension or the horizontal distance between two vertical tangents to the lateral extremities of the lens shape

B: The vertical box dimension or the vertical distance between two horizontal tangents to the vertical extremities of the lens shape

DBL: Distance between lenses (measured between two vertical tangents to the nasal extremities of the lens bevels)

DBC: Distance between centers (the distance between the two geometric centers of the frame eyewires) (see GC)

GC: The geometric center of the box, eyewire, or lens shape

NPD: Near interpupillary distance on the horizontal distance between segment geometric centers

DPD: Distance interpupillary distance or the horizontal distance between major reference points

θ: Angle of the cylinder axis, measured in a counter-clockwise direction from 0°. Zero degrees, by convention , always is the right extremity of the box when viewing the patient.

MRP: Major reference point

OD: Right eye

OS: Left eye

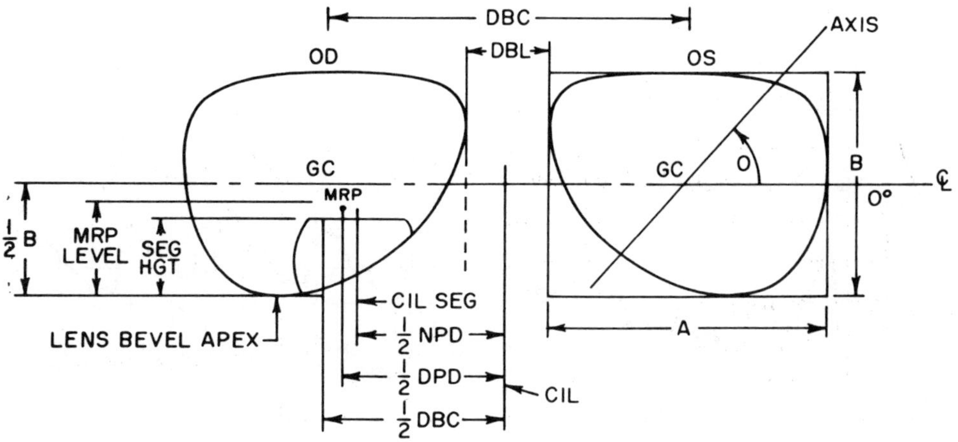

This material is reproduced with permission from American National Standard Z80.5: Requirements for Dress Ophthalmic Frames, copyright 1979 by the American National Standards Institute, copies of which may be purchased from the American National Standards Institute at 1430 Broadway, New York, New York 10018.

10.5. Physiological Optics

Table A. Hue Discrimination

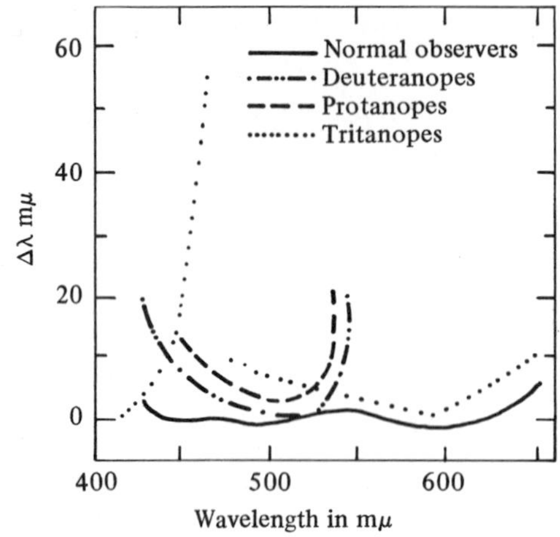

Table B. VEP

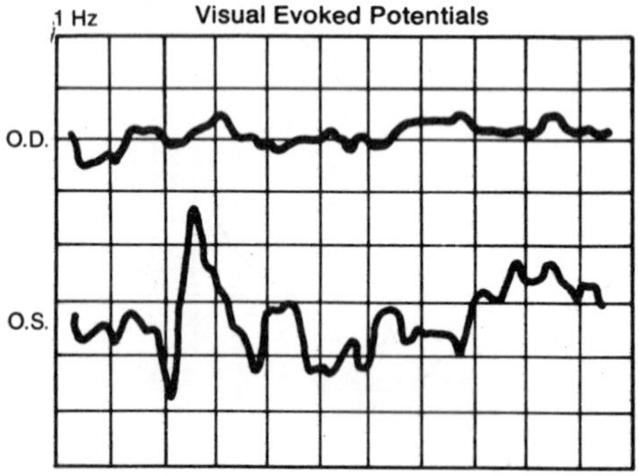

The VEP from the right eye (above) is very reduced. The response from the left eye is normal (below)

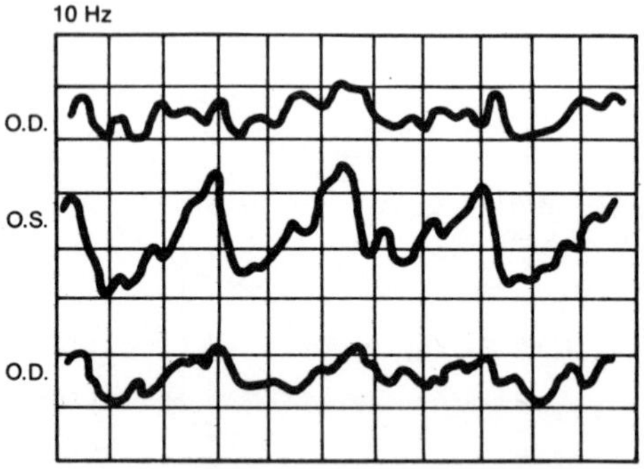

The VEP from the right eye is shown above and below. The middle VEP is the normal left eye's. Note the reduced amplitude response from the right eye as compared to the left eye.

The illustrated VEP's for the left eye are normal. The responses for the right eye are markedly reduced.

Table C. Fixation Disparity

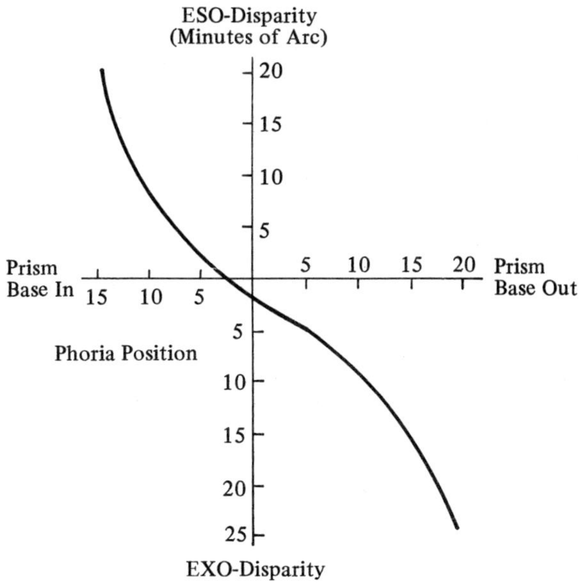

*Disparity In Minutes Of Arc

Table D. Dark Adaptation

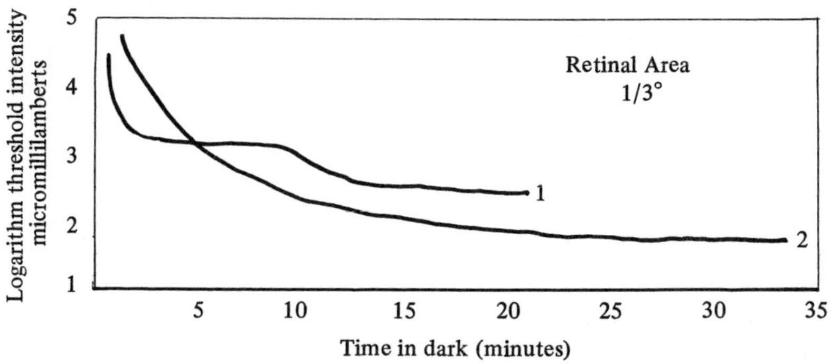

Representative curves showing the course of dark adaptation for the macula (curve 1) and for an area 10 degrees above the macula (curve 2) after light adaptation to 160 foot-candles for three minutes.

Table E. Photopic and Scotopic Luminosity

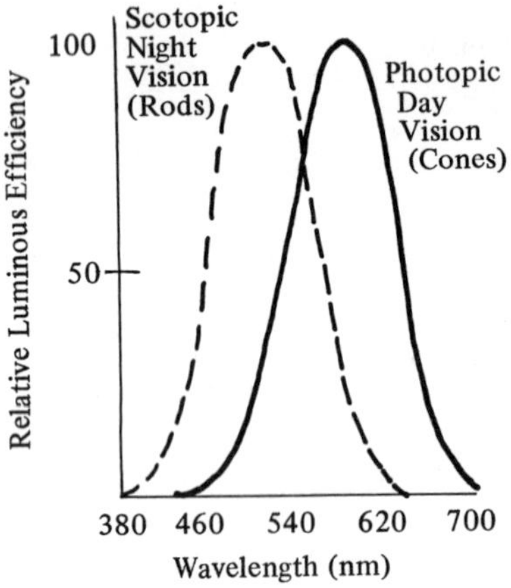

Index 11